NIHAR GALA

Neurosurgical Intensive Care

D1120636

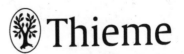

NIHAR GALA

Neurosurgical Intensive Care

Javed Siddiqi, H.B.Sc., M.D., D.Phil (Oxon), F.R.C.S.C., F.A.C.S.
Division of Neurosurgery
Arrowhead Regional Medical Center
Colton, California

Thieme
New York • Stuttgart

Thieme Medical Publishers, Inc.
333 Seventh Ave.
New York, NY 10001

Associate Editor: Ivy Ip
Editor: Birgitta Brandenburg
Vice President, Production and Electronic Publishing: Anne T. Vinnicombe
Vice President, International Marketing and Sales: Cornelia Schulze
Chief Financial Officer: Peter van Woerden
President: Brian D. Scanlan
Compositor: Alden Group Limited
Printer: The Maple-Vail Book Manufacturing Group

Library of Congress Cataloging-in-Publication Data

Neurosurgical intensive care / [edited by] Javed Siddiqi.
    p. ; cm.
    Includes bibliographical references and index.
    ISBN-13: 978-1-58890-390-7 (TMP : pbk. : alk. paper)
    ISBN-10: 1-58890-390-7 (TMP : pbk. : alk. paper)
    ISBN-13: 978-3-13-141911-8 (GTV : pbk. : alk. paper)
    ISBN-10: 3-13-141911-3 (GTV : pbk. : alk. paper)   1. Neurological intensive care.
2. Surgical intensive care. I. Siddiqi, Javed, 1962-
    [DNLM: 1. Intensive Care. 2. Neurosurgical Procedures. WL 368 N49551 2007]
    RC350.N49N485 2007
    616.8'0428—dc22   2006103505

Copyright ©2008 by Thieme Medical Publishers, Inc. This book, including all parts
thereof, is legally protected by copyright. Any use, exploitation, or commercialization
outside the narrow limits set by copyright legislation without the publisher's consent
is illegal and liable to prosecution. This applies in particular to photostat reproduction,
copying, mimeographing or duplication of any kind, translating, preparation of
microfilms, and electronic data processing and storage.

Important note: Medical knowledge is ever-changing. As new research and clinical
experience broaden our knowledge, changes in treatment and drug therapy may be
required. The authors and editors of the material herein have consulted sources
believed to be reliable in their efforts to provide information that is complete and in
accord with the standards accepted at the time of publication. However, in view of
the possibility of human error by the authors, editors, or publisher of the work herein
or changes in medical knowledge, neither the authors, editors, nor publisher, nor any
other party who has been involved in the preparation of this work, warrants that the
information contained herein is in every respect accurate or complete, and they are
not responsible for any errors or omissions or for the results obtained from use of
such information. Readers are encouraged to confirm the information contained
herein with other sources. For example, readers are advised to check the product
information sheet included in the package of each drug they plan to administer to
be certain that the information contained in this publication is accurate and that
changes have not been made in the recommended dose or in the contraindications
for administration. This recommendation is of particular importance in connection
with new or infrequently used drugs.

Some of the product names, patents, and registered designs referred to in this
book are in fact registered trademarks or proprietary names even though specific
reference to this fact is not always made in the text. Therefore, the appearance of a
name without designation as proprietary is not to be construed as a representation
by the publisher that it is in the public domain.

Printed in United States of America

5 4 3 2

The Americas ISBN: 978-1-58890-390-7
Rest of World ISBN: 978-3 13 141911 8

Contributors

Ganna L. Breland, D.O.
Division of Neurosurgery
Arrowhead Regional Medical Center
Colton, California

John D. Cantando, D.O.
Neurosurgery Resident
Division of Neurosurgery
Arrowhead Regional Medical
   Center
Colton, California

Dennis Cramer, D.O.
Fontana, California

Nguyen Do, D.O., M.S.
Division of Neurosurgery
Arrowhead Regional Medical
   Center
Colton, California

Silvio F. Hoshek, M.D.
Department of Neurosurgery
Riverside County Regional Medical
   Center
Moreno Valley, California

Evan A. Houck, B.S., D.O.
Resident
Division of Neurosurgery
Arrowhead Regional Medical Center
Colton, California

Daniel Hutton, D.O.
Redlands, California

Jeffery M. Jones, D.O.
Neurosurgical Resident
Division of Neurosurgery
Arrowhead Regional Medical Center
Colton, California

Theresa Longo, M.D.
Department of Neurosurgery
Riverside County Regional Medical
   Center
Moreno Valley, California

Rosalinda M. Menoni, M.D.
Clinical Assistant Professor
   of Surgery
Division of Neurosurgery
Arrowhead Neurosurgical Group
Colton, California

Dan Miulli, D.O., M.S., F.A.C.O.S.
Associate Neurosurgery Program
   Director
Assistant Professor of Surgery
Department of Neurosurgery
Western University
Arrowhead Regional Medical Center
Colton, California

Nicholas Qandah, D.O.
Rancho Cucamonga, California

Lynn M. Serrano, B.S., D.O.
Neurosurgery Postgraduate Training
Philadelphia College of Osteopathic
   Medicine
Philadelphia, Pennsylvania

Javed Siddiqi, H.B.Sc., M.D., D.Phil (Oxon), F.R.C.S.C., F.A.C.S.
Division of Neurosurgery
Arrowhead Regional Medical
    Center
Colton, California

Paula Snyder, R.N., C.C.R.N.
Neurosurgical Nurse Clinician
Department of Neurosurgical
    Sciences
Riverside County Regional Medical
    Center
Moreno Valley, California

Gayatri Sonti, B.A., D.O., M.S., Ph.D.
Resident Physician
Division of Neurosurgery
Arrowhead Regional Medical Center
Colton, California

John R. Spitalieri, D.O., M.S.
Division of Neurosurgery
Arrowhead Regional Medical Center
Colton, California

Charles H. Tator, C.M., M.D., Ph.D.
Professor of Neurosurgery
University of Toronto and
    Toronto Western Hospital
Toronto, Ontario, Canada

Jon Taveau, D.O., M.S.
Moreno Valley, California

Margaret R. Wacker, M.D., M.S.
Division of Neurosurgery
Arrowhead Regional Medical Center
Colton, California

Darryl M. Warner, D.O.
Division of Neurosurgery
Arrowhead Regional Medical Center
Colton, California

David T. Wong, M.D., F.A.C.S.
Assistant Professor of Surgery
Surgery and Critical Care
Loma Linda University
Arrowhead Regional Medical Center
Colton, California

1
Introduction to the Neurosurgical Intensive Care Unit

Javed Siddiqi

Neurosurgery is, at the same time, the oldest form of surgery and the newest. We know that trephining, for instance, was done thousands of years ago and represents the earliest form of surgery. In recent decades, the addition of microsurgery techniques and the development of technology, including neuroimaging modalities and frameless stereotaxy, have revolutionized neurosurgery. Historically, the operative mortality was tremendously high for neurosurgical operations; now, with the exception of trauma, intraoperative mortality is extremely rare. The most serious morbidity and mortality our patients currently face are really in the postoperative phase, in the intensive care unit (ICU). The subtlety and finesse of ICU management significantly contributes to patient outcomes, with trauma being the most dramatic example.

In the drive to be better physicians, neurosurgeons continue to evolve in their education. Whereas historically it was the anesthesiologist or internist who served as an intensivist for our patients in the ICU, a field of neurointensive care is evolving, with subspecialists who acknowledge that the nervous system is unique and cannot and should not be treated as an extrapolation of other organ systems. An increasing number of neurosurgery residency programs in North America are insisting on a thorough grounding for their residents in direct hands-on neurointensive care management of their patients. This emphasis is expanding the focus of neurosurgery education beyond the technical. Fluid and electrolyte management, blood pressure control, and ventilator management of the postoperative patient are clearly within the domain of the neurosurgeon today; and the intensive care of the neurosurgical patient has now become a genuine multidisciplinary effort in a way it never was only two decades ago (when the surgeon largely handed over the postoperative patient to the intensivist to manage).

In neurointensive care, as in other areas of medicine, the stakes are high. Unfortunately, in this relatively new field of neurocritical care, most of the known treatments and interventions are based on convention, not on science. The field aspires to evidence-based medicine, but the severity of the patients' conditions and the complexity of their diseases render rigorous scientific study very difficult. The number of prospective double-blind randomized studies that guide our clinical management in all medicine is limited; this is no less true in neurointensive care. In this early stage in the development of neurocritical care, all precepts are open to question, and there is ample room for chaos; it is also a time of great optimism, as we have much to learn from our patients. For those of us with a keen eye and a sharp mind, we find ourselves in a position to make significant contributions to the field.

Walking into an ICU can be overwhelming for patients, families, and physicians. For the neurosurgeon taking care of his or her patients in the neurologic ICU, an understanding that the nervous system cannot be treated in isolation of the rest of the body is critical. Having said that, I must emphasize that we need to understand our role in the modern neurosurgical ICU (NICU) in the context of a multidisciplinary team. Within this team, it is no exaggeration to say that all neurosurgery patients in the ICU will be affected, to varying degrees, by one or more of six key problems. In this book, we offer a checklist to these key problems, as well as others that are faced in the NICU.

The six most important areas for neurosurgical critical care are

1. Cerebral perfusion pressure (CPP) and intracranial pressure (ICP) management
2. Fluid and electrolyte management
3. Ventilator management
4. Sedation/pain control
5. Diagnosis and treatment of seizures
6. Emotional support of the patient and family

In this book, we hope to present some factors that are involved in the care of patients in the neurointensive care unit. The art of medicine has not been, and probably never will be, fully quantitated; accordingly, much of what is expressed in this work has not been proven scientifically. We hope to offer rationales of current management of neurosurgery patients in the ICU and raise questions about ongoing controversies that we will not settle here. Most importantly, we wish to make the point that neurosurgeons are ideally suited to deal with neurointensive care management of their own patients, in collaboration with colleagues from anesthesia, general surgery, internal medicine, and so on. Let's become active participants in the care of our ICU patients, as opposed to passive observers.

. Several respiratory patterns may be observed in patients with severe neurologic injury and may indicate the level of dysfunction.

Cheyne-Stokes respirations are characterized by "crescendo-decrescendo" patterns of breathing. This is nonspecific, but it may indicate bilateral hemispheric injury or diencephalic damage.[10]

Cluster breathing entails rapid, irregular breathing with a period of apnea between clusters. This is seen with lower pons or upper medulla lesions.

Biot's (ataxic) breathing is asynchronous of varying depths and signifies medullary dysfunction.

Hyperventilation is also seen often with neurosurgical patients. It is often due to aspiration or in response to metabolic acidosis or pulmonary edema (**Table 2–5**).

Table 2–5   Breathing Patterns

Type of breathing with rostral to caudal progression of lesions	Breathing pattern	Location of lesion
Cheyne-Stokes	Periodic crescendo-decrescendo, amplitude longer than variable pause, then repeat yielding respiratory alkalosis	Generalized cerebral forebrain or midbrain lesion, metabolic encephalopathy without brainstem injury; impending herniation, congestive heart failure
Reflex hyperventilation	Hyperventilation with hypocapnia	Pons tegmentum, midbrain, reticular formation; psychiatric, metabolic acidosis, pulmonary congestion, hepatic encephalopathy
Apneustic	Irregular full inspiration, then irregular pause	Pons, dorsal medulla, metabolic coma, transtentorial herniation
Cluster	Rapid irregular, then pause	Pons, upper medulla, posterior fossa lesion; greatly increased ICP
Ataxic	No pattern	Medulla, acute posterior fossa lesion
No autonomic respiration (Ondine's curse)	Loss of autonomic respirations; awake normal breathing, no breathing during sleep or distraction	Reticular nucleus of medulla (respiratory center)
Apnea	No breathing	Bilateral damage to caudal reticular nucleus of medulla
Kussmaul	Deep regular inspiration	Metabolic acidosis

ICP, intracranial pressure.

◆ Hepatorenal

This system is of particular importance with respect to fluid balance. Postoperative pituitary patients or patients nearing brain death typically develop diabetes insipidus.[11] Hour-by-hour monitoring of patient's fluid balance and salt excess is of utmost concern. Other metabolic derangements may also be present. Syndrome of inappropriate antidiuretic hormone (SIADH) and cerebral salt wasting syndrome are also extremely common. Examination of patient's daily weight, mucous membranes, and skin turgor may prove beneficial when the diagnosis is in question.

Metabolic etiologies for altered level of consciousness should be excluded. Patients admitted with head trauma often have illicit drugs and/or ethanol in their system. Urine drug screening and serum ethanol levels are helpful. Patients with a history of hepatitis, cirrhosis, or renal failure may have altered metabolism of certain drugs. Liver function tests, serum chemistry, blood urea nitrogen (BUN), and creatinine and serum ammonia will assist in the diagnosis of hepatic and renal disease.

References

1. Teasdale G, Jennett B. Assessment of coma and impaired consciousness: a practical scale. Lancet 1974;2:81–84
2. Osborn AG. Diagnosis of descending transtentorial herniation by cranial CT. Radiology 1977;123:93–96
3. Stovring J. Descending tentorial herniation: findings on computerized tomography. Neuroradiology 1977;14:101–105
4. President's Commission for the Study of Ethical Problems in Medicine. Guidelines for the determination of death. JAMA 1981;246:2184–2186
5. Quality Standards Subcommittee of the American Academy of Neurology. Practical parameters for determinating brain death in adults (summary statement). Neurology 1995;45:1012–1014
6. Wijdicks EF. Determining brain death in adults. Neurology 1995;45:1003–1011
7. Benzel EC, Gross CD, Hadden TA, et al. The apnea test for the determination of brain death. J Neurosurg 1989;71:191–194
8. Benzel EC, Mashburn JP, Conrad S, et al. Apnea testing for the determination of brain death: a modified protocol. J Neurosurg 1992;76:1029–1031
9. Greenberg MS. Handbook of Neurosurgery. 5th ed. New York: Thieme; 1991
10. Wijdicks EF. The Clinical Practice of Critical Care Neurology. 2nd ed. Oxford: Oxford University Press; 2003
11. Winn R. Youmans Neurological Surgery. 5th ed. New York: Elsevier; 2004

3
Cranial Nerve Injuries and Their Management

Nguyen Do and Dan Miulli

Case Study

A 22-year old male short-order cook is assaulted while walking to work. He is punched in the face several times, suffering facial bruising and "minor facial fractures"; he has no loss of consciousness during the incident. He is discharged from the emergency room in good condition after a thorough workup and no obvious surgical lesions. Two weeks later, he returns to the neurosurgery clinic complaining of diminished ability to taste the food he cooks, affecting his livelihood.

See page 32 for Case Management.

◆ Olfactory Nerve Injuries

Site of Trauma

The overall incidence of olfactory nerve dysfunction is 7%, increasing to 30% with severe head injuries or anterior cranial fossa fractures. Injury is difficult to establish in an acute trauma phase where nasal bleed and swelling confound the examination. In ~50% of cases, anosmia is only of temporary duration. The reason for the return of olfaction is not entirely clear. Recovery of the sense of smell can be expected at any time from a few days up to 5 years.[1]

Clinical Features

The primary feature is decreased or absent sense of smell. Two objective tests of olfaction are olfactory respiratory reflex and olfactory electroencephalography (EEG). The former helps in ruling out malingering, and the latter provides a nonspecific α response to an odoriferous substance. The olfactory respiratory reflex is performed with the subject seated and blindfolded. This test is based on the principle that sudden inhalation of an odor will cause a temporary arrest in the normal respiratory rhythm. This is a fairly good test to detect malingering. The olfactory EEG is performed with the eyes closed. Once the α rhythm is well established, which may take some time, an odoriferous substance is introduced. If olfaction is present, the α rhythm is abolished. This is a nonspecific response but is of value in identifying malingerers.[2]

Evaluation

A high-resolution computed tomography (CT) scan of the ethmoids and frontal fossa is essential in the workup of anosmia, especially with cerebral spinal fluid (CSF) rhinorrhea, which frequently accompanies trauma to the anterior cranial fossa and nasal sinuses. Magnetic resonance imaging (MRI) of the brain can be useful in showing injury to the orbital surface of the frontal lobe, often observed in association with injury to the olfactory bulbs.[3]

Management

Because there is no specific treatment, patients with post-traumatic anosmia can only be counseled with the known statistical information regarding their potential for recovery.[4]

Prognosis

Recovery occurs in up to 50% of cases, usually during the first 3 months, but it may be up to 5 years after injury.[2]

◆ Optic Nerve Injuries

Trauma to the orbit, with or without significant craniocerebral trauma, is rarely neatly circumscribed, and a severe injury to the eye may involve varying admixtures of optic nerve, extraocular muscle and nerve, and optic globe insults.[1]

Site of Trauma

The optic nerve is tethered in the optic canal and is subject to stretch, causing injury during brain shifts.

Trauma to the Intrabulbar Portion of the Optic Nerve

Injury to this part of the optic nerve occurs in association with direct trauma to the globe as the nerve is pushed posteriorly and suffers a partial or complete avulsion at the back end of the globe. The ophthalmoscopic picture consists of a marginal hemorrhage extending to the disk. On visual field examination, there is a sector defect extending from the blind spot to the periphery.[5]

Trauma to the Intraorbital Portion of the Optic Nerve

Although fractures of the orbit are common, isolated injury to the intraorbital portion of the optic nerve is rare. With severe trauma to the apex of the orbit, there can be a disruption of the sphenoid fissure with loss of function of the third, fourth, and sixth nerves, and the ophthalmic branch of the fifth nerve, accompanied by monocular blindness and proptosis secondary to hemorrhage into the muscle cone.[5]

Trauma to the Intracanalicular Portion of the Optic Nerve

The most vulnerable component of the optic nerve is that portion of the nerve located within the optic canal. Although the intracanalicular portion of the nerve may be injured directly by penetrating foreign objects, the majority of cases follow closed head injuries, primarily those involving frontal, temporal, and orbital trauma.[5]

Clinical Features

The chief clinical feature is decreased or loss of vision. Scotomas, sector, and altitudinal defects can occur. Most traumatic optic neuropathies result from severe head trauma, and altered consciousness in the patient delays the diagnosis. An afferent pupillary defect in an unconscious patient is useful in the detection of the optic nerve injury, whereas in conscious patients, testing for visual fields and acuity usually establishes the diagnosis.[3] With a complete injury to the optic nerve within the canal, there is monocular blindness, a dilated pupil with an absent direct pupillary response, and a brisk consensual response to light. The funduscopic appearance is unremarkable initially, but atrophy of the disk develops in several weeks. The pupil on the affected side is larger than the uninvolved one, and there is some diminution in the pupillomotor response to consensual stimulation.[6]

Evaluation

CT scan and/or MRI is useful to assess for possible basal skull fractures or compressive lesions. Clinical evaluation and investigations such as electroretinography and visual evoked potentials must be combined when evaluating visual impairment.[4]

Management

Treatment is controversial for indirect optic neuropathy and includes observation, high-dose steroids, and surgery. In patients with delayed-onset loss of vision from compression of the optic nerve and failed steroid treatment, operative approaches for optic nerve decompression include transcranial, transethmoidal, transmaxillary, and transorbital routes.[5]

Prognosis

The prognosis for restoration of vision in a patient with an optic nerve injury is poor. Forty to 50% of patients remained blind, and up to 75% showed no improvement in their reduced visual acuity or in a documented field defect. If improvement is to take place spontaneously, it does so within the first several days and continues for 4 to 6 weeks, at which time the condition becomes stationary. The prognosis is said to be better in those patients whose visual acuity is diminished but who retain a good pupillary response to light.[3]

◆ Oculomotor Nerve Injuries

Site of Trauma

The oculomotor nerve projects from the anterior part of the midbrain to the tentorial incisura at the level of the posterior clinoid processes in an open V-shaped fashion. The third nerve probably becomes damaged by a frontal blow to the accelerating head that results in stretching and contusion of the nerve. The most common site of trauma is believed to occur at the point where the nerve enters the dura mater at the posterior end of the cavernous sinus. Bilateral third nerve injuries are extremely uncommon.[7]

Clinical Features

There is paralysis of medial rectus, superior rectus, inferior rectus, inferior oblique, levator palpebrae superior, and constrictor ciliary muscles.[3] Clinical features include ptosis, outward eye deviation, dilated pupil, and no reaction to light or accommodation. The diagnosis of oculomotor nerve injury in conscious and cooperative persons is not difficult. In unconscious patients, especially those with orbital bruising and hematoma, a good history with regard to previous oculomotor status and the findings of the immediate post-traumatic examination are of great help in making an early diagnosis.[7]

Evaluation

Diplopia fields, CT, and/or MRI scans should be used to look for a compressive lesion.

Management

The treatment is initially symptomatic and consists of wearing a patch over the eye to prevent troublesome diplopia. If recovery does not occur in 4 to 6 months, then local muscle shortening procedures can be performed in the affected eye in certain situations.[7]

Prognosis

Recovery begins within 2 to 3 months when the nerve is in continuity. Aberrant regeneration often occurs with findings such as lid elevation and pupillary constriction with attempted adduction or depression.[3]

◆ Trochlear Nerve Injuries

Site of Trauma

The fourth cranial nerve is the least frequently injured ocular motor nerve. When involved, the nerve is damaged by contusion or stretching as it exits the dorsal midbrain near the anterior medullary velum. In severe frontal blows against the accelerating head, the midbrain is displaced against the posterolateral edge of the tentorial incisura, causing contusion, hemorrhage, and damage to one or both fourth nerves.[1]

Clinical Features

There is paralysis of the superior oblique muscle resulting in the impaired ability to turn the eye down and in. Injury to the trochlear nerve is rarely diagnosed. Often a complaint of diplopia after recovery from a severe head injury leads to this diagnosis. Typically, the double vision is vertical, especially when the patient walks down a flight of stairs.[3]

Evaluation

CT and/or MRI scans should be used to look for a compressive lesion.

Management

Treatment is symptomatic, such as an eye patch, semitransparent tape to glasses, and prisms for diplopia. Muscle-shortening procedures may be helpful for permanent diplopia.[4]

Prognosis

Only 50% of patients recover because of frequent avulsion of the trochlear nerve in the traumatic process.[1]

◆ Abducens Nerve Injuries

Site of Trauma

The abducens nerve is injured, along with the seventh and eighth cranial nerves, in fractures of the petrous bone. Vertical movement of the brainstem during trauma can severely stretch or avulse the sixth nerve as it leaves the pons before it enters the clival dura.[8] Increased intracranial pressure or herniation can cause delayed secondary paralysis of the cranial nerve (CN) VI. The abducens nerve can also be injured along with CN III and IV at the superior orbital fissure.[9]

Clinical Features

There is paralysis of the lateral rectus muscle, resulting in inward eye deviation. Diplopia occurs in all gaze directions. Lateral rectus palsy in its minor form may not correlate well with abducens nerve injury, and conjugate movements that are controlled by the brainstem sometimes make the diagnosis of abducens nerve palsy difficult to establish.[1] The diagnosis of abducens palsy in the unconscious patient can be made when the affected eye fails to wander outward spontaneously, abduct when the head is passively turned away from the side of the sixth nerve paralysis, and abduct in response to ipsilateral cold caloric irrigation.[3]

Evaluation

CT and/or MRI scans should be used to look for a compressive lesion or underlying fractures.

Management

The treatment is initially symptomatic and consists of wearing a patch over the eye to prevent troublesome diplopia. If recovery does not occur in 4 to 6 months, then local muscle-shortening procedures can be performed in the affected eye in certain situations. Botulinum toxin, injected into the ipsilateral medial rectus muscle, has also been proposed as a treatment option for a faster recovery.[8]

Prognosis

Many cases of abducens palsy recover spontaneously after ~4 months, a period of time consistent with axonal regeneration.[4]

◆ Internuclear Ophthalmoplegia and Medial Longitudinal Fasciculus Syndromes

Lesions affecting the medial longitudinal fasciculus (MLF) cause failure of the adducting eye to move, whereas the abducting eye deviates laterally to its full extent but has accompanying nystagmus during conjugate deviation. The medial rectus adducts without difficulty during convergence, distinguishing the paresis from a CN III or muscle lesion. This pattern of disconjugate eye movements is referred to as internuclear ophthalmoplegia (INO) because the lesion disconnects the nuclei of cranial nerves III and VI by causing failure of neural conduction in the internuclear pathway, the MLF.[4] The monocular nystagmus can be either transitory (1 or 2 beats) or sustained. When the degree of dysfunction in the MLF is mild, the adducting eye may deviate fully but cannot attain the proper velocity during a saccadic refixation. In this case, there is a noticeable dissociation between the two eyes during the saccade, because the abducting eye completes the movement earlier than the adducting eye.[1]

The clinical importance of diagnosing the MLF syndrome is its localizing value for lesions deep in the substance of the brainstem tegmentum. This general area in the brainstem contains the ascending reticular activating system, which is necessary for consciousness, along with several adjacent cranial nerve nuclei, and various ascending and descending sensory and cerebellar pathways.[4] Therefore, the isolated occurrence of an MLF syndrome in an alert individual without other brainstem signs or symptoms suggests the presence of a highly discrete lesion. This is caused by small demyelinating plaques of multiple sclerosis or by small infarctions due to small vessel disease; very occasionally it can be encountered in the setting of head trauma.[3]

◆ Trigeminal Nerve Injuries

Site of Trauma

Trigeminal nerves and branches are commonly injured with facial trauma, especially supraorbital and supratrochlear nerves as they emerge from the supraorbital notch and superomedial aspect of the bony orbit. The infraorbital nerve is often injured in orbital floor blow-out fractures.[8]

Clinical Features

There is paralysis of muscles of mastication with deviation of the jaw to the side of the lesion; loss of sensation for touch, temperature, or pain in the face; and loss of corneal reflexes.[4]

Evaluation

CT and/or MRI scans should be used to exclude underlying fractures.

Management

Treatment consists of decompression of the infraorbital nerve in orbital floor fractures. However, symptomatic relief of hyperpathia due to supra- and infraorbital neuropathies can be accomplished with medications such as carbamazepine, baclofen, pimozide, phenytoin, capsaicin, clonazepam, and amitriptyline. Carbamazepine is most commonly used with complete or acceptable relief achieved in up to 69% of cases. Baclofen may be more effective as an adjunct to carbamazepine.[8] Surgical options include peripheral nerve blocks by phenol or alcohol or neurectomy, percutaneous rhizotomy, Spiller-Frazier retrogasserian rhizotomy, microvascular decompression, and stereotactic radiosurgery. Percutaneous trigeminal rhizotomy is preferred in patients who are at high risk for major surgery and low life expectancy (<5 years). Rhizotomy is performed using radiofrequency or balloon compression, and results are comparable. Microvascular decompression provides long-lasting relief and a low incidence of facial anesthesia. Up to 90% of recurrences are in the distribution of the previously involved nerve divisions; 10% involve a new one.[1]

Prognosis

Hyperpathia in the distribution of the nerve may be permanent.

◆ Facial Nerve Injuries

Site of Trauma

Trauma is the second most common cause of facial paralysis after Bell's palsy. The long, tortuous, intraosseous course of the facial nerve in the temporal bone makes it highly susceptible to injury in temporal bone fractures. In ~50% of cases of transverse temporal bone fractures, the facial nerve within the internal auditory canal is damaged. With longitudinal fractures, the nerve is not directly involved, but a delayed paralysis may ensue secondary to edema.[10] Trauma involving the internal auditory canal injures both facial and vestibulocochlear nerves, resulting in facial nerve symptoms, loss of hearing, and vertigo. Lacerating injuries of the face can cause total or partial paralysis of the face depending on the branches involved.[1]

Clinical Features

There is paralysis of facial muscles with or without loss of taste on the anterior two thirds of the tongue or altered secretion of the lacrimal and salivary glands (nervus intermedius). Lesions near the origin of the nerve or near the geniculate ganglion lead to loss of motor, gustatory, and autonomic functions. If lesions occur between the geniculate ganglion and the origin of the chorda tympani, lacrimal secretion will not be affected. If the trauma occurs near the stylomastoid foramen, there will only be facial paralysis.[4]

Evaluation

A systematic clinical examination of the facial nerve and its branches can be performed to pinpoint the location of damage to the nerve in the fallopian canal. The testing should include tear production by the Schirmer test (greater superficial petrosal nerve), saliva secretion, taste in the anterior two thirds of the tongue (chorda tympani), and the reflex reaction of the stapedius muscle.[1] Electrodiagnostic studies of the injured facial nerve should be done promptly in every case to serve as a baseline for subsequent follow-up examinations. Electromyography (EMG) of the face, the transcutaneous nerve excitability test (NET), and evoked EMG are the most favored methods at present. Radiologic studies should include high-resolution CT scanning with appropriate bone windows to show the fracture in greatest detail.[11]

Management

Monitoring is the preferred treatment, because an excellent spontaneous recovery can be expected with delayed-onset paralysis. With no surgical management, 90% of patients experience good recovery within 6 months. The peripheral supportive devices in the form of hooks and dental bars to support the sagging face do not achieve their goal and are not recommended, especially in the waiting period. Reassurance regarding the chances of recovery and active exercises in front of a mirror, in case of partial paralysis, are helpful. Artificial tears and an eye patch at night are mandatory to prevent exposure keratitis.[4]

Absent facial nerve stimulation after 4 days may indicate surgical explorations, especially with transverse fractures of the temporal bone and a discontinuous fallopian canal. The surgical methods used include decompression of the nerve and nerve suturing, either directly or with a cable graft to bridge the nerve defect. In the delayed type of facial paralysis, only decompression is required. In immediate types of facial nerve injury when the nerve is found to be transected, meticulous micro-suturing should be performed to approximate the nerve fascicles.[3] Various grafting techniques have also been used with good results. When the nerve is transected outside the stylomastoid foramen, grafting has been done with the sural or great auricular nerves. Hypoglossal-facial anastomosis and a sural nerve graft from the premeatal facial nerve stump to the facial nerve distal to the stylomastoid foramen are other available methods. Plastic surgical procedures on the face in the form of slings and facelift operations can be performed in selected cases when the facial paralysis has been determined to be permanent or when neural repair is not feasible.[1]

Prognosis

Spontaneous recovery is usual after longitudinal fractures. When due to transverse fractures, 50% recovery after decompression has been found (**Table 3–1**).[11]

Table 3–1 House and Brackmann Clinical Grading of Facial Nerve Function[11]

Grade	Descriptor	Detailed description
1	Normal	Normal facial function in all areas
2	Mild dysfunction	• Gross: Slight weakness noticeable on close inspection; may have very slight synkinesis • At rest: Normal symmetry and tone • Motion ○ Forehead: Slight to moderate movement ○ Eye: Complete closure with effort ○ Mouth: Slight asymmetry
3	Moderate dysfunction	• Gross: Obvious but not disfiguring asymmetry: noticeable but not severe synkinesis • Motion ○ Forehead: Slight to moderate movement ○ Eye: Complete closure with effort ○ Mouth: Slightly weak with maximal effort
4	Moderate to severe dysfunction	• Gross: Obvious weakness and/or asymmetry • Motion ○ Forehead: None ○ Eye: Incomplete closure ○ Mouth: Asymmetry with maximum effort
5	Severe dysfunction	• Gross: Only barely perceptible motion • At rest: Asymmetry • Motion ○ Forehead: None ○ Eye: Incomplete closure
6	Total paralysis	No movement

◆ Vestibulocochlear Nerve Injuries

Site of Trauma

Hearing and labyrinthine dysfunction occur in head injuries due to damage to the auditory or vestibular nerves and their end organs, or trauma to the middle ear and conducting elements such as the ossicular chain. Conductive hearing loss follows longitudinal temporal bone fractures in over 50% of cases. Transverse fractures result in vestibular and cochlear nerve laceration in over 80% of cases. In transverse fractures of the petrous bone, the anterior portion of the vestibule and the basilar turn of the cochlea are often damaged, and many of these patients will have an accompanying facial paralysis. Patients with a fracture involving the optic capsule will often develop total degeneration of the cochlear and vestibular end organs.[1]

Clinical Features

Findings associated with a fracture of the petrous portion of the temporal bone include hemotympanum or tympanic membrane perforation with blood in the external canal, hearing loss, vestibular dysfunction, peripheral facial nerve palsy, CSF otorrhea, and ecchymosis of the scalp over the mastoid bone (Battle's sign). Benign positional vertigo occurs in ~25% of patients following head trauma. Vestibular symptoms are often not evaluated with caloric stimulation in the acute phase for fear of introducing infection in the presence of a perforated drum. These tests should be done once the patient is stable and any perforation of the tympanic membrane has healed if vestibular symptoms still persist. In a conscious individual, the absence of nystagmus on caloric testing indicates damage to the vestibular nerve or end organ.[4] Tinnitus has been reported in 30 to 70% of patients with head injuries. Hearing loss of some degree after head trauma has been reported in over one half of patients with serious head injuries. In the majority of cases, hearing loss is of a sensorineural type, with the conductive variety accounting for only ~3% of cases.[3]

Evaluation

To evaluate injury, the external canals and tympanic membranes must be examined. An audiogram including pure-tone and speech audiometry, brainstem auditory evoked potential, acoustic reflexes, and middle ear function is used to assess hearing loss. The main radiologic investigation consists of high-resolution CT of the posterior fossa with appropriate window levels to visualize the bony anatomy of the petrous bone. Labyrinthine function is best assessed by caloric stimulation and electronystagmography.[3]

Management

Conductive hearing loss due to ossicular chain disruption can be treated surgically by correcting the middle ear, and it has a good prognosis. There is no specific treatment for sensorineural deafness. A hearing aid may help. Some improvement ensues with partial injuries. Cochlear implants are undergoing clinical trials and hold promise in the treatment of sensorineural deafness.[3] Labyrinthine sedatives, such as prochlorperazine, along with avoidance of sudden change of posture and firm reassurance, are the recommended treatment of the minor types of dizziness, vertigo, and nausea that are seen so frequently after trivial head injuries. Positioning maneuvers, such as Epley's, Hallpike's, or Semont's, which move the debris out of

Table 3–2   Gardener and Robertson Modification of Silverstein and Norrell's Hearing Classification[13,14]

Class	Description	Pure tone audiogram (dB)	Speech discrimination (%)
I	Good–excellent	0–30	70–100
II	Serviceable	31–50	50–59
III	Not serviceable	51–90	5–49
IV	Poor	91–max	1–4
V	None	Not testable	0

the semicircular canal and into the utricle, can be curative for benign positional vertigo.[4] Perilymph fistula with loss of eighth nerve function indicates surgical exploration. In refractory post-traumatic vertigo, a labyrinthectomy or translabyrinthine vestibulocochlear nerve section or selective vestibular nerve section (in cases with preserved hearing) may provide relief.[1]

Prognosis

The prognosis for impaired hearing of the conductive type due to hemotympanum or ossicular chain disruption is usually good. Hemotympanum usually resolves spontaneously, and ossicular chain disruption can be corrected surgically in most cases. The prognosis of sensorineural deafness is poor. Some improvement may occur with partial lesions. Labyrinthine symptoms of dizziness, nausea, and vertigo usually subside in 6 to 12 weeks (**Table 3–2**).[4]

◆ Injuries to the Glossopharyngeal, Vagus, Spinal Accessory, and Hypoglossal Nerves

Cranial nerves IX, X, and XI, together with the internal jugular vein, pass through the jugular foramen at the base of the skull. The hypoglossal foramen, through which cranial nerve XII passes, lies just medial to the jugular foramen. Unilateral paralysis of the last four cranial nerves, which may be traumatic, inflammatory, or secondary to neoplastic compression, is referred to as the Collet-Sicard syndrome.[12]

Site of Trauma

Gunshot or stab wounds occasionally cause injury. A fracture of the occipital condyle, or Collet-Sicard syndrome, can injure all four nerves. The peripheral portion of CN XI can be injured in surgical procedures such as posterior cervical lymph node biopsies. The hypoglossal and recurrent laryngeal nerves can be traumatized in anterior neck operations such as carotid endarterectomy.[1]

Clinical Features

The symptomatology produced by an injury in this region can be inferred from the anatomy and function of the lower four cranial nerves. It consists of cardiac irregularities, excessive salivation, loss of sensation and gag reflex of the ipsilateral palate, loss of taste sensation of the posterior one third of the tongue, a hoarse voice with paralysis of the ipsilateral vocal cord, some dysphagia, and hemiatrophy of the tongue with deviation to the side of the injury. Additional symptoms and signs may be present if neighboring structures (e.g., the carotid artery, internal jugular vein, styloid process, and facial nerve) are also involved in the traumatic process.[4]

Lower cranial nerve findings associated with signs of brainstem compression are consistent with an intracranial lesion, whereas the presence of Horner's syndrome is consistent with an extracranial lesion.[1]

Evaluation

A careful clinical examination is mandatory. CT and MRI scans are both useful, depending on the case.

Management

Treatment of Collet-Sicard syndrome is supportive with elevation of the head for drainage of excess saliva and intravenous (IV) or nasogastric nutrition until normal swallowing returns. Accessory nerve injuries in the neck may require exploration with neurolysis or resection and repair or grafting, depending on the degree of injury.[1]

Prognosis

Collet-Sicard syndrome may show slow partial recovery. Patients with vagal, spinal accessory, and hypoglossal nerve injuries associated with carotid endarterectomy often recover.[4]

Case Management

The patient's difficulty with tasting his food is related to an injury to the olfactory nerves, CN I, during the assault. The sense of smell is intimately involved with taste, and patients with head injury are at risk for this condition. In this patient, there is really nothing wrong with his taste buds, or other cranial nerves involved with taste sensation. The patient's deficit may improve over time depending on the extent of the injury to his olfactory nerves.

References

1. Winn HR. Youman's Neurological Surgery. 5th ed. Philadelphia: WB Saunders; 2004
2. Reiter ER. Effects of head injury on olfaction and taste. Otolaryngol Clin North Am 2004;37:1167–1184
3. Keane JR, Baloh RW. Posttraumatic cranial neuropathies. Neurol Clin 1992;10: 849–867
4. Greenberg MS. Handbook of Neurosurgery. 5th ed. New York: Thieme; 2000
5. Cook MW, Levin LA, Joseph MP, Pinczower EF. Traumatic optic neuropathy: a meta-analysis. Arch Otolaryngol Head Neck Surg 1996;122:389–392
6. Kline LB, Marawetz RB, Swaid SU. Indirect injury of the optic nerve. Neurosurgery 1984;14:756–764
7. Elston JS. Traumatic third nerve palsy. Br J Ophthalmol 1984;68:538–543
8. Summers CG, Wirtschafter JD. Bilateral trigeminal and abducens neuropathies following low-velocity, crushing head injury. J Neurosurg 1979;50:508–511
9. Advani RM. Bilateral sixth nerve palsy after head trauma. Ann Emerg Med 2003;41:27–31
10. Cannon CR, Jahrsdoerfer RA. Temporal bone fractures: review of 90 cases. Arch Otolaryngol 1983;109:285–288
11. House WF, Brackmann DE. Facial nerve grading system. Otolaryngol Head Neck Surg 1985;98:184–193
12. Hashimoto T, Watanabe O, Takase M, et al. Collet-Sicard syndrome after minor head trauma. Neurosurgery 1988;23:367–370
13. Gardener G, Robertson JH. Hearing preservation in unilateral acoustic neuroma surgery. Ann Otol Rhinol Laryngol 1988;97:55–66
14. Silverstein H, McDaniel A, Norrell H, et al. Hearing preservation after acoustic neuroma surgery with intraoperative direct eighth cranial nerve monitoring, II: A classification of results. Otolaryngol Head Neck Surg 1986;95:285–291

4

Altered Level of Consciousness: Pathophysiology and Management

Jeffery M. Jones and Dan Miulli

Case Study

A 50-year-old Caucasian female was involved in a motor vehicle accident, during which she suffered a severe head injury, with initial Glasgow Coma Scale (GCS) score of 10, and worsening. She was intubated at the accident scene, and brought to the emergency room (ER), where the computed tomography (CT) scan of the head showed a 2-cm right-sided subdural hematoma with 1 cm of midline shift. The Patient was immediately taken to the operating room for a craniotomy for evacuation of the subdural hematoma. Despite an uneventful surgery, postoperatively the patient was apparently worse clinically (with GCS score of 3) even in the face of a postoperative CT scan of the head showing the clot gone and the midline shift resolved.

See page 40 for Case Management.

Before discussing the causes, categories, workup, or treatment of an altered level of consciousness (ALOC), it is necessary to give a brief description of the term *consciousness*. Although this subject frequently lends to long philosophical debates, consciousness exists to perceive that which exists. That which exists includes subjects such as people, places, things, the actions of that which exists, time, and a multitude of other mental functions such as concept formation and the ability to manipulate these concepts. Consciousness is the awareness of self and the environment in which we live.

It is the physician's responsibility to evaluate these mental processes and compare them within the context of the patient's age, medical condition, baseline level of mental functioning, and numerous other factors, including comparison to the average mental functioning of the general population. What follows is the evaluation process, along with the differential diagnosis and initial management, of these patients in the neurosurgical intensive care unit (NICU).

◆ Definitions

There are three major categories of ALOC that should be defined: delirium, dementia, and coma. Coma will be discussed in Chapter 5. The main differences between dementia and delirium are etiology and time course of the disease process. Delirium is generally due to more acute, reversible processes, whereas dementias tend to be due to chronic irreversible diseases. **Table 4–1** summarizes the characteristics of each.[1]

◆ Evaluation of Mental Status

The most common methods for evaluating a patient's mental status as an inpatient are the Glasgow Coma Scale (GCS) and the Mini–Mental State Examination (MMSE). Other methods of evaluation of mental status and disability are available, but they are rarely used in the inpatient setting due to limited time and use in following the patient's day-to-day progress. This being said, it may be of some utility to use more comprehensive functional scales to follow the patient's progress over time. An in-depth functional predischarge assessment can be reviewed and contrasted for each clinic follow-up appointment. It will also provide rehabilitation services with an idea of the patient's baseline following the neurologic insult. The rehabilitation physician, neurointensivist, neurologist, and neurosurgeon should determine, and, if possible, agree upon the best choice of in-depth functional assessment and grading scale for tracking progress. Coma is considered to be a GCS score of 8 or less (see Chapter 5). An additional measurement, the National Institutes of Health (NIH) Stroke Scale, may also be used, particularly if the patient has focal or lateralizing motor or sensory deficits (see **Tables 4–2** and **4–3**).[2–4]

◆ Causes of Altered Level of Consciousness

The causes of altered mentation in the NICU are slightly different than in the ER. Most NICU patients have head trauma, cerebrovascular accident (CVA), neurosurgery, or other known sources of intracranial insult that could lead to an ALOC. Many times the neurointensivist is faced with a patient who was previously alert and aware and has deteriorated. The challenge to the neurointensivist is to identify the cause of the ALOC and institute the appropriate intervention. It is beyond the scope of this book to give an exhaustive list of the possible causes of ALOC, but **Table 4–4** represents the categories of causes and some of the most common causes of ALOC in each category.

Table 4–1 Comparison of Altered States of Consciousness[1]

State of consciousness	Definition	Pathophysiology	Time course	Disposition
Delirium	Acute confusional state, with impaired attention, perception, thinking, and memory	Always has an organic cause • Primary intracranial disease • Systemic disease • Exogenous toxins • Drug withdrawal	Acute	Often reversible when underlying etiology is addressed
Dementia	Implies a loss of mental capacity; short-term memory is particularly affected, as well as cognitive abilities	Most are idiopathic (e.g., Alzheimer's, Parkinson's, vascular dementia)	Usually chronic and progressive	Usually not reversible, but can be treated symptomatically to a limited extent; only 10–20% have a reversible condition
Coma	Reduced state of alertness and responsiveness in which the patient cannot be aroused	Complex with many different sources	Usually acute or subacute	May be reversible if source is rapidly identified; the more time a patient spends in a coma, the less favorable the prognosis

Table 4–2   Glasgow Coma Scale, Age 4 Years and Up*

Points*	Best motor response	Best verbal/ speech response	Best eye response
6	Obeys commands	–	–
5	Localizes to pain	Oriented conversation	–
4	Withdraws from pain	Confused conversation	Open spontaneously
3	Decorticate: flexes abnormally	Inappropriate words	Open to name or verbal stimuli
2	Decerebrate: rigid extension	Incomprehensible sounds	Open to pressure/pain
1	No movement	No speech response	No eye opening

Source: Adapted from Teasdale G, Jennett B. Assessment of coma and impaired consciousness: a practical scale. Lancet 1974;2:81–84. Reprinted by permission.
* Add the totals of best responses from each column. Range of total points: 3 (worst) to 15 (normal).

Table 4–3   Elements of the Mini-Mental State Examination*

- Orientation to time and place
- Registration of spoken information
- Attention and calculation—following directions and doing mathematical calculations
- Recall of information from registration task
- Language tests—naming objects, repeating phrases, following a 3-stage command, reading a command and following it, writing a sentence
- Construction—copying a shape

Source: From Psychological Assessment Resources, Inc., 16204 North Florida Avenue, Lutz, Florida 33549, from the Mini–Mental State Examination by Marshal Folstein and Susan Folstein, by special permission of the publisher. Copyright 1975, 1998, 2001 by Mini Mental LLC, Inc. Published 2001 by Psychological Assessment Resources, Inc. Further reproduction is prohibited without permission of PAR, Inc. The MMSE can be purchased from PAR, Inc., by calling (813) 968-3003.
*The MMSE is a series of questions and tasks that the physician administers to a patient and scores in about 10 minutes and is designed to assess cognitive function.

5
Coma

Jeffery M. Jones and Dan Miulli

Case Study

A 69-year-old African American female is brought to the emergency room (ER) by ambulance after an acute loss of consciousness, prior to which the patient was complaining of a headache. The patient had a prior history of ischemic heart disease, diabetes, hypercholesterolemia, and uncontrolled hypertension. Neurosurgery was consulted prior to the patient's arrival to the ER, as the patient had been intubated by the paramedics at her home.

See page 47 for Case Management.

Consciousness is defined for medical purposes as the awareness of self and environment. Coma is a more severe form of depressed consciousness in which the patient's view of self and environment is not only inaccurate or misperceived, but is a state in which the brain is not able to receive stimuli from the environment without aggressive stimulation. Even with aggressive stimulation the patient is not awake enough to process environmental stimuli to any significant extent, and awareness of self is only on the very basic sensory levels (e.g., pain). The patient's interaction with the environment during coma is, at best, reflexive.

The most commonly used grading system of consciousness (or coma) is the Glasgow Coma Scale (GCS). Coma is usually defined as a GCS score of 8 or less. Comatose patients, at best, open their eyes to painful stimulation and will localize to pain. Anatomically, coma can be caused by diffuse cortical dysfunction or by a dysfunction of the reticular activating system located in the brainstem (midbrain) (see **Table 4–1** on page 35).[1]

◆ Initial Care of the Coma Patient

Most neurosurgical services do not become involved in the initial evaluation of a patient presenting to the ER in a coma of unknown etiology; however, it is useful to review the proper initial management of a comatose patient who has not received any laboratory or radiographic workup (**Table 5–1**).

Table 5–1   Initial Management Steps[1,2]

Goal	Method
Ensure patent airway and adequate oxygenation	Start mechanical ventilation or O_2 by mask if patient is breathing on his or her own
Protect C-spine	Immobilize C-spine with cervical collar
Maintain MAP above 100	Use fluids and vasopressors as necessary
Treat possible metabolic cause(s) after initial blood draw	Thiamine 100 mg IV, then glucose 25 g IV (d50)
Treat increased ICP if there is strong suspicion	Mannitol 0.25–1 g/kg bolus
Treat seizures	Benzodiazepine IV (Ativan 2 mg IV)
Restore acid–base balance	Judicious use of fluids (0.9% saline preferred)
Treat any suspected drug overdose	Naloxone 0.2 mg IV and repeat; physostigmine 1 mg IV; flumazenil 0.2 mg IV
Rule out space-occupying lesion	Stat CT scan of head
Normalize body temperature	Warm fluids and warming blankets
Treat any suspected meningitis or systemic infection	Wide-spectrum antibiotics
Specific therapy ASAP	

ASAP, as soon as possible; CT, computed tomography; d50, dextrose 50; ICP, intracranial pressure; IV, intravenous; MAP, mean arterial pressure.

◆ Causes of Coma

Causes of coma can be broken down into two main categories, structural and metabolic. Structural causes are due to lesions physically interfering with nervous system pathways by trauma, compression due to the lesion, or increased pressure. Metabolic causes are due to chemical imbalances leading to improper functioning of the nervous system or some of its components (**Table 5–2**).[1]

Table 5–2   Structural and Metabolic Causes and Types of Coma[1]

Structural coma	Metabolic coma	
Hematoma	Hypoglycemia	Hypothermia/hyperthermia
Trauma	Adrenal failure	Hypo-/hyperosmolarity
Tumor	Liver disease	Diabetic ketoacidosis
Hydrocephalus	Renal disease	Encephalopathy
Abscess	Pulmonary disease	Drugs
	Dialysis disequilibrium	Toxins

A frequently overlooked cause of coma is silent status epilepticus, which should be considered when structural and other metabolic causes of coma have been excluded.

Structural lesions can cause coma through three general mechanisms: compression of the brainstem, direct damage to the brainstem, or diffuse dysfunction of the cerebral hemispheres. Damage to the brainstem can occur through a primary effect on the brainstem such as a tumor, hemorrhage, or infarct of the brainstem, or it can be due to external pressure on the brainstem by another part of the brain that contains the pathology. This can be due to pathology that causes transtentorial herniation of the diencephalon or medial temporal lobe, or it can be due to a posterior fossa lesion causing compression of the brainstem. Supratentorial pathology tends to lead to one of the herniation syndromes listed in **Table 5–3**. The herniation syndromes, especially uncal and central herniation, pass through the diencephalic, mesencephalic-pontine, pontomedullary, and medullary stages. The tonsillar and cingulate herniation syndromes may be progressive, but their progression is less well defined. Posterior fossa lesions may also lead to supratentorial herniation by causing an obstructive hydrocephalus, which can also result in herniation (**Tables 5–4** and **5–5**).[2]

Table 5–3   Supratentorial Herniation Syndromes[3]

	Central herniation	Uncal herniation	Tonsillar herniation	Cingulate herniation
Lesion location	Diffuse supratentorial increase in ICP with no pressure gradient from right to left	Usually unilateral lesions, especially those located in the temporal lobes	Posterior fossa space-occupying lesion	Usually unilateral lesions, especially those located above the temporal lobes
Structures involved	Diencephalic compression progressing to pressure on the reticular activating system	Ipsilateral CN III, ipsilateral PCA, contralateral cerebral peduncle	Medullary respiratory center	Anterior cerebral artery
Signs/ symptoms	Altered level of consciousness	Ipsilateral pupil dilation, ipsilateral hemiparesis (Kernohan's notch phenomenon)	Respiratory arrest	Leg weakness

CN, cranial nerve; ICP, intracranial pressure; PCA, posterior cerebral artery.

Table 5–4 Stages of Central Herniation[3]

	Diencephalic stage	Mesencephalic-pontine stage	Pontomedullary stage	Medullary stage
Consciousness	Agitation or drowsiness	Comatose	Comatose	Comatose
Respiration	Sighs and yawns	Cheyne-Stokes or tachypnea	Regular or shallow or rapid	Slow, irregular rate and depth, possible hyperpnea with apneic periods
Systemic responses	Diabetes insipidus (DI)	Hypothalamic dysfunction (DI, poikilothermia)		Fluctuating pulse, drop in blood pressure
Pupils	Small (1–3 mm) reactive	Midposition (3–4 mm), fixed	Small to midposition and fixed	Dilated and fixed
Eye movements	Roving eye movements; vestibulo-ocular reflex may be weak or brisk; no caloric response; no vertical eye movement	Vestibulo-ocular reflex impaired with possible disconjugate response	No vestibulo-ocular reflex, no oculocephalic response	No vestibulo-ocular reflex, no oculocephalic response
Motor	Worsening of existing hemiplegia, decorticate posturing	Decerebrate posturing	Flaccid flexor response	Flaccid; no deep tendon reflexes

Table 5–5 Stages of Uncal Herniation[2]

	Early third nerve stage	Late third nerve stage
Consciousness	Agitated or drowsy	Obtunded
Respiration	Normal	Hyperventilation
Pupils	Relative dilation of ipsilateral pupil	Fully dilated pupil
Eye movements	Oculocephalic or normal disconjugate	
Motor	Appropriate to pain (localizes), contralateral Babinski's sign	Possible ipsilateral hemiplegia (Kernohan's notch), decerebrate

◆ Evaluation of Coma Patient

Respiratory Patterns in Coma

The pattern of respiration can give some insight as to the source of coma and possibly indicate where in the brain the dysfunction lies. **Table 5–6** summarizes the different types of respiration and their meaning. Both metabolic and structural lesions can give rise to abnormal respiratory patterns.[3,4]

Ocular Findings in Coma

Ocular findings are most informative in comatose patients, especially in those who do not have a motor response to noxious stimuli. Some generalizations can also be made concerning the pupillary responses:

1. Normal pupillary responses strongly favor a metabolic process in a coma of unknown origin.
2. The size of the pupils can give a clue as to the type of metabolic process that may be involved (e.g., narcotic overdose, anticholinergic toxicity).
3. Pupillary responses can be the most useful information regarding metabolic versus structural lesion short of imaging (**Table 5–7**).[5]

◆ Outcome of Coma[6]

- Twenty percent of comatose patients (GCS = 3) survive; 10% have functional survival.
- Age > 60 years significantly reduces the chances of a good outcome.
- Hypotension and hypoxia double morbidity and mortality.

Table 5–6 Abnormal Respirations in Coma[4,5]

Respiration type	Description	Anatomical structure	Causes
Cheyne-Stokes	Periodic breathing; tachypnea alternates regularly and gradually with apnea	Unknown	Prolonged circulation time, bilateral suprapontine neurologic injury
Hyperventilation	Rapid, regular breathing	Not associated with a particular lesion site	Metabolic and physiologic disorders, acidosis
Apneustic	Inspiration cramp; excessive inspiration relative to expiration	Structure responsible remains unclear; pontine transaction just rostral to the trigeminal motor nuclei and to the nucleus parabrachiales (case reports)	Brainstem demyelinating lesions and cervicomedullary compression have been associated with this ventilatory pattern
Ataxic	Breathing varies irregularly in depth as well as frequency	Pons and medulla	Medullary lesions are probably the only reliable predictor of lesion site

Table 5–7 Ocular and Periocular Findings and Their Meaning[1,2]

Structure	Finding	Meaning
Eyelids	Widened palpebral fissure	Facial paralysis
	Absent corneal reflex	Dysfunction of CN5 or CN7 or their connection
Ocular movements	Ping-pong gaze	Bilateral cerebral dysfunction
	Horizontal gaze deviation	Ipsilateral frontal eye field dysfunction, contralateral seizure; unilateral pons lesion gives ipsilateral gaze palsy
	Vertical gaze disturbance	Posterior diencephalic and midbrain dysfunction
	Ocular bobbing	Extensive structural pontine damage
	Disconjugate ocular bobbing	Pontomesencephalic damage
	Reverse bobbing (fast phase upward)	Metabolic encephalopathy, most prominently in anoxia

CN, cranial nerve.

♦ Traumatic subarachnoid hemorrhage (SAH) is a significant independent prognostic indicator of poor outcome. It occurs in 26 to 53% of traumatic brain injuries, and mortality is increased twofold.

♦ Midline shift of 0.5 to 1.5 cm in patients > 45 years of age is correlated with poor outcome.

Case Management

Upon arrival to the ER, the patient was found to be nonresponsive, albeit she had been sedated and paralyzed for intubation. Despite the paralytics, her pupils could still be examined, and were found to be unequal. The right pupil was 3 mm and reactive to light, and the left pupil was nonreactive at 8 mm. The patient was immediately taken to the CT scanner, being hyperventilated on the way. The CT head showed a massive left-sided basal ganglia bleed and radiologic evidence for left uncal herniation. Clearly, the patient had had a hypertensive hemorrhage as the cause of her coma. The patient was not felt to be surgical due to the location of the bleed.

References

1. Plum F, Posner J. The Diagnosis of Stupor and Coma. Philadelphia: FA Davis; 1980
2. Fisher C. Brain herniation: a revision of classical concepts. Can J Neurol Sci 1995;22:83–91
3. Simon R. Respiratory manifestations of neurologic disease. In: Goetz C, Tanner C, Aminoff M, eds. Handbook of Clinical Neurology. Vol 19. Amsterdam: Elsevier Science Publishers; 1993:477–501
4. North J, Jennett S. Abnormal breathing patterns associated with acute brain damage. Arch Neurol 1974;31:338–344
5. Greenberg M. Handbook of Neurosurgery. 4th ed. New York: Thieme; 1996:553–563
6. Levy DE, Knill-Jones RP, Plum F. The vegetative state and its prognosis following nontraumatic coma. Ann N Y Acad Sci 1978;315:293–306

6
Neuroimaging and the Neurosurgical Intensive Care Unit Patient

Ganna L. Breland and Dan Miulli

Case Study

A 14-year-old boy sustains a head injury during a head-on collision with a tree while snow boarding without a helmet. He is brought to the ER, still awake and alert, but with a 4-cm laceration over his right temple, and obvious cerebrospinal fluid (CSF) leaking from the injury site. Computed tomography (CT) scan of the head shows a right temporal region skull fracture under the laceration with the inner table of the skull depressed 1.5 cm into the cranial cavity.

See page 58 for Case Management.

All patients should be stabilized according to the "A, B, Cs" (A, airway; B, breathing; C, circulation). Most important in determining neurological injuries are the history and neurological examination. After the initial evaluation, the secondary survey includes lateral cervical spine x-rays. Some institutions have supplemented lateral cervical x-rays with CT scans with reconstructed views to rule out obvious fractures and malalignments. The quality of the lateral reconstructed cervical spine views depends on the thickness of the slice and their overlap; the smaller the thickness, the better the quality of reconstruction. Additional x-rays or films are taken as needed.

◆ Plain Films

Skull x-rays may show nontraumatic abnormalities, such as congenital skull defects, skull lesions, or even foreign bodies.[1]

Traumatic linear fractures must differentiate from vessel grooves and suture lines. Vessel grooves are thicker, and may curve and branch. Suture lines are wide and jagged and follow the course to meet other sutures.[2] Traumatic linear fractures are often associated with epidural hematoma (EDH) or subdural hematoma (SDH).[3]

Table 6–1   Classification of Types of Fractures[1]

Type	Characteristics
Linear	Differentiate from vessel grooves and suture lines; often associated with EDH or SDH
Depressed	Best evaluated by CT bone window; depression is greater than thickness of the skull or 8–10 mm
Diastatic	Widens the suture line
Growing	Wide fracture associated with dural tear; confirm with repeat imaging; rarely seen in pediatric patients and less so in adult population
Ping-pong fracture	Most likely seen in newborn; nonsurgical except for cosmetic purposes

CT, computed tomography; EDH, epidural hematoma; SDH, subdural hematoma.

Traumatic depressed skull fractures are best evaluated by CT scan using bone windows. It is important to determine if there is trauma to underlying brain if the depression is greater than the thickness of the skull, or 8 to 10 mm.

The fracture may appear within the suture of the calvarium called diastasis, or widening of the suture line. On follow-up films, the fracture may grow if associated with dural tear. This is rarely seen in pediatric patients and less so in the adult population (**Table 6–1**).

Skull x-rays also demonstrate foreign bodies, postoperative changes, and extracranial material, such as reservoirs, plates, or screws, and intracranial material, such as shunt tubing, coils, or clips.

Spine x-rays may show nontraumatic abnormalities, such as congenital defects, degenerative processes, or pathological fractures.

Traumatic findings include fractures, dislocation, subluxation, and rotation. The completed cervical spine evaluation must be seen from the craniocervical junction through T1. If the entire view is not seen, then a swimmer's view must be obtained with the arm above the head so that there is less tissue to shoot through. A consistent process must be adhered to every time a cervical spine x-ray is obtained. On a lateral x-ray, look for smooth contours of the anterior and posterior marginal line, as well as the alignment of the spinolaminar line. The alignment of the posterior spinous line is an approximation. When reviewing the posterior elements, attention should be paid to the fanning of the spinous processes. After the bone is inspected, the soft tissue should be reviewed. Prevertebral soft tissue swelling may be an indicator of damage as well. Approximations of normal width of the prevertebral tissue is 6 mm at C3 and 12 mm at C6.[2] The lateral cervical spine x-ray should include measurement of the atlantodental interval as an indicator of atlantoaxial subluxation; it should be 2.5 to 3 mm in adults. Other areas of concern are the normal cervical lordotic curvature and loss of vertebral height, or fracture lines, or change in disk height. The same areas should be reviewed in the thoracic and lumbar spine. If there is a mechanism of injury that leads to cervical spine radiographs, then it is usually a good idea to x-ray the thoracic and lumbar spines (**Table 6–2**).

Table 6–2   Plain Film Imaging Views and Their Uses[1-3]

X-ray view	Characteristics
Lateral cervical	Contours of anterior and posterior marginal line, spinolaminar line, and posterior spinous line
	Fanning of the spinous processes
	Prevertebral soft tissue swelling
	Atlantodental interval of 2.5–3 mm in adults
	Normal lordotic curvature
	Loss of vertebral height, fracture lines, disk height
Anteroposterior	Evidence of rotation and compression
Open mouth odontoid	Evaluation of odontoid fractures
	Occipitoatlantal joints
	Lateral masses overhang of C1 and C2 not more than 7 mm
	Atlantoaxial alignment
Oblique	Neural foramina, lamina, and pedicles
Anteroposterior and lateral	Measure angulation caused from compression or burst fractures
Oblique	Pedicles, lamina, facet joint, and pars interarticularis
	Useful to rule out spondylolysis

X-rays in the neurosurgical intensive care unit (NICU) may be done after the application of a halo or tongs for traction to evaluate reduction after each addition of weights or each manipulation of the device. X-rays will look for postoperative instrumentation placement. Dynamic films, or flexion and extension films, evaluate motion. These are most often used for cervical spine clearance, but they are also used to evaluate subluxation with spondylolisthesis and compression fractures. For cervical spine clearance, the patient must be alert and cooperative. Dynamic films cannot be used if there is more than 3.5 mm subluxation seen on the lateral film or if the patient is not neurologically intact.

◆ CT Scan of the Brain

CT scan is the best imaging tool for studying bone or other calcific structures. It is based on attenuation of the electron density of the material in the path of the x-ray beam. It is good for the initial assessment of head injury and neurological deficits, as well as for patients who cannot have magnetic resonance imaging (MRI). However, CT scan is prone to artifact from the densest material and cannot differentiate between soft tissues of similar densities; therefore, it is less advantageous for posterior fossa evaluation. It is contraindicated with contrast enhancement if the patient is in renal failure and blood urea nitrogen (BUN) > 2.0, or if there is a first-trimester pregnancy. CT scans can be completed with or without contrast. If you suspect a bleed inside the skull, do not use contrast on initial exam. Noncontrasted CT scans can also be utilized to evaluate hardware placement and function with deep brain stimulators, intracranial pressure (ICP) monitors and drains, external ventricular drain, and subdural catheters and as follow-up for residual or reaccumulation of hemorrhage. Contrasted CT scans are helpful when evaluating residual tumor or abscess, when MRI is not accessible or tolerated by the patient.

The CT scan measures exposures in Hounsfield units from –1000 to 4000, progressing from dark (hypodense) to bright (hyperdense), for example, air→fat→water→CSF→brain tissue→subacute blood→liquid blood→clotted blood→bone→contrast→metals.[4]

CT scans can demonstrate deleterious changes for the neurological patient. This is useful when the neurological exam is compromised by sedation or overmedication. Some CT scan signs of increased intracranial pressure are the following:[5]

◆ Loss of sulci
◆ Compressed ventricles, loss of fourth ventricle
◆ Loss of cisterns
◆ Midline shift

As the condition worsens, the patient may progress to herniation (**Table 6–3**).

Brain CT scans are useful for the evaluation of neurological deficits, both new onset and progressive, and for following the progression of known pathology, such as hydrocephalus, infarction, edema, and intra- and extra-axial hemorrhage. Contrasted CT scans evaluate neurological deficits when there is a suspected mass or infection.

Table 6–3   Types of Herniation[3–6]

Type of herniation	Characteristics
Subfalcine	Cingulated gyrus shifts under the falx
Central transtentorial	Diencephalon is forced through the incisura; obliteration of the quadrigeminal and perimesencephalic cisterns
Uncal	Uncus and hippocampal gyrus forced over the edge of the tentorium; decrease in suprasellar cistern followed by parasellar and interpeduncular cisterns
Upward	Cerebellar vermis ascends above tentorium; may cause hydrocephalus by compression of sylvian aqueduct and quadrigeminal cistern
Tonsillar	Cerebellar tonsils descend through foramen magnum (more likely seen on sagittal section of MRI)

MRI, magnetic resonance imaging.

Some characteristic CT scan findings for bleeds are:[6]

- *Epidural hematoma*   Biconvex or lentiform appearance, often underlying fractures, located between skull and dura; may be limited by suture lines; usually seen in acute phase when lesion is hyperdense; areas of hypodensity indicate active bleeding
- *Subdural hematoma*   Crescent shaped, between brain and dura; may be acute (hyperdense), subacute (nearly isodense), or chronic (hypodense); areas of hypodensity indicate active bleeding in an acute SDH; may see areas of calcification in chronic SDH
- *Subarachnoid hemorrhage (SAH)*   Seen within the cisterns and sulci
- *Intracerebral hemorrhage (ICH)*   Seen in putamen, caudate, cerebellum, and brainstem where hypertensive hemorrhages are likely to occur spontaneously

EDHs are seen less frequently than SDHs and are usually the result of bleeding from the lacerated middle meningeal artery or the dural venous sinus.

SDH is usually the result of bleeding from bridging cortical veins.

SAH should be suspected before or after an accident or in association with the worst headache of the patient's life. Most CT scans should be repeated in 12 to 24 hours. ICHs tend to reoccur after 6 to 12 hours.

CT Scan of the Spine

When used by itself, a CT scan of the spine provides limited data. It is useful for the evaluation of the bone and its alignment, such as when considering canal stenosis, degeneration, spontaneous hemorrhage, bony lesions, pathological fractures, traumatic fractures, or subluxation, or when planning for the surgical approach and instrumentation. When suspecting a fracture, obtain sagittal and coronal reconstructions for maximum benefit. There are also three-dimensional reconstructions that assist even further with fracture and malalignment identification.

A CT scan of the spine provides only limited data about soft tissue. When done after myelography, it becomes extremely useful, particularly when instrumentation obscures the view with MRI, the patient cannot tolerate MRI, or the patient has a history of multiple back surgeries. However, when concerned about changes within the spinal canal, other than stenosis, consider using MRI as the first advanced test. Contrasted CT scans can help identify osteomyelitis and tumor.

Other Types of CT Scans

CT scan information can be formatted in newer ways that have proven to be extremely beneficial, such as CT angiography (CTA). CTA is a less invasive test than conventional angiogram and offers comparable results for many clinical situations. It aids with the diagnosis of arterial dissections, acute stroke, and aneurysms.

◆ MRI

MRI is based on the relaxation characteristics of protons in different chemical states. For the optimal scan, the patient must not have any ferromagnetic material in the area to be scanned and must remain immobile in a narrow, loud scanning tube for 20 to 40 minutes; if not, the image will be severely degraded. The MRI is quite different from the CT scan in that different information can be sought based on the radiofrequency pulsations and magnetic gradients programmed prior to scanning. MRI does not use ionizing radiation, unlike CT scan. In the past, MRI has been more expensive, because it was a newer technology. Now the costs of MRI and CT are comparable, so the initial advanced test after the history and physical exam should be an MRI when appropriate. It is not cost-effective to use CT first.

MRI Protocols

- ◆ T1-weighted image
    - ◇ Echo time (TE) < 50, repetition time (TR) < 1000
    - ◇ Progressing in intensity from hypointense, to isointense, to hyperintense (from dark to bright): bone→calcium→CSF→gray matter→white matter→fat/ melanin/blood > 48 hours old[4]
    - ◇ Most pathology is dark (hypointense = low signal).
    - ◇ Good for detecting gadolinium contrast enhancement

- ◆ T2-weighted image
    - ◇ TE > 80, TR > 2000
    - ◇ Progressing from dark to bright: fat→bone→white matter→gray matter→CSF→edema/water
    - ◇ Notice that fat becomes dark on a T2-weighted image, whereas it is bright on a T1-weighted image.
    - ◇ Most pathology is light.
    - ◇ Gadolinium contrast enhancement does not cause much change in intensity of signal.
    - ◇ Good for detecting pathological areas with edema, inflammation, or water (**Table 6–4**)

- ◆ Diffusion-weighted image
    - ◇ Based on movement of water in tissues
    - ◇ Freely diffusing water (CSF) appears dark, whereas restricted diffusion seen with intracellular edema–associated cell swelling from infarction appears bright.
    - ◇ Acute infarction appears bright within minutes.

Table 6–4   Characteristics of T1- and T2-Weighted MRI[1-3]

	TR (msec)	TE (msec)	Bright to dark	Pathology
T1-weighted image	<50	<1000	Fat/melanin/blood >48 h White matter Gray matter Calcium CSF Bone	Dark
T2-weighted image	>80	>2000	Edema/water CSF Gray matter White matter Bone/fat	Light

CSF, cerebrospinal fluid; MRI, magnetic resonance images; TE, echo time; TR, repetition time.

- ◆ Perfusion-weighted image
  - ◇ Uses a bolus of gadolinium
  - ◇ Provides information on microcirculation and further insight into tissue infarction
  - ◇ Used in combination with a diffusion-weighted image to define the area of ischemic penumbra (tissue near the infarction zone that may be salvageable by thrombolytic therapy)

Other MRI protocols include fast spin echo, gradient echo, fluid attenuation inversion recovery (FLAIR), short T1 inversion recovery (STIR), and proton density.

MRI of the Brain

In general, MRI is good for evaluation of soft tissue, posterior fossa lesions, small lesions, and seizure workup when quantifying the amount of specific tissue present, such as the size of the hippocampus. Gadolinium contrast can be used in renal failure when CT contrast may not be used. MRI is still not the most accepted study when evaluating acute bleeding in the brain or for bone evaluation. The MRI scan is much slower than a CT scan, the former taking 20 to 40 minutes, the latter, mere seconds. It should not be used when patients have active pacemakers, known life-sustaining ferromagnetic implants, or any ferromagnetic implants directly in the area to be examined. Gunshot is not ferromagnetic unless a steel-jacket bullet is used, such as in the military.

MRI of the brain should be the first advanced scan in numerous conditions, such as

* Plain MRI

  ◇ Demyelinating disease
  ◇ Degenerative disease
  ◇ Edema
  ◇ Infarct (to distinguish between old and new strokes)
  ◇ Diffuse axonal injury caused by shearing from rotational or deceleration/acceleration, seen at the gray matter–white matter junction, the corpus callosum, and the dorsolateral aspect of the upper brainstem, in order of frequency
  ◇ Midbrain and pontine injury
  ◇ Orbital compartment syndrome

* Contrasted MRI

  ◇ Tumor
  ◇ Infection
  ◇ Inflammation of nerves

MRI of the Spine

MRI is also very useful in the spine, especially when soft tissue evaluation is essential. It is the evaluation of choice after taking the patient's history and performing a physical exam for herniated disc and nerve root impingement, congenital abnormalities, stroke, hemorrhage, ligamentous injury, spinal cord injury, and spinal cord hemorrhage. In the spine, MRI contrast and noncontrasted films are the imaging modality of choice for tumors, including drop metastases; infection, including paravertebral lesions; fistulas; the extent of tumor removal; and postoperative infection.[6]

In facilities with a neurosurgical intensive care unit, an MRI scanner must be available 24 hours a day. It is used emergently in patients with incomplete spinal cord injury or worsening neurological deficit, as well as clinical evidence without radiographic proof of spinal cord injury.[5]

Other Uses of MRI

MRI is used without contrast in determining peripheral nerve injury. Just as CT angiography provides detailed anatomy of the vessels in the brain and the large vessels of the spine, MRI angiography (MRA) demonstrates normal and pathological vascular anatomy such as carotid-cavernous fistulas, as well as vascular malformations, including aneurysms and arteriovenous malformations (AVMs). The venous phase of circulation can also be specifically probed when looking for venous sinus thrombosis. MRI has been employed in neuroscience for decades. It was once referred to as nuclear magnetic resonance (NMR), but the term was changed because of the connotation attached to *nuclear*. MRI examines the characteristic molecules in tissue samples. Magnetic resonance spectroscopy does the same thing on a much larger scale; it produces a graph based on the chemical shift and is used primarily in the brain to help distinguish tumor from infection.[2]

◆ Additional Imaging in the NICU

The angiogram is an invasive test having a 0.5 to 2% risk of major morbidity or mortality.[3] It also carries the risk of ionizing radiation. Although still the "gold standard" in many vascular cases, it has been replaced in some large institutions with CTA and MRA. In the community neurosurgical setting, it remains the procedure of choice to investigate cerebral AVM, aneurysm, and carotid-cavernous fistulas, to determine tumor blood supply and embolization of arterial feeders, to administer an injection for vasospasm, and to evaluate vessel injury (e.g., with gunshot wounds) and pseudoaneurysm development. In the spine the angiogram can be used to evaluate spinal AVM and dural fistulas.

Nuclear medicine scans, such as bone and tagged white blood scans, are used to evaluate osteoblastic activity seen in infection, tumor, and abnormal metabolism. They also can be used to differentiate between old and new fractures.

Transcranial Doppler scans have become extremely useful tools in both trauma and cerebral vascular disease. Such a scan can be performed at bedside to determine if there is vasospasm in the intracranial circulation, as well as the efficacy of thrombolysis in acute stroke. A transcranial Doppler is used to determine brain death.

Ultrasound has become critical in the evaluation of extracranial circulation, both carotid and vertebral, for the degree of stenosis, as well as in the evaluation of the neonatal brain.

◆ Radiology in the NICU

The brain and spinal cord cannot be directly visualized in the intact patient. The most important pieces of information needed to determine the disease process and treatment modalities in the neurocritical patient are the patient's history and physical exam. After obtaining these, the physician must develop an informed opinion of what is wrong and how to treat the patient. Only after this opinion is formed should a radiographic examination be performed to confirm the physician's hypothesis. Radiographic information is not a substitute for good clinical skills.

Case Management

The patient has an open depressed skull fracture. In light of the CSF leak from the laceration over the fracture, almost certainly this patient has an associated dural tear. Despite the good clinical condition of the patient, this is a serious condition with high infection risk, requiring early irrigation and debridement, elevation of the skull fracture, and repair of the dural laceration. The patient was taken to the OR soon after arrival in the ER.

References

1. Novelline RA. Squire's Fundamentals of Radiology. 5th ed. Cambridge, MA, and London: Harvard University Press; 1997
2. Osborn AG. Diagnostic Neuroradiology. St. Louis: Mosby; 1994
3. Greenberg M. Handbook of Neurosurgery. 5th ed. New York: Thieme; 2001
4. Flaherty A. The Massachusetts General Hospital Handbook of Neurology. Philadelphia: Lippincott Williams & Wilkins; 2000
5. Layon AJ, Gabrielli A, Friedman W. Textbook of Neurointensive Care. Philadelphia: WB Saunders; 2004
6. Winn HR. Youmans Neurological Surgery. 5th ed. Philadelphia: WB Saunders; 2004

Table 7–1   Common Laboratory Panels *(Continued)*

Toxicology screen
Acetaminophen
Carbon monoxide
Barbiturate
Ethanol
Ethylene glycol
Cocaine
Cyanide
Benzodiazepines
Tricyclic antidepressants
Methanol
Insulin

ACTH, adrenocorticotropic hormone; ALT, alanine aminotransferase; AST, aspartate aminotransferase; BUN, blood urea nitrogren; CBC, complete blood count; CK, creatine kinase; CK-MB, creatine kinase–MB mass; CMP, cytidine monophosphate; CSF, cerebrospinal fluid; DNA, deoxyribonucleic acid; ESR, erythrocyte sedimentation rate; FTA, fluorescent treponema absorption; HLA, human leukocyte antigen; Ig, immunoglobulin; INR, International Normalized Ratio; LDH, lactate dehydrogenase; MCH, mean corpuscular hemoglobin; MCHC, mean corpuscular hemoglobin concentration; MCV, mean corpuscular volume; PCR, polymerase chain reaction; RBC, red blood cell; TSH, thyroid-stimulating hormone; VDRL, venereal disease research laboratory; WBC, white blood cell.

total and direct bilirubin, γ-glutamyl transterase, glucose, lactate dehydrogenase (LDH), phosphorus, potassium, sodium, protein, magnesium, and uric acid.)

Accuracy of laboratory values is also complicated by sex, age, diet, malnutrition, medications, time of day, and patient position. For example, plasma volume increases when the patient changes from upright to supine; age results in declining cardiac, pulmonary, renal, and metabolic functions; high serum potassium may be simply due to cellular release after prolonged tourniquet constriction or may be the result of hemolysis; low serum glucose may result in patients with high white blood cell (WBC) counts; or low serum sodium and high plasma hemoglobin may result in patients with hyperlipidemia.

Also, automated testing methods tend to be more subject to errors than manual methods, perhaps due to traces of sample remaining in instruments.[1]

◆ Preoperative Testing

Routine preoperative laboratory tests should include a hemogram with differential (WBC, hemoglobin, hematocrit, and platelets), an electrolyte panel (sodium, potassium, chloride, carbon dioxide, BUN, creatinine, and serum

Table 7–2 Normal Laboratory Values[1–7]

Test	Specimen	Method	Normal range conventional units	SI units
Acetylcholine receptor antibody	Serum	Immunoassay	<0.5 nmol/L	<0.5 nmol/L
Acetylcholinesterase	RBC	Enzymatic colorimetry	11,000–15,000 U/L	11–15 kU/L
Adrenocorticotropic hormone (ACTH)	Plasma	Immunoassay	<70 pg/mL	<15 pmol/L
Alanine aminotransferase (ALT)	Serum	Enzymatic colorimetry	<48 U/L	<0.80 mkat/L
Albumin	Serum	Colorimetry	3.5–5.0 g/dL	35–50 g/L
Aldolase	Serum	Enzymatic colorimetry	<8.1 U/L	<135 nkat/L
Aldosterone	Serum	Immunoassay	Supine: <16 ng/dL Upright: 4–31 ng/dL (Normal sodium intake: 100–200 mEq/day)	Supine: < 444 pmol/L Upright: 111–860 pmol/L (Normal sodium intake: 100–200 mmol/day)
Alkaline phosphatase				
Isoenzymes	Serum	Electrophoresis	Intestinal: <18% of total activity Bone: 23–62% of total activity Liver: 38–72% of total activity	Intestinal: <0.18 of total activity Bone: 0.23–0.62 of total activity Liver: 0.38–0.72 of total activity
Total	Serum	Enzymatic colorimetry	20–125 U/L	0.33–2.08 mkat/L
Ammonia	Plasma	Enzymatic colorimetry	0.17–0.80 mg/mL	10–47 μmol/L
Amylase	Serum	Enzymatic colorimetry	30–170 U/L	0.50–2.83 mkat/ L

Androstenedione	Serum	Immunoassay	65–270 ng/dL Postmenopausal: <180 ng/dL	2.3–9.4 nmol/L Postmenopausal: <6.3 nmol/L
Angiotensin converting enzyme (ACE)	Serum	Enzymatic colorimetry	8–52 U/L	133–867 nkat/L
Antidiuretic hormone (ADH)	Plasma	Extraction/immunoassay	<2.2 pg/mL (serum Osm <285 mOsm/kg) < 2.2 ng/L (serum Osm < 285 mOsm/kg)	2.2–8.5 pg/mL (serum Osm >290 mOsm/kg) 2.2 – 8.5 ng / L (serum Osm >290 mOsm/kg)
Anti-DNA antibody (double-stranded)	Serum	Immunoassay	<30 U/mL	<30 kU/ L
Antimicrosomal antibody (thyroid)	Serum	Immunoassay	<0.3 U/mL	<300 U/L
Antimitochondrial antibody	Serum	Immunofluorescence	Negative (<1:20)	
Antineutrophil cytoplasmic antibody (ANCA)	Serum	Immunofluorescence	Negative (<1:20)	
Antinuclear antibody (ANA)	Serum	Immunofluorescence	Negative (<1:40)	
Antithrombin III activity	Plasma	Nephelometry	85–130% of normal activity	0.85–1.3 of normal activity
Antithrombin III antigen	Plasma	Enzymatic colorimetry	25–33 mg/dL	250–330 mg/L
Antithyroglobulin antibody	Serum	Immunoassay	<1 U/mL	<1 kU/L
α1–antitrypsin	Serum	Nephelometry	80–200 mg/dL	0.8–2.0 g/L
Apolipoprotein A-I	Serum	Nephelometry	Male: 94–176 mg/dL Female: 101–198 mg/dL	Male: 0.94–1.76 g/L Female: 1.01– 1.98 g/L
Apolipoprotein B	Serum	Nephelometry	Male: 52–109 mg/dL Female: 49–103 mg/dL	Male: 0.52–1.09 g/L Female: 0.49–1.03 g/L
Apolipoprotein E	Serum	Nephelometry		

(Continued)

Table 7-2 Normal Laboratory Values (Continued)

Test	Specimen	Method	Normal range conventional units	SI units
Apolipoprotein E4	Serum	Nephelometry		
Arsenic	Urine	ICP-MS	<50 mg/day	<0.65 mmol/day
Aspartate aminotransferase (AST)	Serum	Enzymatic colorimetry	<42 U/L	<0.7 mkat/L
Bilirubin				
Direct	Serum	Colorimetry	<0.4 mg/dL	<7 mmol/L
Indirect	Serum	Colorimetry	<1.3 mg/dL	<22 mmol/L
Total	Serum	Colorimetry	<1.3 mg/dL	<22 mmol/L
Bleeding time, template	Not applicable	Template method	2.5–9.5 minutes	
Cancer antigen (CA) 15.3	Serum	ABBOTT AXSYM CA 15–3 MEIA	<32 U/mL	<32 kU/L
CA 19.9	Serum	CIS ELSA-CA 19–9 IRMA	<33 U/mL	<33 kU/L
CA 27.29	Serum	BIOMIRA TRUQANT BR RIA	<38 U/mL	<38 kU/L
CA 125	Serum	CENTOCOR CA 125 II RIA	<35 U/mL	<35 kU/L
Calcitonin	Serum	Immunoassay	Male: <13.8 pg/mL	Male: <13.8 ng/L
Calcitonin	Serum	Immunoassay	Female: <6.4 pg/mL	Female: <6.4 ng/L
Calcium	Serum	Colorimetry	8.5–10.3 mg/dL	2.12–2.57 mmol/L
	Urine	Colorimetry	Male: <300 mg/day	Male: <7.5 mmol/day
			Female: <250 mg/day	Female: <6.2 mmol/day
Carbon dioxide	Serum	Colorimetry	20–32 mmol/L	20–32 mmol/L
Carboxyhemoglobin	Blood	Spectrophotometry	<2% of total Hb (nonsmoker)	<0.02

Carcinoembryonic antigen (CEA)	Serum	CHIRON ACS: 180 ICMA	<2.5 ng/mL (nonsmoker)	<2.5 mg/L (nonsmoker)
Catecholamines				
Fractionated	Plasma	HPLC	Dopamine	Dopamine
			Supine: <90 pg/mL	Supine: <588 pmol/L
			Standing: <90 pg/mL	Standing: <588pmol/L
			Epinephrine	Epinephrine
			Supine: <50 pg/mL	Supine: <273 pmol/L
			Standing: <90 pg/mL	Standing: <491 pmol/L
			Norepinephrine	Norepinephrine
			Supine: 110–410 pg/mL	Supine: 650–2423 pmol/L
			Standing: 125–700 pg/mL	Standing: 739–4137 pmol/L
Total	Plasma	HPLC	Supine: 120–450 pg/mL	Supine: 709–2660 pmol/L
			Standing: 150–750 pg/mL	Standing: 887–4433 pmol/L
Ceruloplasmin	Serum	Nephelometry	25–63 mg/dL	250–630 mg/L
Chloride	Serum	ISE	95–108 mmol/L	95–108 mmol/L
Cholesterol, total	Serum	Colorimetry	Desirable: <200 mg/dl.	Desirable: <5.17 mmol/L
			Borderline–high:	Borderline–high:
			200–239 mg/dl	5.17–6.18 mmol/L
			High: >240 mg/dl	High: >6.21 mmol/L
Complement				
C3	Serum	Nephelometry	75–161 mg/dL	0.75–1.61 g/L
C4	Serum	Nephelometry	16–47 mg/dL	0.16–0.47 g/L
Total (CH 50)	Serum	Liposome lysis	31–66 U/mL	31–66 kU/L

(Continued)

Table 7-2 Normal Laboratory Values (*Continued*)

Test	Specimen	Method	Normal range conventional units	SI units
Complete blood count (CBC) Hemoglobin (Hb)	Blood	Automated analyzer	Male: 13.8–17.2 g/dL Female: 12.0–15.6 g/dL	Male: 138–172 g/L Female: 120–156 g/L
Hematocrit (Hct)			Male: 41–50% Female: 35–46%	Male: 0.41–0.50 Female: 0.35–0.46
RBC count			Male: $4.4–5.8 \times 10^6$/mL Female: $3.9–5.2 \times 10^6$/mL	Male: $4.4–5.8 \times 10^{12}$/L Female: $3.9–5.2 \times 10^{12}$/L
RBC indices			Mean corpuscular volume: 78–102 fL Mean corpuscular Hb: 27–33 pg Mean corpuscular Hb concentration: 32–36 g/dL RBC distribution width: <15%	Mean corpuscular volume: 78–102 fL Mean corpuscular Hb: 27–33 pg Mean corpuscular Hb concentration: 320–360 g/L RBC distribution width: <0.15
WBC count			$3.8–10.8 \times 10^3$/µL	$3.8–10.8 \times 10^9$/L
WBC differential			Absolute neutrophils: 1500–7800 cells/mL Absolute eosinophils: 50–550 cells/mL Absolute basophils: 0–200 cells/mL Absolute lymphocytes: 850–4100 cells/mL	Absolute neutrophils: $1.5–7.8 \times 10^9$/L Absolute eosinophils: $0.05–0.55 \times 10^9$/L Absolute basophils: $0–0.2 \times 10^9$/L Absolute lymphocytes: $0.85–4.10 \times 10^9$/L

				Absolute monocytes: 0.2–1.10⁹/L
Platelet count			Absolute monocytes: 200–1100 cells/mL	Absolute monocytes: $0.2–1.10^9$/L
			130–400 × 103/mL	130–400 × 10^9/L
Cortisol, free	Urine	Immunoassay	20–90 mg/day	55–248 nmol/day
Cortisol	Serum	Immunoassay	4–22 mg/dL (morning specimen)	110–607 nmol/L (morning specimen)
			3–17 mg/dL (afternoon specimen)	83–469 nmol/L (afternoon specimen)
C - peptide	Serum	Immunoassay	0.8–4.0 ng/mL	0.26–1.32 nmol/L
C - reactive protein (CRP)	Serum	Nephelometry	<0.8 mg/dL	<8 mg/L
Creatine kinase (CK) Isoenzymes	Serum	Electrophoresis	CK-MM: 97–100% of total, CK-MB: <3% of total, CK-BB: 0% of total	CK-MM: 0.97–1.00 of total, CK-MB: <0.03 of total, CK-BB: 0 of total
Total	Serum	Enzymatic colorimetry	Male: <235 U/L, Female: <190 U/L	Male: <3.92 mkat/L, Female: <3.17 mkat/L
Creatinine	Serum	Enzymatic colorimetry	<1.2 mg/dL	<106 mmol/L
	Urine	Enzymatic colorimetry	Male: 0.8–2.4 g/day, Female: 0.6–1.8 g/day	Male: 7.1–21.2 mmol/day, Female: 5.3–15.9 mmol/day
Creatinine clearance	Serum, urine	Calculation:	Male: 82–125 mL/min, Female: 75–115 mL/min	Male: 1.37–2.08 mL/sec, Female: 1.25–1.92 mL/sec
Cyanide	Blood	Colorimetry	<0.1 mg/L	<3.8 mmol/L
D-dimer	Plasma	Slide latex agglutination	<250 mg/L	<250 mg/L
Dehydroepiandrosterone (DHEA), unconjugated	Serum	Immunoassay	130–1200 ng/dL	4.5–41.6 nmol/L

(Continued)

Table 7–2 Normal Laboratory Values (*Continued*)

Test	Specimen	Method	Normal range conventional units	SI units
Dehydroepiandrosterone sulfate (DHEA-S)	Serum	Immunoassay	Male (age): 29 years 1.4–7.9 mg/mL 30–39 years 1.0–7.0 mg/mL 40–49 years 0.9–5.7 mg/mL 50–59 years 0.6–4.1 mg/mL 60–69 years 0.4–3.2 mg/mL 70–79 years 0.3–2.6 mg/mL Female (age): 29 years 0.7–4.5 mg/mL 30–39 years 0.5–4.1 mg/mL 40–49 years 0.4–3.5 mg/mL 50–59 years 0.3–2.7 mg/mL 60–69 years 0.2–1.8 mg/mL 70–79 years 0.1–0.9 mg/mL	Male (age): 29 years 3.8–21.4 mmol/L 30–39 years 2.7–19.0 mmol/L 40–49 years 2.4–15.5 mmol/L 50–59 years 1.6–11.1 mmol/L 60–69 years 1.1–8.7 mmol/L 70–79 years 0.8–7.1 mmol/L Female: 29 years 1.9–12.2 mmol/L 30–39 years 1.4–11.1 mmol/L 40–49 years 1.1–9.5 mmol/L 50–59 years 0.8–7.3 mmol/L 60–69 years 0.5–4.9 mmol/L 70–79 years 0.3–2.4 mmol/L
11-deoxycortisol	Serum	Immunoassay	<0.8 µg/dl	<23 nmol/L
Erythrocyte sedimentation rate (ESR)	Blood	Modified Westergren	Male: <20 mm/h Female: <30 mm/h	Male: <20 mm/h Female: <30 mm/h
Erythropoietin	Serum	Immunoassay	<25 U/L	<25 U/L
Estradiol	Serum	Immunoassay	Male: <50 pg/mL Female: Follicular phase 10–200 pg/mL	Male: <184 pmol/L Female: Follicular phase 37–734 pmol/L

Test	Specimen	Method		
17-ketosteroids, total	Urine	Colorimetry	Female: 3–15 mg/day Male: 9–22 mg/day Female: 5–15 mg/day	Female: 10–52 mmol/day Male: 31–76 mmol/day Female: 17–52 mmol/day
Lactate dehydrogenase (LD) Isoenzymes	Serum	Electrophoresis	LD1: 20–36% of total LD2: 32–50% of total LD3: 15–25% of total LD4: 2–10% of total LD5: 3–13% of total	LD1: 0.20–0.36 of total LD2: 0.32–0.50 of total LD3: 0.15–0.25 of total LD4: 0.02–0.10 of total LD5: 0.03–0.13 of total
Total	Serum	Enzymatic colorimetry	<270 U/L	<4.5 mkat/L
Lactic acid	Plasma (venous)	Enzymatic colorimetry	9–16 mg/dL	1.0–1.8 mmol/L
Lead	Blood	Atomic spectroscopy	<25 mg/dL	<1.21 mmol/L
Lipase	Serum	Enzymatic colorimetry	7–60 U/L	0.12–1.00 mkat/L
Low-density lipoprotein (LDL) cholesterol, direct	Serum	Immunoseparation	Desirable: <130 mg/dL	Desirable: <3.36 mmol/L
Luteinizing hormone (LH)	Serum	Immunoassay	Borderline–high: 130–159 mg/dL High: >160 mg/dL Male (age): 20–70 years 1.3–12.9 U/L >70 years 11.3–56.4 U/L Female: Follicular phase 0.8–25.8 U/L Midcycle 25.0–57.3 U/L	Borderline–high: 3.36–4.11 mmol/L High: >4.14 mmol/L Male (age): 20–70 years 1.3–12.9 U/L >70 years 11.3–56.4 U/L Female: Follicular phase 0.8–25.8 U/L Midcycle 25.0–57.3 U/L

(Continued)

Table 7–2 Normal Laboratory Values (*Continued*)

Test	Specimen	Method	Normal range conventional units	SI units
			Luteal phase 0.8–27.1 U/L	Luteal phase 0.8–27.1 U/L
			Pregnancy < 1.4 U/L	Pregnancy < 1.4 U/L
			Postmenopausal 5.0–52.3 U/L	Postmenopausal 5.0–52.3 U/L
Lymphocyte surface markers (T cell)				
CD3	Blood	Flow cytometry	Absolute: 840–3060 cells/mL	Absolute: 0.84–3.06 × 109 cells/L
			Percentage: 57–85%	Percentage: 0.57–0.85 (57–85%)
CD4	Blood	Flow cytometry	Absolute: 490–1740 cells/mL	Absolute: 0.49–1.74 × 109 cells/L
			Percentage: 30–61%	Percentage: 0.30– 0.61 (30–61%)
CD8	Blood	Flow cytometry	Absolute: 180–1170 cells/mL	Absolute: 0.18–1.17 × 109 cells/L
Helper/suppressor (CD4/CD8) ratio	Blood	Flow cytometry	Percentage: 12–42%	Percentage: 0.12–0.42 (12–42%)
			0.86–5.00	0.86–5.00
Magnesium	Serum	Colorimetry	0.6–1.0 mmol/L	0.6–1.0 mmol/L
Mercury	Blood	Atomic spectroscopy	<1 mg/dl	<50 nmol/L
Metanephrines				
Fractionated	Urine	HPLC	Metanephrine: <0.4 mg/day	Metanephrine: <2.2 mmol/day
			Normetanephrine: <0.9 mg/day	Normetanephrine: <4.9 mmol/day
Total	Urine	HPLC	<1.3 mg/day	<7.1 mmol/day

Methemoglobin	Blood	Spectrophotometry	<2% of total Hb	<0.02 of total Hb
β2-microglobulin	Serum	Immunoassay	<3 mg/L	<3 mg/L
Muramidase (lysozyme)	Serum	Turbidimetry	2.8–8.0 mg/L	0.20–0.56 mmol/L
Myelin basic protein	CSF	Immunoassay	<4 ng/mL	<4 mg/L
Myoglobin	Serum	Immunoassay	<55 ng/mL	<55 mg/L
Nitrogen, total	Feces	Acid digestion/titrimetry	<2 g/day	<143 mmol/day
Osmolality	Serum	Freezing point depression	278–305 mOsm/kg	278–305 mmol/kg
	Urine	Freezing point depression	50–1200 mOsm/kg	50–1200 mmol/kg
Oxalate	Urine	Colorimetry	<40 mg/day	<456 mmol/day
Parathyroid hormone (PTH), intact	Serum	Immunoassay	11–54 pg/mL	1.2–5.8 pmol/L
Partial thromboplastin time, activated (aPTT)	Plasma	Photo-optical clot detection	20–36 seconds	20–36 seconds
Phosphorus	Serum	Colorimetry	2.5–4.5 mg/dL	0.81–1.45 mmol/L
Platelet count	Blood	Automated analyzer	$130-400 \times 10^3$/mL	$130-400 \times 10^9$/L
Porphobilinogen	Urine	Column chromatography/spectrophotometry	<2 mg/day	<8.8 mmol/day
Porphyrins, fractionated (protoporphyrin)	Feces	HPLC	Dicarboxyporphyrin <1830 mg/day (protoporphyrin) Heptacarboxyporphyrin <20 mg/day Octacarboxyporphyrin <80 mg/day (uroporphyrin)	Dicarboxyporphyrin <3.26 mmol/day Octacarboxyporphyrin <96 nmol/day (uroporphyrin)

(Continued)

Table 7–2   Normal Laboratory Values (*Continued*)

Test	Specimen	Method	Normal range conventional units	SI units
			Tetracarboxyporphyrin <640 mg/day (coproporphyrin)	Tetracarboxyporphyrin <977 nmol/day (coproporphyrin)
Potassium	Serum	ISE	3.5–5.3 mmol/L	3.5–5.3 mmol/L
Prealbumin	Serum	Nephelometry	18–45 mg/dL	180–450 mg/L
Progesterone	Serum	Immunoassay	Male: <1.2 ng/mL	Male: <3.8 nmol/L
			Female:	Female:
			Follicular phase <1.4 ng/mL	Follicular phase <4.5 nmol/L
			Luteal phase 2.5–28.0 ng/mL	Luteal phase 8.0–89.0 nmol/L
			Pregnancy	Pregnancy
			1st trimester	1st trimester
			9.0–47.0 ng/mL	28.6–149.5 nmol/L
			2nd trimester	2nd trimester
			17.0–146.0 ng/mL	54.1–464.3 nmol/L
			3rd trimester	3rd trimester
			55.0–255.0 ng/mL	174.9–810.9 nmol/L
			Postmenopausal < 0.7 ng/mL	Postmenopausal < 2.2 nmol/L
Prolactin	Serum	Immunoassay	Male: 2–18 ng/mL	Male: 2–18 mg/L
			Female:	Female:
			Nonpregnant 3–30 ng/mL	Nonpregnant 3–30 mg/L
			Pregnant 10–209 ng/mL	Pregnant 10–209 mg/L
			Postmenopausal 2–20 ng/mL	Postmenopausal 2–20 mg/L

Prostate-specific antigen (PSA)	Serum	Immunoassay	<4 ng/ml (male)	<4 mg/L (male)
Protein, total	Serum	Colorimetry	6.0–8.5 g/dL	60–85 g/L
	Urine	Colorimetry	<150 mg/day	<150 mg/day
Protein C activity	Plasma	Photo-optical clot detection	70–140% of normal	0.7–1.4 of normal
Protein C antigen	Plasma	Immunoassay	70–140% of normal	0.7–1.4 of normal
Protein electrophoresis	Serum	Electrophoresis	Albumin: 3.5–5.5 g/dL α_1-globulins: 0.1–0.3 g/dL α_2-globulins: 0.2–1.1 g/dL β-globulins: 0.5–1.2 g/dL γ-globulins: 0.5–1.5 g/dL	Albumin: 35–55 g/L α_1-globulins: 1–3 g/L α_2-globulins: 2–11 g/L β-globulins: 5–12 g/L γ-globulins: 5–15 g/L
Protein S activity	Plasma	Photo-optical clot detection	Male: 70–150% of normal Female: 58–130% of normal	Male: 0.7–1.5 of normal Female: 0.58–1.30 of normal
Protein S antigen	Plasma	Immunoassay	Male: 70–140% of normal Female: 70–140% of normal	Male: 0.7–1.4 of normal Female: 0.7–1.4 of normal
Prothrombin time (PT)	Plasma	Photo-optical clot detection International Normalized Ratio (INR): 0.9–1.1 (patients not on anticoagulant therapy)	10.0–12.5 seconds	10.0–12.5 seconds
Protoporphyrin				
Free erythrocyte	Blood	Fluorometry	<35 mg/dL RBCs	<0.62 mmol/L RBCs
Zinc	Blood	Fluorometry	<70 mg/dL	<700 mg/L
Pyruvate	Blood	Enzymatic colorimetry	0.3–0.9 mg/dL	34–102 mmol/L
Pyruvate kinase	Blood	Fluorometry	Enzyme activity detected	

(Continued)

Table 7–2 Normal Laboratory Values (*Continued*)

Test	Specimen	Method	Normal range conventional units	SI units
RBC count	Blood	Automated analyzer	Male: 4.4–5.8 × 10⁶/mL Female: 3.9–5.2 × 10⁶/mL	Male: 4. 4–5. 8 × 10¹²/L Female: 3.9–5.2 × 10¹²/L
RBC indices	Blood	Automated analyzer	Mean corpuscular volume: 78–102 fl Mean corpuscular Hb: 27–33 pg Mean corpuscular Hb concentration: 32–36 g/dL RBC distribution width: <15%	Mean corpuscular volume: 78–102 fl Mean corpuscular Hb: 27–33 pg Mean corpuscular Hb concentration: 320–360 g/l RBC distribution width: <0.15
Renin activity	Plasma	Immunoassay	1.3–4.0 ng/mL/h (upright) (Normal sodium intake: 100–200 mEq/day)	1.00–3. 07 nmol/L/h (upright) (Normal sodium intake: 100–200 mmol/day)
Reticulocyte count	Blood	Automated analyzer	0.5–2.3% of RBCs	0.005–0.023 of RBCs
Rheumatoid factor	Serum	Nephelometry	<40 U/mL	<40 kU/L
Schilling test	Urine	Radio-isotopic measurement	>7% of administered dose in 24-hour urine	>0.07 of administered dose in 24-hour urine
Scleroderma antibody (Scl-70)	Serum	Immunoassay	Negative	
Serotonin	Blood	HPLC	46–319 ng/mL	0.26–1.81 mmol/L
Sodium	Serum	ISE	135–146 mmol/L	135–146 mmol/L
Somatomedin-C	Serum	Immunoassay	Male: 90–318 ng/mL Female: 116–270 ng/mL	Male: 90–318 mg/L Female: 116–270 mg/L
T3 (triiodothyronine)				
Free	Serum	Immunoassay	230–420 pg/dL	3.5–6.5 pmol/L
Reverse	Serum	Immunoassay	2.6–18.9 ng/dL	0.04–0. 29 nmol/L

Test	Specimen	Method	Conventional units	SI units
Total	Serum	Immunoassay	60-181 ng/dL	0.9-2.8 nmol/L
T4 (thyroxine)				
Free	Serum	Immunoassay	0.8-1.8 ng/dL	10-23 pmol/L
Total	Serum	Immunoassay	4.5-12.5 mg/dL	58-161 nmol/L
Testosterone, total	Serum	Immunoassay	Male: 194-833 ng/dL Female: 62 ng/dL	Male: 6.7-28.9 nmol/L Female: <2.1 nmol/L
Thrombin time	Plasma	Photo-optical clot detection	10.0-13.5 seconds	10.0-13.5 seconds
Thyroglobulin	Serum	Immunoassay	<60 ng/mL	<60 ng/mL
Thyroid-stimulating hormone (TSH), ultrasensitive (third generation)	Serum	Immunoassay	0.50-4.70 mU/mL	0.50-4.70 mU/L
Thyroxine-binding globulin (TBG)	Serum	Immunoassay	16-34 mg/L	16-34 mg/L
Transferrin	Serum	Nephelometry	188-341 mg/dL	1.88-3.41 g/L
Triglycerides	Serum	Enzymatic colorimetry	<200 mg/dL	<2.26 mmol/L
Urea nitrogen, blood (BUN)	Serum	Colorimetry	7-30 mg/dL	2.5-10.7 mmol urea/L
Uric acid	Serum	Enzymatic colorimetry	Male: 4.0-8.5 mg/dL Female: 2.5-7.5 mg/dL	Male: 238-506 mmol/L Female: 149-446 mmol/L
	Urine	Enzymatic colorimetry	200-750 mg/day	1.2-4.5 mmol/day
Urinalysis, complete	Urine	Reagent-impregnated strips Microscopy	Appearance: clear, yellow Specific gravity: 1.001-1.035 pH: 4.6-8.0 Protein: negative Glucose: negative	

(Continued)

Table 7–2   Normal Laboratory Values (*Continued*)

Test	Specimen	Method	Normal range conventional units	SI units
			Reducing substances: negative	
			Ketones: negative	
			Bilirubin: negative	
			Occult blood: negative	
			WBC esterase: negative	
			Nitrite: negative	
			WBC: <5/high-power field	
			RBC: <3/high-power field	
			Renal epithelial cells: <3/high-power field	
			Squamous epithelial cells: none or few/high-power field	
			Casts: none	
			Bacteria: none	
			Yeast: none	
Vanillylmandelic acid (VMA)	Urine	HPLC	<10 mg/day	<50 mmol/day
Viscosity	Serum	Viscometer	1.5–1.9 viscosity units (relative to water)	
Vitamin A	Serum	HPLC	30–95 mg/dL	1.05–3.32 mmol/L
Vitamin B$_6$	Plasma	HPLC	5–24 ng/mL	30–144 nmol/L
Vitamin B$_{12}$	Serum	Immunoassay	200–800 pg/mL	>150–590 pmol/L
Vitamin C	Plasma	Colorimetry	0.2–2.0 mg/dL	11–114 mmol/L

Test	Sample	Method	Value	SI Units
1,25-dihydroxy-vitamin D	Serum	Chromatography	24–65 pg/mL	58–156 pmol/L
25-hydroxy-vitamin D	Serum	Acetonitrile extraction/immunoassay	10–55 ng/mL	25–137 nmol/L
Vitamin E	Serum	Fluorometry	5–20 mg/mL	12–46 mmol/L
WBC count	Blood	Automated analyzer	$3.8–10.8 \times 10^3$/mL	$3.8–10.8 \times 10^9$/L
WBC differential	Blood	Automated analyzer	Absolute neutrophils: 1500–7800 cells/mL	Absolute neutrophils: $1.5–7.8 \times 10^9$/L
			Absolute eosinophils: 50–550 cells/mL	Absolute eosinophils: $0.05–0.55 \times 10^9$/L
			Absolute basophils: 0–200 cells/mL	Absolute basophils: $0–0.2 \times 10^9$/L
			Absolute lymphocytes: 850–4100 cells/mL	Absolute lymphocytes: $0.85–4.10 \times 10^9$/L
			Absolute monocytes: 200–1100 cells/mL	Absolute monocytes: $0.2–1.10^9$/L
Zinc	Plasma	Atomic spectroscopy	60–130 mg/dl	9.2–19.9 mmol/L

CSF, cerebrospinal fluid; DNA, deoxyribonucleic acid; HPLC, high-performance liquid chromatography; HRT, hormone replacement therapy; ICMA, immunochemiluminometric assay; ICP-MS, inductively coupled mass spectroscopy; IRMA, immunoradiometric assay; ISE, ion-selective electrode; MEIA, microparticle enzyme immunoassay; RBC, red blood (cell) count; RIA, radioimmunoassay; SI, International System of Units; WBC, white blood (cell) count.

glucose), and coagulation studies (prothrombin time [PT], International Normalized Ratio [INR], and partial thromboplastin time [PTT]). Depending on age and clinical suspicion, electrocardiogram (EKG) and chest x-ray may be appropriate. For all intracranial procedures and extensive spine procedures, blood should be typed and crossed for possible transfusion. For other neurosurgical procedures, blood should at least be typed and screened. Ancillary laboratory tests should be ordered based on the preoperative assessment and according to American Society of Anesthesiologists (ASA) guidelines.

The 2002 ASA Preoperative Testing Advisory[1] is a loose set of guidelines that may be summarized as follows:

1. No laboratory study may clear a patient for surgery. A physician must review the patient and state that "the patient is in optimal shape to undergo surgery."
2. Evaluation must occur prior to the day of surgery.
3. Routine laboratory testing should be performed.
4. Pregnancy testing should be routine for women of childbearing age (ages 11–55), irrespective of the patient's belief that "there is no way" that she could be pregnant.

On the whole, not much benefit appears to result from nonindicated routine laboratory testing. There is little evidence to suggest that patients classified as ASA I or II benefit from laboratory testing. Furthermore, in the absence of laboratory tests in ASA I patients, medical care is not shown to be adversely affected.[2]

◆ Testing for Tumors

Radiologic studies and surgical biopsy are the primary methods used to diagnose central nervous system (CNS) tumors; however, diagnostic laboratory studies may assist with diagnosis and therapeutic monitoring. Pituitary tumors may produce endocrine abnormalities that may be measured in serum. Polycythemia is associated with hemangioblastoma, a posterior fossa tumor. Some parasellar and pineal region embryonal tumors secrete hormones and proteins: α-fetoprotein (AFP), β subunit of human chorionic gonadotropin (β-hCG), and placental alkaline phosphatase (PLAP). Cerebrospinal fluid (CSF) cytology may be used to diagnose tumor type. CSF analysis may reveal polyamines (putrecine) that localize tumors to ventricles or subarachnoid space, or a pleocytosis that may increase suspicion for lymphoma.

Neuroepithelial Tumors

Astrocytomas, oligodendrogliomas, ependymomas, mixed gliomas, neuronal tumors, and other neoplastic processes of the CNS may be identified in CSF by cytology.

Choroid plexus papillomas and carcinomas typically feature xanthochromia and high red blood cell (RBC) count in CSF due to spontaneous hemorrhage. These patients may have high opening pressure due to excess CSF production and/or deficient CSF absorption, and, in up to 20% of cases, dissemination of tumor cells within the CSF.

Pineal parenchymal tumors produce a characteristic clinical picture due to their proximity to the ventricular system. Opening pressure during lumbar puncture may be high due to obstructive hydrocephalus. Laboratory values reflecting endocrine dysfunction may be present in tumors invading the hypothalamus: diabetes insipidus, hypopituitarism, and precocious puberty. Biochemical tumor markers may suggest tumor type. Serum and CSF AFP, β-hCG, and PLAP levels are most commonly ordered to discriminate between choriocarcinoma or mixed germ cell tumors containing choriocarcinomatous elements (high β-hCG levels); germinomas, pineal parenchymal tumors, and teratomas (neither AFP nor β-hCG elevations); and germinomas (very high elevations of PLAP). However, tumor markers lack sufficient specificity and sensitivity to accurately predict tumor histology.

Medulloblastomas arise from the inferior medullary velum, then fill and expand into the fourth ventricle. High opening pressure during lumbar puncture may reflect obstructive hydrocephalus, and cytology from CSF analysis in 30% of patients will be positive for metastatic dissemination at the time of diagnosis (this is an indication of either drop metastasis or rostral dissemination supratentorially). Because medulloblastoma is characterized as the CNS neoplasm that most frequently metastasizes systemically (extraneural deposits occur in 5% of patients), diagnostic laboratory studies of bone and liver (alkaline phosphatase, γ-glutamyltransferase [GGT], and liver function test [LFT]) may result in vague, positive studies.[3,4]

Sellar Region Tumors

Pituitary tumors present clinically by symptoms of pituitary hypersecretion (70% of cases), symptoms of pituitary hyposecretion, or neurologic symptoms of compression of the pituitary or other adjacent sellar structures.

Hypersecretory syndromes include acromegaly, Cushing's disease, amenorrhea-galactorrhea syndrome, and secondary hyperthyroidism from hypersecretion of growth hormone (GH), adrenocorticotropic hormone (ACTH), prolactin (PRL), and thyroid-stimulating hormone (TSH).

Hypopituitarism results in fatigue, weakness, hypogonadism, regression of secondary sexual characteristics, and hypothyroidism. Pituitary insufficiency also occurs acutely in pituitary apoplexy.

Chronic progressive compression of the pituitary is accompanied by decline in functional reserve of secretory elements: gonadotrophs are most vulnerable and are affected first, next thyrotrophs, somatotrophs, and finally corticotrophs (the most resilient among pituitary hormones). Acute processes produce the opposite effect. Panhypopituitarism results in compromise of all of the pituitary hormones, but hypocortisolism from ACTH deficit produces life-threatening adrenal insufficiency. Large adenomas may result in compression of the hypothalamus or in obstruction of CSF outflow and subsequent noncommunicating hydrocephalus. Also, inhibition of dopamine transport from the hypothalamus via the portal vessels to the anterior lobe of the pituitary results in loss of suppression of PRL output (the "stalk section effect"). This phenomenon may result in PRL levels elevating to 150 ng/mL or greater (normal levels are <25 ng/mL).

Diagnostic laboratory studies are very sensitive indicators of endocrine dysfunction and are focused on measuring pituitary and/or target-organ hormones in basal and provoked states to discriminate between various pituitary adenoma subtypes. Screening tests include (1) adrenal axis: morning serum cortisol, 24-hour urine free cortisol, dexamethasone suppression test, cosyntropin stimulation test, and insulin tolerance test; (2) thyroid axis: TSH, T4, and thyrotropin-releasing hormone (TRH) stimulation test; (3) gonadal axis: serum luteinizing hormone/follicle-stimulating hormone (LH/FSH); (4) prolactin levels: PRL; (5) growth hormone: somatomedin-C (insulin-like growth factor I [IGF-I]), growth hormone releasing hormone (GH-RH) stimulation test, and glucose suppression test; and (6) neurohypophysis: water deprivation test and serum antidiuretic hormone (ADH).

Craniopharyngiomas produce effects seen using endocrine studies. They may reflect arrested pituitary function in children (growth failure, diabetes insipidus, and primary amenorrhea) and some degree of hypopituitarism in adults. Also, opening pressures during lumbar puncture may be elevated due to mass-effect.[3–5]

Hematopoietic Tumors (Primary Central Nervous System Lymphoma)

Primary CNS lymphoma (PCNSL) is lymphoma of the CNS in the absence of systemic lymphoma. Systemic lymphoma disseminates to the meninges and rarely to the brain parenchyma, whereas primary CNS lymphoma frequently start as periventricular lesions.

PCNSL is rare and accounts for only 1 to 2% of intracranial tumors. It occurs primarily in the elderly; however, patients having human immunodeficiency virus (HIV) and congenital immunodeficiencies, collagen vascular disease, and organ transplants are particularly at risk for primary CNS lymphoma.

CSF cytology may detect high-grade disease and involvement of leptomeninges. The CSF analysis may reveal elevations in protein and pleocytosis (immunohistochemical stains reveal monoclonal populations of cells); β_2-microglobulin, lactic acid dehydrogenase isoenzymes, and β-glucuronidase are elevated as well. Tissue biopsy is the preferred method of diagnosis of PCNSL. However, an unequivocally positive CSF cytology eliminates the need for brain biopsy.

Systemic lymphoma must be differentiated from PCNSL and is detected by analysis of the hemogram: polymorphonuclear leukocytosis may be present, lymphocytopenia occurs early and becomes pronounced with advanced disease, eosinophilia is present in ~20% of patients, and thrombocytosis and microcytic anemia develop with advanced disease. Also, elevated serum alkaline phosphatase levels indicate bone marrow or liver involvement, or both, and increases in leukocyte alkaline phosphatase, serum haptoglobin, erythrocyte sedimentation rate (ESR), serum copper, and other acute-phase reactants reflect active disease.[3]

Germ Cell Tumors

Germ cell tumors account for more than 50% of all pineal tumors. They range from low- or intermediate-grade to very aggressive high-grade tumors. For example, germinomas may metastasize within the spinal axis in 10% of patients and systemically in 3%, compared with aggressive pineal choriocarcinomas that disseminate throughout the craniospinal axis in 25% of cases and systemically in less than 5%. Cytology from CSF analysis may assist in diagnosis. However, highly aggressive germ cell tumors carry a grave prognosis and are frequently disseminated at the time of diagnosis.[3]

Nonmeningothelial Tumors of Uncertain Histogenesis (Hemangioblastomas)

Hemangioblastomas are benign neoplasms of uncertain origin. They are associated with a multisystem genetic disorder (Von Hippel-Lindau syndrome), pheochromocytomas, pancreatic and renal cysts, and renal cell carcinoma. Associated diagnostic laboratory studies may include complete blood count (CBC, for polycythemia from liberation of erythropoietin), measuring free catecholamines in a 24-hour urine specimen with a specific analysis for epinephrine (most sensitive) and vanillylmandelic acid excretion (often normal early on), LFT, amylase, lipase, creatinine clearance, and urinalysis (UA) (for hematuria), respectively.[3]

Local Extensions from Regional Tumors (Chordomas)

Chordomas may arise at any site along the axial skeleton. Preferred locations are the clivus (35%), sacrum (50%), and spine (15%). Regardless of location, all chordomas are locally invasive. They begin with destruction of bone at the site of origin, followed by infiltration of the dura, and eventually spread intracranially to encase vital cranial structures. Late dissemination (in 10–20% of cases) occurs to liver, lungs, heart, peritoneum, lymph nodes, and bone. Vague elevations in laboratory studies targeting these systems may be present, but only tissue biopsy is diagnostic.[3]

Metastatic Tumors

Metastasis to the brain and spinal cord is common among cancer patients. Brain metastasis occurs in 20% and spinal cord metastasis in 10% of patients having primary malignancies of the lung (bronchogenic carcinoma, especially small-cell carcinomas), breast cancer, renal cell carcinoma, melanoma, and gastrointestinal malignancies.

Primary lung cancers may present with several paraneoplastic syndromes, including carcinoid syndrome (symptoms caused by secretion of serotonin, prostaglandins, and other biologically active substances), Cushing's syndrome (hyperadrenocorticism), hypercalcemia, and antidiuretic hormone secretion. Appropriate screening studies for paraneoplastic syndromes may assist in confirmation of disease but are not diagnostic.

Sputum cytology can also be used to confirm the presence of central lesions but is not helpful for evaluation of peripheral solitary pulmonary nodules.

Renal cell carcinoma is usually silent; symptoms of hematuria, palpable flank mass, and flank pain denote advanced disease. Renal cell carcinomas secrete hormones (parathyroid hormone and erythropoietin) that cause hypercalcemia and erythrocytosis. Stauffer's syndrome is a reversible hepatorenal condition with abnormal results on liver function studies.

Melanoma frequently spreads to lymphatics, liver, bone, brain, and lungs. In addition to comprehensive radiographic evaluation, serum alkaline phosphatase, γ-glutamyltransferase, and lactic dehydrogenase levels are ordered to evaluate for possible spread to bone and liver.[3-5]

◆ Cysts and Tumor-Like Lesions (Epidermoid and Dermoid Cysts)

Epidermoid and dermoid cysts have a predilection for basal regions of the brain and tend to enlarge along CSF pathways. Common locations include the cerebellopontine angle, suprasellar region, fourth ventricle, and inside the diploë of the skull. Epidermoid tumors can cause local mass effect or recurrent bouts of aseptic meningitis due to leakage of irritative cyst contents (i.e., cholesterol and fatty acids) into the CSF. Lumbar puncture may result in high opening pressures as expected if hydrocephalus is present. CSF analysis may result in nonspecific leukocytosis. Alkaline phosphatase may be elevated due to destruction of bone.[3]

◆ Trauma

Following trauma, several delayed conditions may present. Diagnostic laboratory studies may be implemented to diagnose and/or prevent delayed hemorrhage, post-traumatic diffuse cerebral edema, seizures, metabolic abnormalities, and meningitis.

Intracranial Hematoma

Initial or delayed hemorrhage may be anticipated in 75% of patients with traumatic brain injury. Epidural hematoma (EDH), subdural hematoma (SDH), or traumatic intracerebral hemorrhage (TICH) may be present in either initial or delayed fashions.

Following initial management (intubation, sedation, elevation of head of bed [HOB], and management of hypertension), the focus is turned toward correction of coagulopathy, administration of antiepileptic drugs (AEDs), and monitoring of electrolytes and osmolarity in anticipation of the onset of syndrome of inappropriate antidiuretic hormone (SIADH).

Coagulopathy is identified using PT, INR, PTT, bleeding time, and platelet count. Coagulopathy is treated with fresh frozen plasma (FFP) and vitamin K (phytonadione) and is carefully monitored using coagulation studies every 4 hours until it is corrected.

Phenytoin is the first-line antiseizure medication, and levels are observed as per the above protocol.

Serum and urine electrolytes, serum and urine osmolarity, and urine-specific gravity is ordered every 6 hours to screen for SIADH. It is important to record hourly fluid input and output. Serum uric acid may also be a helpful study to rule in the presence of SIADH (serum uric acid is decreased in SIADH).[5–8]

Diffuse Cerebral Edema

Increased cerebral blood volume may result from loss of cerebral vascular autoregulation. It occurs in children more frequently than in adults and when associated with severe head injury carries close to 100% rate of mortality.

Aggressive management of intracerebral pressure (ICP) is required. Along with general measures to lower ICP (elevation of HOB, sedation, normotension, and euvolemia), patients may be considered for hypertonic therapy with hypertonic saline or osmotic therapy using mannitol and Lasix. High tonicity (>320 mOsm/L) and hypovolemia ("running dry") have little advantage to prevent cerebral edema and may result in renal dysfunction. Prevention of hypoglycemia is also important, as it aggravates cerebral edema.

Diagnostic studies should be geared toward monitoring of serum electrolytes and glucose, BUN, creatinine, and serum osmolarity. Also, hemoglobin and hematocrit should be measured to allow for optimization of volume status and oxygenation.[5–7]

Post-traumatic Seizure

Post-traumatic seizures may occur early (<7 days) or late (>7 days) following head trauma and may precipitate adverse events as the result of elevation of ICP, alterations in systolic blood pressure (SBP), changes in oxygenation, and excessive neurotransmitter release. Anticonvulsants may be used to prevent early post-traumatic seizures in patients that meet high-risk criteria: (1) presence of SDH, EDH, ICH, TICH, or delayed traumatic intracerebral hemorrhage (DTICH); (2) open-depressed skull fracture with parenchymal injury; (3) penetrating brain injury; or (4) seizure within the first 24 hours following trauma.

Patients meeting criteria should be started on phenytoin, carbamazepine, valproic acid, or phenobarbital for 1 week. Diagnostic laboratory studies to monitor AED levels are per specific agent:

- *Phenytoin* Peak serum drug concentrations are achieved between 3 and 12 hours after administration of an oral dose. Therapeutic drug concentrations can be obtained in 1 to 2 hours when the drug is administered intravenously. Time to steady state is highly variable, ranging from 7 to 10 days. Therapeutic range is 10 to 20 µg/mL.

♦ *Carbamazepine* Single oral dose, the carbamazepine tablets and chewable tablets yield peak plasma concentrations of unchanged carbamazepine within 4 to 24 hours. Carbamazepine suspension is absorbed faster than the tablet; peak plasma levels are reached within 2 hours. Time to steady state is 2 to 4 weeks. The therapeutic range is 6 to 12 µg/mL.

♦ *Valproic acid* Peak serum drug concentrations are achieved between 1 and 4 hours with oral dosing. Time to steady state is between 2 and 4 days. Therapeutic range is 50 to 100 µg/mL.

♦ *Phenobarbital* Peak serum drug concentrations are achieved between 1 and 6 hours after oral or intramuscular dosing. Time to steady state is 16 to 30 days. Therapeutic range is 15–30 µg/mL.[5–7]

Metabolic Disorders

Several metabolic disorders may result from trauma (directly or indirectly) that affect the CNS: hypoxia, hyponatremia, hypoglycemia, renal failure, and adrenal insufficiency, as well as hepatic encephalopathy.

Acute Renal Failure

Acute renal failure (ARF) is categorized as prerenal, postrenal, and intrinsic renal. Prerenal and postrenal causes are potentially reversible if diagnosed and treated early; some intrinsic renal causes that result in acute glomerular vascular and tubulointerstitial nephropathy are also treatable (malignant hypertension, glomerulonephritis, vasculitis, bacterial infections, electrolyte disorders [hypercalcemia], and drug reactions).

Prerenal azotemia (50–80% of ARF cases) results from inadequate renal perfusion caused by extracellular fluid volume depletion or cardiovascular disease. Postrenal azotemia (5–10% of ARF cases) results from various types of obstruction in the voiding and collecting systems. Intrinsic renal causes of ARF are the result of prolonged renal ischemia (hemorrhage, surgery) or a nephrotoxin.

Symptoms and signs relate to the loss of excretory function and depend on the degree of renal dysfunction, the rate of renal failure, and the cause (trauma, surgery). Preserved urine output of 1 to 2.4 L/day is common. Oliguria may occur; anuria suggests bilateral renal artery occlusion, obstructive uropathy, acute cortical necrosis, or rapidly progressive glomerulonephritis.

Prerenal azotemia may be suggested by any disorder lowering renal perfusion (excessive diuresis, dehydration, hemorrhage, pericardial tamponade, sepsis, liver failure, congestive heart failure [CHF], pulmonary embolism, transcellular fluid accumulation, ascites, peritonitis, pancreatitis, or burns). Postrenal azotemia should be sought in the absence of prerenal factors. Intrinsic renal disease causing acute tubular injury may have three phases. The prodromal phase varies in duration depending on causative factors (amount of toxin ingested, the duration and severity of hypotension). In prerenal azotemia, serum creatinine increases by 1 to 2 mg/dL/day (90–180 mmol/L) and BUN by 10 to 20 mg/dL (3.6–7.1 mmol urea/L). However, BUN levels by themselves may be misleading as an early index of renal function because they are elevated due to increased protein catabolism resulting from surgery, trauma, burns, transfusion reactions, or gastrointestinal or internal bleeding. Therefore, the ratio of BUN to creatinine must be known and should be no higher than 15 to 20:1. The oliguric phase lasts an average of 10 to 14 days, but it varies from 1 to 2 days to 6 to 8 weeks. Urine output varies between 50 and 400 mL/day. Nonoliguric patients have a lower mortality, morbidity, and need for dialysis. In the postoliguric phase, urine output gradually returns to normal; however, serum creatinine and urea levels may not fall for several more days. Tubular dysfunction may persist and is manifested by sodium wasting, polyuria unresponsive to vasopressin, or hyperchloremic metabolic acidosis.

The first step to diagnosing renal failure is to determine whether the renal failure is acute, chronic, or acute superimposed on chronic. Progression to chronic renal failure (CRF) is common when the serum creatinine concentration is >1.5 to 2 mg/dL. This may occur even if the underlying disorder is not active. The definitive diagnostic tool is renal biopsy. Urea and creatinine levels are elevated. Plasma sodium concentrations may be normal or reduced. The serum potassium is normal or only moderately elevated (<6 mmol/L) unless potassium-sparing diuretics, angiotensin converting enzyme (ACE) inhibitors, β-blockers, or angiotensin receptor blockers are taken. Abnormalities of calcium, phosphorus, parathyroid hormone (PTH), vitamin D metabolism, and renal osteodystrophy can occur; hypocalcemia and hyperphosphatemia are found regularly. Acidosis (plasma CO_2 content, 15–20 mmol/L) and anemia occur. The anemia of CRF is normochromic-normocytic, with a hematocrit of 20 to 30%. It is usually caused by deficient erythropoietin production due to a reduction of functional renal mass. Urinary volume does not respond readily to variations in water intake. Urinary osmolarity is close to that of plasma (300–320 mOsm/kg). Urinalysis may reveal casts.[5,6,9]

Adrenal Insufficiency

Secondary adrenal insufficiency may occur in panhypopituitarism, in isolated failure of ACTH production, in patients receiving corticosteroids, or after acute discontinuance of longer use of corticosteroid therapy without appropriate tapering.

Panhypopituitarism occurs in a trauma setting resulting directly from destruction of pituitary tissue or secondarily from infection. Also, patients receiving corticosteroids for more than 4 weeks, or who have discontinued their use after a period of weeks to months, may have insufficient ACTH secretion during metabolic stress to stimulate the adrenals to produce adequate quantities of corticosteroids, or they may have atrophic adrenals that are unresponsive to ACTH.

Patients with secondary adrenal insufficiency are not hyperpigmented, as are those with Addison's disease. They have relatively normal electrolyte levels. Hyperkalemia and elevated BUN are not present because of the near-normal secretion of aldosterone. Hyponatremia may occur on a dilutional basis. Patients with panhypopituitarism have depressed thyroid and gonadal function and hypoglycemia; coma may result when symptomatic secondary adrenal insufficiency occurs.

Function of the hypothalamic-pituitary-adrenal axis during long-term steroid treatment can be determined by the cosyntropin stimulation test: injection of 5 to 250 mg cosyntropin intravenously results in plasma cortisol level >20 mg/dL 30 minutes following the injection. Also, morning specimen cortisol, 24-hour urine free cortisol, dexamethasone suppression test, and insulin tolerance test may be used to test adrenal function.[5,6,9]

Hepatic Encephalopathy

Hepatic encephalopathy may result from hepatic failure resulting from trauma. The liver metabolizes and detoxifies digestive products brought from the intestine by the portal vein. In hepatic failure, these products escape into the systemic circulation if portal blood bypasses parenchymal cells or if the function of these cells is severely impaired. The resulting toxic effect on the brain produces the clinical syndrome.

Personality changes (inappropriate behavior, altered mood, impaired judgment) are common early manifestations. Psychomotor testing can detect such abnormalities not suspected clinically. Usually, impaired consciousness occurs. Initially, subtle sleep pattern changes or sluggish movement and speech may be present. Drowsiness, confusion, stupor, and frank coma indicate increasingly advanced encephalopathy. Constructional apraxia, in which the patient cannot reproduce simple designs (a star), is a characteristic early sign. A musty sweet odor of the breath, fetor hepaticus, occurs. A peculiar, characteristic flapping tremor due to lack of attention, called asterixis, is elicited when the patient holds his or her arms outstretched with wrists dorsiflexed; as coma progresses, this sign disappears, and hyperreflexia and the Babinski response may occur. Agitation or mania may occur. Seizures and localizing neurologic signs may also occur.

Diagnostic laboratory studies for hepatic function include serum total protein, albumin, alkaline phosphatase, ALT, AST, total bilirubin, ammonia (NH_3), (GGT), prothrombin time, platelet count, and serum protein electrophoresis.

The diagnosis of hepatic encephalopathy is clinical. There is no correlation with liver function tests. Blood ammonia levels are elevated, but values correlate poorly with clinical status. The CSF is unremarkable except for mild protein elevation.

An electroencephalography (EEG) usually shows diffuse slow-wave activity, even in mild cases, and may be useful in questionable early encephalopathy.[5,9]

Post-traumatic Meningitis

Post-traumatic meningitis occurs in up to 20% of patients with moderate to severe head injuries. Most cases occur within 2 weeks of trauma; 75% of cases have demonstrable basal skull fracture, and 50% have obvious CSF rhinorrhea.

Antibiotic coverage for active infection should empirically be broad-spectrum, targeting gram-positive, gram-negative, and anaerobic organisms until culture and sensitivity results are known. They should be continued for at least 1 week following CSF sterilization.

Routine CSF analysis should include Gram's stain, culture and sensitivity, protein, glucose, cell count with differential, color, and clarity. Pathogens frequently cultured following basal skull fracture include gram-positive cocci (*Streptococcus haemolyticus, Staphylococcus warneri, Staphylococcus cohnii, Staphylococcus epidermidis,* and *Streptococcus pneumoniae*), and gram-negative bacilli (*E. coli,* Klebsiella *pneumoniae,* and *Acinetobacter anitratus*). Elevations of protein and WBCs (polymorphonuclear neutrophil leukocytes), low glucose, and cloudy/turbid CSF suggest bacterial infection. CSF should be collected for CSF analysis weekly until sterilization is achieved.[5–7]

◆ Cerebrovascular Disease

Cerebrovascular Accident

Cerebrovascular accidents (CVAs) can be divided into ischemic and hemorrhagic. Approximately 80 to 85% of CVAs are ischemic, 15 to 20% are hemorrhagic.

Of patients presenting with focal deficit, 5% of cases are seizure, tumor, or psychogenic in etiology, and 95% vascular. Eighty to 85% of CVAs are attributed to ischemic infarct, whereas only 15 to 20% are from hemorrhage. With the mainstream use of thrombolytic therapy in the management of ischemic infarction, it is important to be familiar with the exclusion criteria used to make decisions regarding their administration. The use of anticoagulants (heparin or Coumadin), and extreme values of serum glucose may exclude a patient from receiving thrombolytic agents. Patients being considered for thrombolytic therapy should have coagulation studies as well as serum glucose screening prior to their administration.

Intracerebral hemorrhage (ICH) accounts for 15 to 20% of strokes. Etiologies of ICH include amyloid angiopathy, trauma, hemorrhagic transformation of an ischemic infarct, tumors, cerebrovascular malformations (cerebral aneurysms, arteriovenous malformations [AVMs], venous malformations, cavernomas, capillary telangiectasias). Several risk factors are associated with ICH: age, gender, race, prior CVA, alcohol consumption and substance abuse, cigarette smoking, and liver dysfunction. Diagnostic laboratory studies may be utilized in both diagnosis and management.

Factors complicating intracerebral hemorrhage are coagulopathy, seizure, and SIADH.

Coagulopathy is identified using PT, INR, PTT, bleeding time, and platelet count. Coagulopathy is treated with FFP and vitamin K (AquaMEPHYTON) and is carefully monitored using coagulation studies every 4 hours until it is corrected.

Phenytoin is the first-line antiseizure medication, and levels are observed as per the above protocol.

Serum and urine electrolytes, serum and urine osmolarity, and urine specific gravity are ordered every 6 hours to screen for SIADH. Serum uric acid may also be a helpful study to rule in the presence of SIADH (serum uric acid is decreased in SIADH).

Toxicology screening may be ordered if there is suspicion of substance abuse.[5,6,8]

Subarachnoid Hemorrhage

Many etiologies for subarachnoid hemorrhage (SAH) exist: rupture of intracranial aneurysms (80%), cerebral AVM (5%), spinal AVM, arterial dissection or rupture, vasculitides, tumors, coagulation disorders, dural sinus thrombosis, drugs, sickle cell disease, and pituitary apoplexy. Risk factors include hypertension, use of oral contraceptives, substance abuse, tobacco abuse, alcohol abuse, pregnancy, lumbar puncture, and advanced age. Along with radiologic studies, diagnostic laboratory studies may assist with diagnosis and are essential for management of SAH.

Patients having high suspicion for SAH will have noncontrast computed tomography (CT) performed. If CT is negative, lumbar puncture may be performed. Lumbar puncture is the most sensitive test for SAH, although false positives may occur as the result of a traumatic tap. Elevations of opening pressure and xanthochromia of CSF present during the lumbar puncture are consistent with SAH. CSF analysis will reveal nonclotting bloody fluid that does not clear with sequential tubes. Xanthochromia, or yellow discoloration, may take 48 hours to develop but may be seen early on. This may be subtle and will require fluid to be spun down to have supernatant evaluated via spectrophotometry (visual inspection is less accurate). Cell count reveals >100,000 RBCs/mm^3, and when the first and last tubes are compared, there should not be a significant drop in counts. Protein elevations are from blood breakdown products. Glucose may be normal or reduced; RBCs present within CSF may metabolize glucose.

Once the diagnosis of SAH has been made, initial management is directed toward preventing rebleeding, detection and treatment of hydrocephalus and vasospasm, monitoring for hyponatremia, deep venous thrombosis (DVT) prophylaxis, seizure prevention, and determining a source of bleeding. Arterial blood gases (ABG), electrolytes, CBC, and PT/INR/PTT should be ordered on admission.

Coagulopathy is expeditiously corrected, and anticoagulants, including aspirin or other nonsteroidal anti-inflammatory drugs (NSAIDs), enoxaparin or other low-molecular weight heparin products, and Coumadin

Section II

Triage

Other Possible Tests or Treatments

Other tests or treatments that may be initiated upon arrival in the ER are

- Arterial blood gas
- Electrocardiogram (EKG) monitoring
- Urinary monitoring (hourly output)
- Gastric catheters (prefer oral placement if brain injury or facial trauma is present in an intubated patient)
- Anteroposterior chest, pelvic, and lateral cervical spine x-rays if needed
- Diagnostic peritoneal lavage or ultrasonography if needed

If treatment is required during any part of the ABCs, the patient's airway, breathing, and circulation must be reassessed to be sure that a fatal injury is not missed.

Secondary Assessment

At the conclusion of the primary assessment, the trauma team must perform a thorough secondary assessment. The secondary assessment is a complete history and a head-to-toe physical exam of the injured patient. Adjuncts to the secondary assessment, if warranted, include computed tomography (CT) scans of the head, chest, abdomen, and pelvis, as well as angiography. Consultation, if warranted, of specialized services, such as neurosurgery, orthopedic, oral-maxillofacial surgery, and/or cardiothoracic surgery, is obtained in a timely manner.

Trauma-induced injury, especially head injury, is a time-dependent pathology. The rapid assessment and stabilization of the multisystem-injured trauma patient requires a well-coordinated prehospital and hospital multidisciplinary system. The initial assessment, performed in minutes, must recognize and correct life-threatening problems to the airway, breathing, and circulatory system. In the face of traumatic injury, the outcome is not only affected by the transition to definitive care but also by hypoxia and hypotension.

Case Management

At the accident scene, the patient's airway is secured by oral intubation with cervical spine stabilization. Needle thoracostomy was performed on the right chest second intercostal space with a rush of air. Bilateral arm large-bore intravenous access was obtained with normal saline infused. The blood pressure increases to 110/60, and the heart rate drops to 98.

On arrival at the ER, the patient's airway is confirmed by direct laryngoscopy. Breath sounds are still diminished on the right side, where a chest tube is placed with 200 cc of blood released. The patient's arterial saturation improves from 80 to 98% on 100% inspired oxygen. Blood pressure and heart rate are unchanged. Body temperature is 94°F. GCS is 6T. Chest and pelvic x-rays are obtained that reveal wide mediastinum, pulmonary contusion, and pelvic fractures. The patient gets head/chest/abdomen/pelvis CT scans that show evidence of cerebral edema with no shift, bilateral pulmonary contusions, and a grade II liver laceration. The patient is transported to the intensive care unit with continued resuscitation and warming measures. Intracranial pressure monitoring is placed with treatment of cerebral edema. Lung protection ventilatory strategies are initiated.

References

1. Advanced Trauma Life Support (ATLS). 6th ed. Chicago: American College of Surgeons; 2002
2. U.S. Department of Transportation, Federal Highway Administration. ITS benefits: continuing successes and operational test results. Pub No FHWA-JPO-98–002,12/97(1.5M)EW; 1997:14
3. Graham DI, Ford I, Adams JH, et al. Ischaemic brain damage is still common in fatal non-missile head injury. J Neurol Neurosurg Psychiatry 1989;52:346–350
4. Chesnut RM, Marshall LF, Klauber MR, et al. The role of secondary brain injury in determining outcome from severe head injury. J Trauma 1993;34:216–222

9

The Spinal Cord–Injured Patient

Jeffery M. Jones and Dan Miulli

Case Study

A 77-year-old female was admitted 5 hours after a fall down three steps, with ³⁄₅ strength of her deltoid, bicep, and brachioradialis; the remaining distal musculature was flaccid. She had pinprick sensation preserved from her lateral elbow up. She had no reflexes, including a bulbocavernosus reflex.

See page 118 for Case Management.

Spinal cord (SPC) injuries that occur emergently may be treated surgically based on the initial clinical exam, depending upon whether the deficit is complete or not. When encountering a person with SPC injury, trauma specialists have several considerations, in order of importance: (1) preservation of life, (2) preservation of intact neurologic function, (3) restoration of spinal stability and prevention of spinal deformity, (4) treatment of associated injuries and prevention of complications while optimizing the potential for recovery of neurologic function, and (5) rehabilitation.

◆ Immobilization

All patients with head trauma, neurologic deficit, or complaints of neck or back pain must be considered to have a spine injury until proven otherwise. Maintaining a high index of suspicion is the key to prevention of further neurologic injury during transport. Frequently, spinal injuries are missed during trauma resuscitation because attention is focused on more obvious or life-threatening injuries. Particular attention must be given to the unconscious patient or patient who is obtunded from substance abuse who may lack protective muscle tone. When such injuries are merely contemplated, fixation of the head to the fracture board can be achieved by placing wedges under the head and immobilizing the motion of the trunk.[1] Immobilization has made a dramatic impact, demonstrating a decline in percentage of complete spinal

cord injuries in the United States from 55% in the 1970s to 39% in the 1980s.*
When an SPC injury is suspected, the patient must have proper oxygenation,
which in many cases can only be achieved with intubation. Tracheal intubation
may require fibroscopic control, with insertion of the tube only after topical
anesthesia of the airways under titrated intravenous sedation. However, in
cases of severe deterioration of vital functions, intubation must be performed
without any delay at the site of the accident or in the emergency room.

After airway, breathing, and circulation have been stabilized, the trauma
team must inspect the patient by log rolling and examining the posterior spine,
feeling for step-offs, tenderness, and deformity along the spine. Vitals signs
should be monitored frequently to detect any decreased sympathetic tone.

◆ Neurologic Exam

A detailed neurologic examination is the most important and sensitive test
for spinal cord injury and must be completed at the time of injury and then
subsequently every 8 to 24 hours to assess improvement or deterioration in
the patient's neurologic status. The areas of SPC injury include quadriplegia,
which is a spinal cord injury from the high cervical to the first thoracic level
with complete loss of motor and sensory function below the level of cord
injury more than 48 hours after injury, and paraplegia, which is a spinal
cord injury below the T1 level involving the thoracic, lumbar, and sacral
segments, sparing the upper extremities.

Level of Lesion

The neurologic exam defines the level of the lesion as the most caudal
segment with normal motor and/or sensory function. Muscle strength is
graded from 0 to 5. C5 motor and sensory quadriplegic patients will have full
strength of deltoids and intact pinprick sensation of distal shoulders. The
neurologic level is the most caudal segment of the spinal cord with normal
sensory and motor function on both sides of the body. The motor level is the
lowest key muscle with at least grade 3, provided the key muscles above that
level are judged to be normal.[1a]

Classification as to Completeness of Spinal Cord Injuries

Once the neurologic exam is completed, the patient can be further classified
into complete or incomplete SPC injury, that is, no residual motor or sensory
function below the level of the lesion. Signs of incomplete SPC injury are (1)
any type of sensation below the level of the lesion (all modes of sensation
should be tested), (2) any type of motor function below the level of the lesion,
and (3) sacral sparring (perianal sensation, voluntary sphincter, toe flexion).

* Data from National Spinal Cord Injury Statistical Cener, University of Alabama
at Birmingham.

Approximately 3% of patients initially diagnosed with a complete injury will have some neurologic recovery within 24 hours. One to 2% are shown to become ambulatory in most large studies. An injury cannot be designated as complete until the initial period of spinal shock has resolved.

Spinal Shock

The hallmark of the end of spinal shock is the return of the bulbocavernosus reflex (BCR). Spinal shock occurs at the time of injury and usually resolves within a few hours to a few days, sometimes several weeks. It consists of loss of sensation, flaccid paralysis, and absent reflexes below the level of the injury. The mechanism of spinal shock is controversial but may involve deafferentation of motor neurons and interneurons in the gray matter. At the cellular level, it may be as a result of excess potassium accumulating in the extracellular space immediately after trauma and blocking conduction. As stated, the BCR is used to determine the absence of spinal shock. It is the first reflex to return. The absence of this reflex documents continuation of spinal shock or spinal injury at the level of the reflex arc itself.[2] It is elicited by genital stimulation and produces anal contraction. No injury may be considered a complete injury until spinal shock has resolved. The treatment for hypotension and bradycardia associated with spinal shock is dopamine, 0.5 to 15 μg/kg/min to desired systolic pressures (max: 20 μg/kg/min). Atropine may also be used for bradycardia (0.5–1.0 mg IV or ET q 3 to 5 min, max: 2 mg).[3]

To test for the BCR, pinch the glans penis or clitoris, or tug on a Foley catheter and feel for reflexive contraction of the anal sphincter. The presence of the BCR does not suggest the potential recovery of motor or sensory function. Patients with a BCR and no motor or sensory function below the injury (including absent perianal pinprick and deep rectal sensation) have a complete injury with less than a 1% chance of significant motor recovery.

◆ Components of the Neurologic Examination

The neurologic exam should be measured using universal motor myotomes and sensory dermatomes. For this reason, the standard scale of the American Spinal Injury Association (ASIA) should be utilized.[4] It is important to stress that only a grading of 4 can have a plus or minus associated with it (**Tables 9–1** and **9–2**).

The sensory pinprick is the most important test for determining the location of injury. It should be done using accepted dermatomes, and each side should be given a sensory grade, up to a total of 112 points per side. The perianal pinprick and anal wink test determine if injury is to the bowel/bladder, the conus, and/or the cauda equina. The presence of perianal pinprick sensation suggests incomplete spinal cord injury and may be the only sign of this incompleteness. Pinprick sensation (spinothalamic tract) is more prognostic than posterior column function because of the proximity of the spinothalamic tract to the corticospinal tract in the acute situation; sparing of sensation to

Table 9–1   American Spinal Injury Association (ASIA) Motor Exam

Segment	Myotome	Right (points)	Left (points)
C5	Elbow flexors	0–5	0–5
C6	Wrist extensors	0–5	0–5
C7	Elbow extensors	0–5	0–5
C8	Finger flexors	0–5	0–5
T1	Finger abductors	0–5	0–5
L2	Hip flexors	0–5	0–5
L3	Knee extensors	0–5	0–5
L4	Ankle dorsiflexors	0–5	0–5
L5	Long toe extensors	0–5	0–5
S1	Plantar flexors	0–5	0–5
S4–S5	Voluntary anal	P	A
Total possible points		50	50

A, anterior; P, posterior.

pinprick in a motor segment with grade 0 power indicates an 85% chance of motor recovery to at least grade 3 (**Tables 9–3** and **9–4**).

The most important method to determine the validity of the neurologic exam is reflex testing. Patients may not be able to cooperate with the motor or sensory exam, or their cooperation may be limited because of pain or medication. Reflexes will be affected by temperature, paralytics, pain, and secondary gain. However, a change from normal reflexes to hyporeflective or absent reflexes is clinically significant (**Table 9–5**).

Not only the extremities are important for reflex testing. In areas of the spine that do not have corresponding limbs, cutaneous reflexes can often be

Table 9–2   American Spinal Injury Association (ASIA) Grading

Sensory grading	
0	No sensation
1	Abnormal/decreased sensation
2	Normal sensation
Motor grading	
0	Total paralysis
1	Palpable or visible contraction
2	Active movement, gravity eliminated
3	Active movement against gravity
4	Active movement against some resistance +/−
5	Active movement against full resistance
NT	Not testable

Table 9–3   Spinal Dermatome Levels[1a]

Level	Dermatome
C4	Shoulder
C5	Lateral elbow
C6	Thumb
C7	Middle finger
C8	Little finger
T4	Nipples
T6	Xiphoid
T10	Umbilicus
L3	Just above patella
L4	Medial malleolus
L5	Webbing between great toe and next
S1	Bottom lateral foot
S4–S5	Perianal

elicited. These reflexes depend on the thickness of the skin and the ability to perceive small muscle movement in the patient (**Table 9–6**).

Once a full reflex exam is completed, the patient's injury can be classified. The classification helps to determine treatment and prognosis (**Table 9–7**).

In all cases of SPC injury, standard management of acute neurologic injury should be instituted. The patient should have adequate blood flow and blood oxygenation, with intravenous fluids initiated and PO_2 maintained at >115 mm Hg to avoid hypotension. Additionally, immobilization should be employed to prevent other injuries, and rehabilitation should be started as soon as feasible.

◆ Indications for Surgery

Absolute indications for emergent surgery:

- ◆ Progressing neurologic deficit
- ◆ Open (compound) fracture
- ◆ Unsuccessful closed reduction of subluxation

Relative indications for early surgery:

- ◆ Spinal canal compromise by bone, blood, and so on
- ◆ Urinary retention as only symptom

Contraindications for early surgery:

- ◆ Medically unstable patient
- ◆ Central cord syndrome

Table 9–4 American Spinal Injury Association (ASIA) Sensory Exam

Dermatome	PP R	PP L	LT R	LT L
C2	0–2	0–2	0–2	0–2
C3	0–2	0–2	0–2	0–2
C4	0–2	0–2	0–2	0–2
C5	0–2	0–2	0–2	0–2
C6	0–2	0–2	0–2	0–2
C7	0–2	0–2	0–2	0–2
C8	0–2	0–2	0–2	0–2
Total possible points	14	14	14	14

Dermatome	PP R	PP L	LT R	LT L
T1	0–2	0–2	0–2	0–2
T2	0–2	0–2	0–2	0–2
T3	0–2	0–2	0–2	0–2
T4	0–2	0–2	0–2	0–2
T5	0–2	0–2	0–2	0–2
T6	0–2	0–2	0–2	0–2
T7	0–2	0–2	0–2	0–2
T8	0–2	0–2	0–2	0–2
T9	0–2	0–2	0–2	0–2
T10	0–2	0–2	0–2	0–2
T11	0–2	0–2	0–2	0–2
T12	0–2	0–2	0–2	0–2
Total possible points	24	24	24	24

Dermatome	PP R	PP L	LT R	LT L
L1	0–2	0–2	0–2	0–2
L2	0–2	0–2	0–2	0–2
L3	0–2	0–2	0–2	0–2
L4	0–2	0–2	0–2	0–2
L5	0–2	0–2	0–2	0–2
S1	0–2	0–2	0–2	0–2
S2	0–2	0–2	0–2	0–2
S3	0–2	0–2	0–2	0–2
S4–S5	0–2	0–2	0–2	0–2
Total possible points	18	18	18	18

L, left; LT, light touch; PP, pinprick; R, right.

Table 9–5   Reflex Exam Grading[1a]

Grade	Reflex quality
0	No reflex
1	Hyporeflexia
2	Normal
3	Brisk
4	Hyper-reflexia

Table 9–6   Important Testable Reflexes[1a]

Reflex	Level	Description
Abdominal cutaneous	T8–T12	• A cortical reflex that is elicited by stroking one quadrant of the abdomen, which causes contraction of the underlying musculature, which in turn causes the umbilicus to migrate toward that quadrant
Bulbocavernosus	S2–S4	• Bulbocavernosus reflex is used to determine the absence of spinal shock • First reflex to return following injury • Absence of this reflex documents continuation of spinal shock or spinal injury at the level of the reflex arc itself • The reflex is elicited by genital stimulation and produces anal contraction • No injury may be considered a complete injury until spinal shock has resolved
Cremasteric	L1–L2	• Superficial reflex that consists of scrotal shrinkage following stroking of the inner thigh
Anal cutaneous	S2–S4	• Known as anal wink • Contraction of the anal sphincter following stimulation of the skin surrounding the anus
Reverse radial	UMN	• Indicates UMN dysfunction
Hoffmann's	UMN	• Indicates dysfunction
Priapism		• Indicates loss of sympathetic tone following cord injury and a predominance of parasympathetic tone

UMN, upper motor neuron.

Table 9–7 Classification of Spinal Cord Syndromes[3]

Syndrome	Mechanism	Motor loss	Sensory loss	Recovery
Brown-Séquard[16,17]	Hemisection of the spinal cord, usually by penetrating objects; tumors or hematomas can also be a source	Ipsilateral loss of motor below level of lesion	Contralateral loss of pain and temperature below level of lesion; ipsilateral loss of light touch, proprioception, vibration	Most promising of the incomplete syndromes in terms of recovery; ~ 90% will regain independent ambulation, anal and urinary sphincter control
Central cord[18,19]	Accidents or minor falls resulting in neck extension are common causes	Motor loss is greater in upper than lower extremities; UE recovery is variable and fine motor control of UEs usually does not recover well	Majority have intact bowel and bladder because of the peripheral arrangement of sacral fibers in the cord	Will usually ambulate but commonly with spasticity
Anterior cord[20]	Usually flexion/compression mechanism, resulting from diving accidents; ischemic injury from compression of anterior spinal artery	Loss of all motor function below lesion	Loss of pain and temperature sensations below lesion and preservation of posterior column sensation; bowel/bladder also affected	The poorest prognosis for any recovery of motor function of all the incomplete syndromes; only 10–20% may regain motor function

		Preservation of motor function	Preservation of pain and temperature function with loss of posterior column function (proprioception, two-point tactile discrimination, vibration modalities)	Patients can walk but rely on visual input for spatial orientation; prognosis is unknown because it is so rare
Posterior cord				
Conus medullaris	Injury to the terminal spinal cord usually just posterior to the bodies from T12 to L1; common causes are trauma, tumor, and infection	Produces loss of bowel and bladder control, poor rectal muscle tone; no motor signs in legs (if pure); if motor function is lost, it is symmetrical, and ankle jerk is absent (S1)	Loss of perirectal sensation; saddle distribution of sensory loss	Prognosis is poor for significant return of bowel and bladder control

UE, upper extremity.

◆ Initial Medical Treatment of Spinal Cord Injuries

The use of corticosteroids (methylprednisolone [MP]) after acute SPC injury remains controversial. There are many animal models that show efficacy. MP works to stabilize membrane structures and the blood–spinal cord barrier, reducing vasogenic edema; to enhance blood flow in the spinal cord; to inhibit endorphin release; to prevent free radical accumulation; and to moderate the inflammatory response. In a review of the literature, it was found that through 2002, there were 639 studies on corticosteroids and human spinal cord injury, of which 46 studies were of high enough scientific value to be used to develop guidelines for their use.[5] The results of these studies are reviewed in **Table 9–8**.[6–21]

Methylprednisolone is prepared as 62.5 mg/mL with 30 mg/kg IV bolus over 15 minutes, then 5.4 mg/kg/hr continuous infusion of methylprednisolone for 23 hours started 45 minutes after bolus. It is not for use in life-threatening morbidities, cauda equina syndrome, gunshot wounds, for those under age 13 years, narcotic addiction, complete SPC injuries, or pregnancy.[6–21]

Rehabilitation

Once the patient has been managed appropriately to prevent any episodes of hypotension and hypoxia, while restoring stability, he or she should progress to rehabilitation. Several classification systems have been used to document SPC injury. Once again, any classification system employed allows health-care providers to track the patient's progress (**Tables 9–9** and **9–10**).

Case Management

A 77-year-old female was admitted 5 hours after falling down three steps, with ³/₅ strength of her deltoid, bicep, and brachioradialis; the remaining distal musculature was flaccid. She had pinprick sensation preserved from her lateral elbow up. She had no reflexes, including no bulbocavernosus reflex. The patient should be started on spinal cord steroid protocol for 48 hours. At this time, her injury cannot be determined because her BCR has not returned. The level of the injury appears to be at C6 because C5 appears intact, but once again the BCR has not returned, and the neurologic examination is expected to change. In addition to the steroids, the patient should have stomach protectants, intravenous fluids to keep her euvolemic to hypervolemic, oxygenation, and measures to prevent hypotension. Additionally, the patient should be immobilized. Most importantly, the patient should have frequent neurologic examinations and magnetic resonance imaging to document her injuries and possible treatments, which will be known as soon as the spinal shock wears off.

Table 9–8 North American Spinal Cord Injury Study (NASCIS)*

Study	Study type	Format	Results	Conclusion
NASCIS I	Multicenter randomized double-blind clinical trial (1979), reported in 1984	Compared MP 100 mg bolus and MP 100 mg/day × 10 days versus 1000 mg bolus and 1000 mg/day for 10 days	There was no difference in neurologic recovery between the groups, but there was no control	MP at the tested levels did not significantly change outcome; was the level of MP too low?
NASCIS II	Multicenter reported in 1990	Compared standard MP dosage of 30 mg/kg bolus, then 5.4 mg/kg/h infusion for 23 hours, with naloxone at 5.4 mg/kg bolus, then 4 mg/kg/h for 23 hours or placebo; randomized within 12 hours	MP administered within 8 hours was associated with a significant improvement in motor function score, sensation at 6-month follow-up; also reported statistically significant improvement of motor function scores at 1 year	Post hoc analyses detected a small gain in the total motor and sensory function scores in a subgroup of patients who had received MP within 8 hours after their injury
NASCIS III	Double-blind, multicenter study; no placebo	Compared a 48-hour infusion of MP with a 24-hour infusion started within 8 hours after injury; found no benefit from extending the infusion beyond 24 hours	48-hour MP group showed improved motor score at 6 weeks and improved motor and sensory function scores at 6 months compared with 24-hour MP, especially if given between 3 and 8 hours	Found no benefit from extending the infusion beyond 24 hours
Cochrane review	Meta-analysis	Based on the controversial subgroup post hoc analyses in NASCIS II and III and the data from a Japanese study		Concluded that a 24-hour high-dose MP infusion within 8 hours after injury is efficacious

* In all three NASCIS studies and other, smaller studies, the incidence of sepsis and pneumonia was higher in the high-dose methylprednisolone groups than in the placebo or other treatment groups.
MP, methylprednisolone.

Table 9–9 Frankel Classification

A	Complete loss of motor and sensory functions below a given level
B	Some preservation of sensation, complete motor function paralysis
C	Sensory function useless, some motor function preserved, but insufficient to be useful
D	Sensory function useful; weak but useful motor function
E	Neurologically intact

Table 9–10 American Spinal Injury Association (ASIA) Impairment Scale

A	Complete	No motor or sensory function is preserved in the sacral segments S4–S5
B	Incomplete	Sensory but not motor function is preserved below the neurologic level and extends through the sacral segments S4–S5
C	Incomplete	Motor function is preserved below the neurologic level, and the majority of key muscles below the neurologic level have a muscle grade < 3
D	Incomplete	Motor function is preserved below the neurologic level, and the majority of key muscles below the neurologic level have a muscle grade ≥ 3
E	Normal	Motor and sensory functions are normal

References

1. Cervical spine immobilization before admission to hospital. Guidelines for Management of Acute Cervical Spine and Spinal Injuries. Neurosurgery 2002; 50(suppl):7–17
1a. American Spinal Injury Association. Standards for the Neurologic Classification of Spinal Injury Patients. Chicago: ASIA; 1982
2. Atkinson PP, Atkinson JLD. Spinal shock. Mayo Clin Proc 1996;71:384–389
3. Schneider RC, Crosby EC, Russo RH, Gosch HH. Traumatic spinal cord syndromes and their management. Clin Neurosurg 1973;20:424–492
4. American Spinal Injury Association. Guidelines for Facility Categorization and Standards of Care: Spinal Cord Injury. Chicago: ASIA; 1981
5. Guidelines for Management of Acute Cervical Spine and Spinal Cord Injuries. Neurosurgery 2002;50(Suppl S1) Neurosurg 2002;50(3 Suppl):S85–S99
6. Bracken MB, Collins WF, Freeman DF, et al. Efficacy of methylprednisolone in acute spinal cord injury. JAMA 1984;251(1):45–52
7. Bracken MB, Shepard MJ, Hellenbrand KG, et al. Methylprednisolone and neurological function 1 year after spinal cord injury: results of the National Acute Spinal Cord Injury Study. J Neurosurg 1985;63(5):704–713
8. Bracken MB, Shepard MJ, Collins WF, et al. A randomized, controlled trial of methylprednisolone or naloxone in the treatment of acute spinal-cord injury: results of the Second National Acute Spinal Cord Injury Study. N Engl J Med 1990;322(20):1405–1411
9. Bracken MB, Shepard MJ, Collins WF, et al. Methylprednisolone or naloxone treatment after acute spinal cord injury: 1-year follow-up data. Results of the Second National Acute Spinal Cord Injury Study. J Neurosurg 1992;76(1):23–31

10. Bracken MB, Shepard MJ, Holford TR, et al. Administration of methylprednisolone for 24 or 48 hours or tirilazad mesylate for 48 hours in the treatment of acute spinal cord injury: results of the Third National Acute Spinal Cord Injury Randomized Controlled Trial, National Acute Spinal Cord Injury Study. JAMA 1997;277(20):1597–1604
11. Bracken MB, Shepard MJ, Holford TR, et al. Methylprednisolone or tirilazad mesylate administration after acute spinal cord injury: 1-year follow up. Results of the Third National Acute Spinal Cord Injury Randomized Controlled Trial. J Neurosurg 1998;89(5):699–706
12. Bracken MB. Pharmacological intervention for acute spinal cord injury [Cochrane review]. Cochrane Library 2001(1)
13. Matsumoto T, Tamaki T, Kawakami M, Yoshida M, Ando M, Yamada H. Early complications of high-dose methylprednisolone sodium succinate treatment in the follow-up of acute cervical spinal cord injury. Spine 2001;26(4):426–430
14. Galandiuk S, Raque G, Appel S, Polk HC Jr. The two-edged sword of large-dose steroids for spinal cord trauma. Ann Surg 1993;218(4):419–425, discussion 425–427
15. Gerndt SJ, Rodriguez JL, Pawlik JW, et al. Consequences of high-dose steroid therapy for acute spinal cord injury. J Trauma 1997;42(2):279–284
16. Nesathurai S. Steroids and spinal cord injury: revisiting the NASCIS 2 and NASCIS 3 trials. J Trauma 1998;45(6):1088–1093
17. Lim E, Wong YS, Lo YL, Lim SH. Traumatic atypical Brown-Séquard syndrome: case report and literature review. Clin Neurol Neurosurg 2003;105(2):143–145
18. Rumana CS, Baskin DS. Brown-Séquard syndrome produced by cervical disc herniation: case report and literature review. Surg Neurol 1996;45(4):359–361
19. Maroon JC, Abla AA, Wilberger JI. Central cord syndrome. Clin Neurosurg 1991;37:612–621
20. Massaro F, Lanotte M, Faccani G. Acute traumatic central cord syndrome. Acta Neurol (Napoli) 1993;15(2):97–105
21. Schneider RC. The syndrome of the Acute Anterior Spinal Cord Injury. J Neurosurg 1955;12:95–122

Progressing Postoperative Neurologic Deficit: Cranial or Spinal

Ganna L. Breland and Dan Miulli

Case Study

A 42-year-old male is in the recovery room after a posterior lumbar fusion following an L4 burst fracture from a fall of 30 feet. Pre-operatively, the patient's strength in his lower extremities was determined to be 5/5 bilaterally, and sensation was intact. The fusion went well, and there were no intraoperative complications or indications of problems, as seen in the spinal cord monitoring. During the postanesthesia recovery period, the patient complains of difficulty in moving his left foot. A significant decrease in muscle strength is found in the patient's left leg from the knee distally compared to his preoperative evaluation. The patient's incisional pain is well controlled, and his efforts are at his maximum.

See page 128 for Case Management.

◆ Determining Neurologic Status

Determining Level of Consciousness

The Glasgow Coma Scale (GCS) is an internationally recognized tool used to assess level of consciousness. It is intended for use in patients over the age of 4 years. A modified scale is used with children under 4 years. The GCS is based on a 15-point grading system, with the minimum score being 3 and the maximum being 15. Patients who score 8 or less are considered to be in a comatose state. The GCS is considered the gold standard in assessing trauma patients; it is also often used to describe any patient with impairment in mental status. The scale is based on the best function in eye, verbal, and motor responses. For a patient who is intubated, the maximum score obtainable is 11 and is denoted as 11T (for intubated, or "tubed").[1]

Using a systematic method, usually the patient's best eye response is evaluated first. A maximum score of 4 indicates the patient's eyes are open upon visual inspection during the initial moments of the examination, or the eyes open spontaneously prior to the initiation of the rest of the examination.

A score of 3 indicates the eyes open to the sound of a voice or voice command. A score of 2 indicates the eyes open to tactile stimulus or painful stimuli, such as a sternal rub or pressure to the nail bed. A score of 1 is the lowest score possible and is given if there is no eye opening at all. At this time, it is also convenient to examine the patient's pupils for size and reactivity.[2-6] Although not part of the GCS, the pupil exam is a critical part of the full neurologic examination of the patient.

The next part of the evaluation is of verbal response. The maximum score of 5 indicates the patient is coherent and able to answer questions appropriately and correctly. For instance, the patient can tell the examiner the year, the location of the patient, and the name of the current U.S. president or can recall certain recent events, including but not limited to the details of the accident. A score of 4 indicates the patient is awake and alert but slightly confused. For example, the patient may be unsure of the year. A score of 3 indicates the patient's responses are inappropriate. For example, when asked a question regarding one subject, the patient may speak of an entirely unrelated subject. A score of 2 indicates the patient's replies are incomprehensible. The patient may be able to mumble or make noises, but no comprehensible sentences are spoken. If there is no verbal response, a score of 1 is given.

The last part of the GCS is the assessment of the patient's motor function. The highest score of 6 indicates the patient is able to follow a physical command, such as "Hold up two fingers" or "Blink twice if you understand me." A score of 5 indicates the patient does not follow commands fully but is able to, for instance, raise an arm (or a leg) in response to an attempt to find a source of painful stimuli. A score of 4 is given if the patient withdraws an extremity to a painful stimulus, such as applying pressure to the nail bed of a finger or toe. Do not confuse withdrawal with a spinal reflex. Withdrawal is held, whereas spinal reflexes return to a normal position while the stimulus is still being applied. The best location to perform a painful stimulus to determine withdrawal versus reflex is on the inner aspect of the upper arm. In withdrawal, the patient will move the arm away from the torso, or abduct the arm. In a reflex response, the patient will bring the arm closer to the torso, or adduct the arm.

In more severe levels of coma, patients reveal "posturing" that results from brainstem involvement. There are two types of posturing: flexion, also known as decorticate posturing, and extension, or decerebrate posturing. A score of 3 is given for flexion or decorticate posturing. As an example of flexion, the patient's arms flex at the elbows, while the legs extend and rotate internally, and the feet plantar flex.

Decerebrate or extensor posturing involves extension rather than flexion of the arms and legs; it is indicated by a score of 2. Posturing may be seen bilaterally but often is seen only in one extremity. The extent of injury can be estimated with decorticate and decerebrate posturing. The level of the damage is above the red nuclei and may be in the bilateral cerebral hemispheres with decorticate posturing. With decerebrate posturing, there is disruption between the superior colliculi or the decussation of the rubrospinal pathway and the rostral portion of the vestibular nuclei. The major response to painful stimulation is the function of the vestibulospinal tract—extension of the neck, back, and limbs, as well as inhibition of flexion of the trunk and limbs. Because the tracts are uncrossed, the response is on the same side. Decerebrate posturing carries a worse prognosis. If a patient has no movement at all to deep central stimuli, then a score of 1 is given.

A depressed or declining GCS deserves emergent evaluation and initiation of management. This is true in both trauma and postsurgical patients in which progression of intracerebral pathology and herniation should be investigated expeditiously. When assessing the GCS, one must keep in mind extracerebral influences such as sedating medications, paralytics, illicit drugs, and alcohol. These confounding factors may drastically change patient management or at least warrant a repeat neurologic examination before any aggressive management is initiated, for example, placing an intracranial pressure monitor or administering mannitol.

Using GCS and Spinal Checks in the NICU and in the Postoperative Period

The postoperative period is an extremely important time in a patient's hospitalization course. Depending on the location and complexity of the procedure performed, the patient may be placed in the neurosurgical intensive care unit (NICU) for frequent neurologic checks by the nursing staff as well as by the neurosurgical team. Most brain surgery patients require neurochecks every hour for at least a 24-hour period. In addition to normal parameters, such as blood pressure, heart rate, and respiratory rate, the staff assesses pupil size and reactivity, GCS score, and, if spinal surgery was performed or there is spinal injury, spinal checks. These hourly comparisons are an effective way to grade any changes in the patient's neurologic condition so that the neurosurgical team can be alerted to any negative changes. This is particularly significant in postoperative patients.[5,6]

Any change in the patient's GCS, pupils, or motor or sensory examinations requires immediate notification of the neurosurgical team so that important decisions regarding the next step in management can be made in a timely manner. This can range simply from turning off a patient's sedating medications and allowing the patient to wake up to a return trip to the operating room for exploration. Often, repeat imaging is necessary to rule out lesions that would require a return to the operating room.

Determining Spinal Deficits

The Royal Medical Research Council of Great Britain developed a scale for grading strength as part of a motor function examination that is the spinal equivalent of the GCS for head injury.[1,5,6] The scale ranges from 0 to 5 and is denoted as 0/5, 1/5, 4+/5, and so on. A grade of 0 means there is no contraction of the muscle fibers. Grade 1 indicates the slightest movement; grade 2, movement from side to side. For instance, the patient may be able to slide an arm or leg on the bed but is unable to lift it off the bed. Grade 3 indicates movement against gravity; grade 4, movement against resistance. Grade 4 is the only grade that is subdivided. The divisions are as follows: 4– slight resistance, 4 moderate resistance, and 4+ strong resistance. Grade 5 indicates normal strength. It is important to bear in mind the strength of the examiner as well. A younger or stronger examiner may easily overpower a frail individual, although the strength is still recorded as 5/5.[1] **Table 2–3** (page 12) outlines the Royal Medical Research Council of Great Britain muscle strength grading scale.

The American Spinal Injury Association (ASIA)[1] developed a motor function scoring system to apply to 10 muscles or groups in conjunction with the Royal Medical Research Council's grading scale so that a rapid assessment of spinal cord function can be achieved. The 10 muscles or groups are the deltoid or biceps, wrist extensors, triceps, flexor digitorum profundus, hand intrinsics, iliopsoas, quadriceps, tibialis anterior, extensor hallucis longus, and gastrocnemius.

The ASIA grading system is usually used only by the neurosurgical team and not the nursing staff unless spinal checks are included as part of the ICU neurocheck. In addition to being part of a complete neurologic examination, the ASIA system can be particularly useful in the postoperative period after spinal surgery for comparison with the preoperative state. Often a subtle change in a patient's motor examination by the staff, or subjectively recognized by the patient, is the first indicator of the development of a spinal epidural hematoma after surgery. Development of a spinal epidural hematoma is a surgical emergency and means a return to the operating room for evacuation. Prompt recognition is crucial when each minute that passes could equal additional loss of spinal cord function from strangulation by the hematoma[1] (**Fig. 10–1**).

Each muscle/group is graded bilaterally using the 0/5–5/5 system as described above. There is a maximum score of 50 for each side, for a total maximum score of 100. The nerve root at C5 is tested by shoulder abduction or elbow flexion to grade the strength of the deltoid or biceps, respectively. Having the patient cock the wrist back using the wrist extensors tests C6. Triceps muscle contraction causing elbow extension tests C7. Squeezing the hand to engage the flexor digitorum profundus tests C8. Abducting the little finger grades the hand intrinsics for T1. Flexing the hip to engage the iliopsoas tests L2. L3 is tested using the quadriceps muscle to straighten the knee. Dorsiflexion of the foot by the tibialis anterior tests L4. Dorsiflexion of the big toe alone using the extensor hallucis longus grades L5. Plantar flexing the foot using the gastrocnemius tests S1.

Equally important as the motor examination is the sensory examination. The sensory examination, especially a patient's "pinprick level," is the most reliable clinical indicator of the level of the spinal cord lesion. However, on initial neurologic examination by the neurosurgical team, all forms of sensory modalities should be tested. The posterior column, specifically the medial lemniscus, is the location of proprioception and vibratory senses. Having the patient balance during eye closure tests proprioception. Falling/leaning to one side indicates poor posterior column function. Applying a vibrating tuning fork to part of the distal extremities, usually the nail or joint of the big toe or thumb, tests vibration sense. Joint position is tested by having the patient close the eyes and indicate the direction that the big toe has been moved toward, either up or down. The technique for this test is to place the examiner's fingers on the sides of the toe, not on top

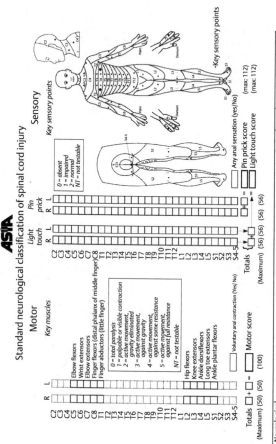

Figure 10–1 American Spine Injury Association standard neurologic classification of spinal cord injury. (Courtesy of the American Spine Injury Association.)

and bottom, because this can lead the patent toward an answer. Pain, temperature, and light touch fibers travel in the spinothalamic tract.

Pain is the most widely tested sensory modality in the NICU setting. Usually this is done by lightly applying pressure with a pin to determine if the patient can feel the pinprick at the key sensory landmarks tested or, in contrast, if the patient has decreased sensation in a specific dermatomal distribution. More specifically, a patient may have complete loss of sensation below a certain level. This is described as the pinprick or sensory level. The insult to the spinal cord is usually about one to three levels above the pinprick level because the spinothalamic fibers continue one to three segments cephaladly before decussating. For instance, in the case study at the beginning of this chapter, a pinprick test was done starting at the patient's neck and traveling caudally. The patient could not feel the pinprick below the level of the umbilicus. The dermatome at the umbilicus is T10. The patient was described as having a T10 sensory level and was determined to have a burst fracture at T8, which was causing severe spinal cord compression.

An ascending sensory level prompts emergent investigation in most settings, especially in the postoperative or post-trauma period. Not only can it indicate increasing spinal cord damage, but it can be life-threatening if C3, C4, and C5 become involved in a patient who is not already mechanically ventilated. Key sensory landmarks to evaluate are listed in **Table 10–1**.

Table 10–1   Key Sensory Landmarks

Sensory examination: tested in each of the 28 dermatomes on the right and left sides for sensation to pinprick and light touch	
Responses are scored as 0 = absent; 1 = impaired (partial or altered including hyperesthesia); 2 = normal	
C3	Supraclavicular fossa
C4	Shoulders, top
C5	Lateral antecubital
C6	Thumb (first finger)
C7	Middle (third) finger
C8	Little (fifth) finger
T4	Nipple line
T6	Xiphoid
T10	Umbilicus
L3	Proximal to patella medial
L4	Medial malleolus
L5	Dorsal webbing between base great toe and second toe
S1	Lateral plantar foot
S2	Popliteal fossa midline
S4–S5	Perianal

Source: Adapted with permission from Greenberg M. Handbook of Neurosurgery. 5th ed. New York: Thieme; 2001.

Case Management

The patient was taken back to the operating room for exploration of the surgical area, where the surgeon found a hematoma compressing the spinal cord. It was evacuated, and a drain was left in place. The patient's motor exam returned to his baseline. Prompt recognition of change in the patient's clinical status by the neurosurgical team and by the patient himself allowed for a quick return to the operating room before permanent damage could be done by compression of the epidural hematoma.

◆ Additional Cases

Case 1

A 23-year-old female returns to the NICU after removal of an epidural hematoma (EDH). A nurse notices that the patient is not returning to her baseline GCS of 9T prior to the surgical evacuation of the hematoma. Her pupils are 3 mm and reactive. The patient is sent for an emergent computed tomography (CT) scan, which shows that the epidural hematoma was nicely evacuated. Upon further investigation, it is determined that another nurse had given a bolus of propofol and morphine prior to the change of shift. This was the reason behind the patient's lower GCS, not a reaccumulation of the EDH. After 1 hour the patient returned to her baseline GCS of 9T.

Case 2

A 23-year-old female returns to the NICU after evacuation of an EDH. A nurse notices that the patient has not returned to her baseline GCS. Her right pupil is larger than the left and sluggish. The patient is sent for a stat CT of the brain, which shows reaccumulation of the EDH. The patient is taken back to the operating room for surgical evacuation of the recurrent EDH.

Case 3

A 22-year-old male is involved in a rollover motor vehicle accident. He was intubated in the field without the administration of sedatives or paralytics. He has not received any additional medications except phenytoin. In the emergency room, his laboratory values are normal; however, his blood alcohol level is beyond the legal range. He scores a 5 on the GCS, with the CT demonstrating no hemorrhage, no compression of the basal cisterns, and no edema. In this situation, it is appropriate to wait and reexamine the patient over the next few hours to see if he improves as the alcohol wears off instead of placing an intracranial pressure monitor right away.

References

1. Greenberg MS. Handbook of Neurosurgery. 6th ed. New York: Thieme; 2006
2. Tsementzis SA. Differential Diagnosis in Neurology and Neurosurgery: A Clinician's Pocket Guide. New York: Thieme; 2000
3. Waxman SG. Correlative Neuroanatomy. 24th ed. New York: Lange; 2000
4. Young PA, Young PH. Basic Clinical Neuroanatomy. Baltimore: Williams & Wilkins; 1997
5. Youmans JR. Neurological Surgery. 4th ed. Philadelphia: WB Saunders; 1996
6. Rengachary SS, Ellenbogen RG. Principles of Neurosurgery. 2nd ed. Edinburgh: Elsevier Mosby; 2005

11

Delayed Intracerebral Hemorrhage

Lynn M. Serrano

Case Study

A 35-year-old male fell from a 6 foot ladder. His family describes a brief 2 to 3 minute loss of consciousness with significant confusion after the event. He was transported by emergency medical services to the hospital. On initial evaluation by paramedics, the patient was noted to have a Glasgow Coma Scale (GCS) of 13 and continued as such at the hospital. He had no focal neurologic deficits at that time. A noncontrasted head CT obtained upon arrival at the hospital showed a 6 mm right frontoparietal subdural hematoma (**Fig. 11–1**).

The radiologist reported no additional intracranial lesions or skull fractures. The patient was admitted for observation. After ~3 hours, the patient developed a fixed and dilated left pupil and a GCS of 9. The patient received an emergent repeat CT scan that showed a 3 cm left frontoparietal epidural hematoma with a 1 cm midline shift (**Fig. 11–2**).

See page 141 for Case Management.

Intracranial hemorrhage has been a topic of significant research in the past several decades and includes multiple etiologies. Delayed hemorrhages previously discovered via angiography were considered relatively rare, yet with the advent of computed tomography (CT) scanning, the ease of diagnosis and follow-up has increased, as well as the incidence. Etiologies include both post-traumatic and nontraumatic. In this chapter we review the pathogenesis, diagnosis, management, and outcome of these lesions using three case examples.

◆ Delayed Traumatic Intracranial Hemorrhage

In 1891 Bollinger et al described delayed traumatic intracranial hemorrhages (DTICHs) as *traumatische Spät-Apoplexie* ("traumatic apoplectic event") events using three criteria:[1]

1. An apoplectic event preceded by a traumatic history
2. A relatively symptom-free period followed by a neurologic decline
3. The lack of preexisting vascular pathology

Duret and other researchers expanded on Bollinger et al's work by delineating the stages of DTICH.[2,3] In the early 1900s, continued research led to theories of pathogenesis for DTICH, which we will discuss. Today, improved imaging has increased detection and diagnosis of DTICH, which was previously limited to operative and autopsy findings, and has enhanced our understanding of the disease. DTICH can be divided into epidural, subdural, and intracerebral hemorrhages.

◆ Delayed Traumatic Epidural Hematoma

A delayed traumatic epidural hematoma (DTEH) exists when there is evidence of an epidural collection of blood on follow-up CT scan, not apparent on initial CT scan. This may occur with or without an underlying skull fracture. It has classically been described as "talk and deteriorate." The symptoms vary according to the size and location of the hematoma and range from

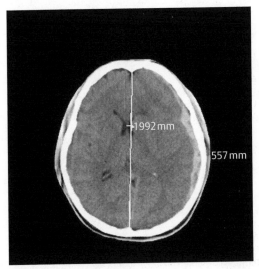

Figure 11–1   Subdural hematoma.

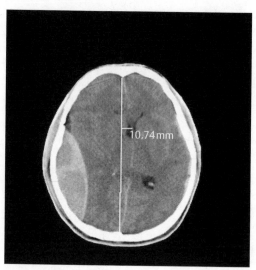

Figure 11–2   Epidural hematoma.

mild headache to focal neurologic deficits to deep comatose states. The delayed decline can occur anywhere from minutes to weeks after the initial traumatic event, most frequently between 6 and 48 hours after the trauma.[3,4]

The incidence of post-traumatic epidural hematoma in the pre-CT era occurred in less than 10% of all traumatic head injuries.[5,6] The recent widespread use of CT scans reveals an incidence as high as 30%.[7–9] DTEH specifically is estimated to occur in 2 to 10% of traumatic head injuries and as such has a predilection in males. It is more frequent in younger adults (average age: 27) relative to the elderly.[10] One possible explanation for the accumulation is lifestyle differences; another is that, in advanced age, the dura mater can frequently adhere to the skull, preventing fluid accumulation.[3]

DTEH occurs most commonly in the temporal area (possibly secondary to thinner bone and the fragility of the middle meningeal artery) and with equal frequency in the frontal, parietal, and occipital areas.[11,12]

Pathogenesis

Delayed elevation of intracranial pressure, which may be caused by arterial bleeding or progressive edema, is a likely cause of the rapid deterioration these patients experience. Damaged vessels, initially in vasospasm, would allow increased blood flow and hematoma formation once the vasospasm has resolved.[5,13–16] Hematomas also occur secondary to damage to superficial veins running along the arteries in the bony grooves, or damage to venous sinuses. Venous bleeding is slower and could account for the delayed detection of these bleeds. Patients initially in shock would be resuscitated, and efforts reversing the hypovolemic state would encourage bleeding from a damaged vessel. Measures taken to treat and relieve elevated intracranial pressure, including surgical and medical techniques, decompress the brain and create new space for subsequent bleeding as the tamponade effect is reversed.[5,6,15] Piepmeier and Wagner[17] showed that 10% of patients with an evacuated traumatic extra-axial hematoma developed a second surgical hematoma at an alternate site within 24 hours of the original surgery. Skull fractures could act as a decompressive device for acute epidural hematoma, allowing blood to seep into the subgaleal space and delaying intracranial symptoms, leading physicians to incorrectly believe the diagnosis to be delayed epidural hematoma.

Treatment

The gold standard is craniotomy for the removal of the hematoma. The patients described by Ashkenazi et al[16] recovered completely after evacuation of the bleed with a craniotomy. They were discharged in excellent condition, and follow-up scans showed no reaccumulation. Smaller bleeds can be observed.

Outcome

Outcome is dependent on the initial presentation, the size and location of the bleed, and the aggressive treatment by the physician. Unsuccessful treatment of elevated intracranial pressure with an initial negative CT occurs in as many as 60% of cases of DTEH and is often used as an indication for follow-up scanning.[6] Overall mortality approaches 12%, yet 91% of initially noncomatose patients and 35% of initially comatose patients taken to the operating room have a good recovery.[10]

◆ Delayed Traumatic Subdural Hematoma

Delayed subdural hematomas have been difficult to diagnose because of the frequently subacute and chronic presentation of this entity. A delayed traumatic subdural hematoma (DTSH) is an acute subdural hemorrhage, not apparent on initial imaging, appearing on follow-up CT scans within 30 days of a traumatic event. It usually presents as a decline in mental status, but significant neurologic deficit, though rarely seen, is a late finding of DTSH. The majority of cases are identified incidentally on follow-up scans or while being evaluated for new onset headaches and mental status changes.

Incidence

Of completely evacuated acute subdural hemorrhages, 0.5% will develop subsequent delayed reoccurrence.[3] DTSH is most commonly associated with other intracranial hemorrhages, mass lesions, and brain edema. As with acute subdural hematoma, DTSH is frequently attributed to the tearing of bridging veins.

Pathogenesis

The detection of subdural hemorrhages is often delayed because initial resuscitation efforts reverse low flow secondary to systemic hypotension or shock from other traumatic injuries.

The tamponade effect caused by elevated intracranial pressure would delay frank bleeding. Generalized traumatic edema and other intracranial lesions (i.e., hemorrhagic or mass effect) would cause just this type of tamponade. The evacuation or reversal of the offending agent, via medication, procedures (e.g., ventriculostomy), or surgery would allow expansion of the subdural hemorrhage appearing as a DTSH. Vascular malformations may also be traumatically induced and have been identified as causes of DTSH.[18]

Treatment

Treatment of DTSH depends on the size, location, overall mass effect, and neurologic status of the patient.

General guidelines for DTSH are similar to acute subdural hematoma. Symptomatic lesions, lesions over 1 cm thick, and lesions with more than 0.5 cm midline shift should be evacuated. Depending on the age of the hematoma and the presence of membrane formation on CT scan, burr hole drainage or bedside drain placement drainage may be an acceptable alternative to a full craniotomy.

Outcome

The outcome for DTSH is highly variable and very case specific, as most studies incorporate patients with different etiologies, hematoma subtypes, symptoms, and presentations.[19]

◆ Delayed Traumatic Intracerebral Hematoma

As previously discussed, the ambiguity and multitude of classification systems surrounding a diagnosis of "delayed" nature, as well as the varied courses of cases and the wide range of possible intracerebral locations, make a clear definition of delayed traumatic intracerebral hematoma (DTIH) difficult. Studies are under way to investigate the practicality of using contrasted CT scans and/or magnetic resonance imaging (MRI) to detect future sites of DTIH.

Lipper and Kishore's suggested definition of DTIH[20] mandates an initial CT scan with lesions smaller than 1 cm (including completely negative CT scans) and subsequent identification of a high-density intraparenchymal lesion on follow-up imaging.

Fukamachi and Nagaseki[21] divided traumatic intracerebral hemorrhages into four subtypes:

- *Type 1*   Hematomas visible on initial CT without changes on further CT scans
- *Type 2*   Hematomas that progressively enlarge
- *Type 3*   Delayed hematoma, which developed in different areas from the original intracerebral hematoma on initial CT scan
- *Type 4*   Hematomas that developed in areas with previous contusions but no intracerebral hemorrhage

The clinical presentation of patients with DTIH can be classified into four groups:

- *Group I*   Patients with a GCS of 8 to 15, mild to moderate head injuries, develop DTIH as identified on routine follow-up CT scans.
- *Group II*   Patients are asymptomatic for hours to weeks after a traumatic event, with subsequent later neurologic decline; DTIH is diagnosed on CT scan or at autopsy.
- *Group III*   Patients have an initial GCS of less than 8 and no evidence of further neurologic decline; initial CT scan shows no intracerebral hemorrhage, but follow-up imaging shows DTIH.
- *Group IV*   Patients have a GCS of less than 8 and progressive neurologic decline and/or medically uncontrollable intracranial pressure.

Incidence

The detection of DTIH has increased significantly with improved imaging techniques. The incidence is highly dependent on patient selection and project inclusion criteria, as well as the timing, availability, and quality of imaging. Delayed post-traumatic intracerebral hemorrhage is the fourth most common cause of all intracerebral hemorrhages after hypertension, vascular malformations, and alcoholism, in that order.[13] As many as 50% of post-traumatic intraparenchymal enhancing lesions will develop into a hematoma.[3] Since the advent of CT scanners, the overall incidence of delayed post-traumatic intracerebral hemorrhage is noted between 1.7 and 7.4% of all closed head injuries. It is generally accepted that ~10 to 20% of patients presenting with a GCS of less than 8 will continue to develop DTIH (group III and IV).[22,23] There is little reliable data on the incidence of DTIH associated with group I and II patients.

Pathogenesis

Although the severity and extent of trauma sustained are variable, head motion at the time of impact is significant for the development of DTIH.[11,24] Bollinger et al initially hypothesized that necrotic brain softening around traumatized blood vessels led to DTIH.[1] Microscopically damaged blood vessels, including traumatic aneurysms, may develop into DTIH. Post-traumatic dysregulation of cerebral blood flow leading to vasodilatation, caused by focal hypoxia and hypotension, and subsequent increased intravascular pressure due to resuscitative efforts, leads to elevated intracranial pressure and possible hemorrhage.[25-27] Coagulopathy will cause poor hemostasis and clotting and can develop into a DTIH in 70 to 80% of patients.[27,28] Locally damaged brain will release thromboplastic substances, which will produce intravascular coagulation. Such coagulation will lead to small areas of infarct, injuring the brain and restarting the cycle. The small infarction also creates additional space for possible expansion of the hematoma or future hemorrhagic conversion.

Treatment

Treatment is not significantly different from other traumatic intracranial hemorrhages. Intracranial pressure (ICP) monitoring is indicated for all groups, as rapid deterioration may be preventable with close monitoring and treatment of ICP. Any coagulopathies or other medical problems should be managed concurrently. Treatment is based on the clinical presentation, as follows:[3]

- ◆ *Group I*   Patients are generally observed and treated medically unless progression occurs.
- ◆ *Group II*   Patients are categorized as such because of their neurologic decline and should be operatively treated unless otherwise contraindicated because of location or comorbidity factors.
- ◆ *Group III*   Patients who have not progressed to group IV criteria warrant close observation and aggressive medical management of ICP.
- ◆ *Group IV*   Patients necessitate immediate operative intervention with aggressive ICP management.

Outcome

Prolonged low cerebral perfusion pressure directly correlates with poor outcome. Mortality rates as high as 75% are noted with group III and IV patients. Poor quality of life and vegetative states are not uncommon. The degree of secondary insult caused by the natural cascade of brain injury only adds to the underlying damage done by the hematoma itself and the associated mass effect. Coagulopathy needs to be corrected as soon as possible to decrease morbidity and mortality.[27-29] Prompt intervention where appropriate is our only current tool to counteract the natural progression of DTIH.

◆ Delayed Nontraumatic Intracranial Hemorrhages

The clinical signs of nontraumatic intracranial hemorrhages usually occur spontaneously and are equally as unexpected as traumatic hemorrhages. Bleeding is usually short-lived and is tamponaded by anatomical and physiological means. Hemorrhages are best described, and treatment planned, based on their location and size, as identified on CT scans. It is estimated that 20% of patients with a previous intracranial hemorrhage will rebleed.[30-32] Etiologies are widespread for spontaneous intracranial hemorrhages. However, delayed or recurrent nontraumatic hemorrhages are not as common and can be categorized as those that are due to anticoagulation treatments, subarachnoid hemorrhage, and other underlying medical conditions, including hypertension, infarction, tumors, migraines, or amyloidosis, and those that occur after invasive procedures.

The general guidelines for evacuation of an ICH are

- GCS 5 to 13 or deterioration of 2 GCS points
- Volume greater than 20 to 30 cc
- No brainstem involvement, no active myocardial infarction (MI)
- 0.5 cm midline shift and location of clot near the surface

Case Example

A 48-year-old woman was found in her automobile in status epilepticus with generalized tonic-clonic seizures and a history of traveling cross-country for 1 month. Past medical history and family medical history were negative except for a 6 week fast for religious reasons. She was intubated and sedated; seizure control was achieved via benzodiazepines. Initially, she had a GCS of 7T with mild (4/5) left-sided hemiparesis. A CT scan of the brain demonstrated a 1.3 cm intraparenchymal hematoma in the right parietal lobe with edematous changes associated with an infarct in the left parietal convexity (**Fig. 11–3**).

Thrombus was directly visualized on CT in the superior sagittal sinus and the right transverse sinus and later confirmed on MRI. The patient was diagnosed with venous sinus thrombosis secondary to severe dehydration with an associated intracerebral hemorrhage and infarction. Aggressive rehydration and anticoagulation therapy with heparin were initiated. On reexamination of the patient 4 hours after beginning the heparin protocol, the patient had improved and was observed to have a GCS of 11T with residual left hemiparesis but moving all extremities. The patient was weaned to extubation and continued to become more alert. Thirty-six hours status postheparinization, the patient was noted to have a flaccid left side, although with a GCS of 15. Emergent CT scan of the brain demonstrated a rebleed into the original intraparenchymal hemorrhage in the right parietal convexity, now measuring 3 cm, with worsening edema bilaterally (**Fig. 11–4**). Heparin protocol was halted, and aggressive rehydration continued as the primary treatment. The patient's left hemiplegia gradually improved over the course of her hospital stay into a hemiparesis, and she was discharged to a rehabilitation center.

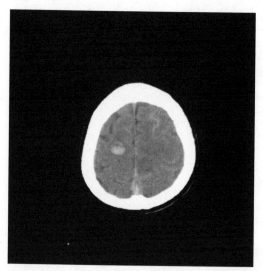

Figure 11–3 A 1.3 cm intraparenchymal hematoma in the right parietal lobe with edematous changes associated with an infarct in the left parietal convexity.

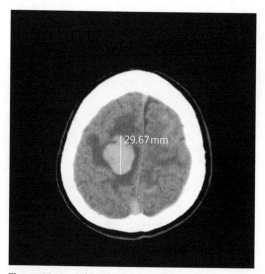

Figure 11–4 Rebleed into the original intraparenchymal hemorrhage in the right parietal convexity, now measuring 3 cm, with worsening edema bilaterally.

◆ Anticoagulation and Intracranial Hemorrhages

Anticoagulation in itself does not predispose patients to intracerebral hemorrhage; however, it does produce complications if a hemorrhage occurs.[33,34] Intracerebral hemorrhages associated with anticoagulation yield higher morbidity and mortality (67%) than those hemorrhage patients without anticoagulation treatment (55%). There is also documentation that the volume of hematoma is larger in those patients receiving anticoagulation treatment, although the volume itself is unrelated to the degree of anticoagulation.[33,35] Emergency reversal of anticoagulation after intracerebral hemorrhage detection is critical to preventing further bleeding. Fredriksson and Norrving[36] suggested that treatment with prothrombin complex concentrate reverses anticoagulation more rapidly than fresh frozen plasma, and therefore is indicated with suspected intracranial hemorrhage.

◆ Rebleeding of Subarachnoid Hemorrhages

The incidence of subarachnoid hemorrhage varies significantly according to underlying pathology. When considering aneurysm rupture, the incidence of rebleeding is as high as 4% in the first 24 hours, then 1.5% per day for the first 2 weeks. A total of 50% will rebleed in the first 6 months. The higher the Hunt and Hess score,[37a] the higher the risk of rebleed.[37] Nonaneurysmal subarachnoid hemorrhage has a lower incidence of recurrent hemorrhage at ~1% each year.[38] Theories suggest the decreased rate of rebleed in these patients is secondary to the initial hemorrhagic rupture eradicating the offending pathology. No known prophylactic treatment options currently exist to prevent rebleeding.

◆ Delayed Intracranial Hemorrhage Secondary to Underlying Medical Pathology

Cerebrovascular Infarction

The frequency of hemorrhagic transformation of cerebrovascular accidents is still under debate, with multiple studies under way. The incidence increases as a function of the frequency at which follow-up neuroimaging studies are performed. A study of 200 patients determined that 68.6% underwent hemorrhagic conversion, most without further clinical deterioration.[39] Hemorrhagic transformation of ischemic strokes in the carotid artery distribution has an incidence of 43%.[40] Higher blood pressures may account for the repeat bleeding regardless of the presence or absence of arterial reopening.

Hypertension

Hypertensive hemorrhages account for 10 to 30% of all strokes. Studies of recurrent intracerebral hemorrhage without other identifiable etiology and a history of hypertension show a relatively infrequent incidence of 2.7%.[41–44] The recurrence rate is theorized to be low due to the lipohyalinosis and transmural necrosis affecting the vessels, leading to hemorrhage. The hemorrhage ultimately destroys the vessels and leads to thrombosis at the time of the event, thereby preventing a future repeat episode. Over 90% of recurrent hypertensive hemorrhages are in a different location from the original bleeding; however, the distribution of locations is similar, with most recurrent hypertensive bleeds occurring in the basal ganglia.

Tumors

Underlying tumors account for 1 to 2% of intracerebral hemorrhage cases, as determined in an autopsy series; however, they can range to as high as 10% in clinic-radiologic series. The majority of hemorrhages into tumor beds occur in malignant tumors or metastatic tumors, rarely meningiomas or oligodendrogliomas.[45] Rebleeding itself is a rare entity, as the primary tumor is itself treated or the patient clinically deteriorates and follow-up studies are forgone. However, in an extensive study of postoperative hematomas, 56% of patients had a primary diagnosis of intracranial tumor that then bled into the resection site. Meningiomas are the most common tumor to hemorrhage after resection, at 40%.[46,47]

Migraines

Migraines have also been documented to be associated with recurrent hemorrhages, albeit rarely. Most cases arise from symptomatic grade IIA migraines or grade IIB migraine mimics. Reported cases are most frequently associated with a preexisting arteriovenous malformation, where hemorrhage occurs into the bed during a migraine attack. Also, lobar hemorrhages can occur after a migraine attack associated with sudden hypertensive episodes.[48]

Cerebral Amyloid Angiopathy

Beta amyloid protein depositions can accumulate in the media of small cerebral vessels with or without accumulation in other systemic vessels. Cerebral amyloid angiopathy (CAA) is present in 50% of those patients over 70 years old, accounts for 10% of all first-time intracerebral hemorrhages, and is the leading cause of angiographically negative recurrent hemorrhages in this age group.[49] Frequently, but not exclusively, apolipoprotein E €4 allele is associated with CAA. Presentation is similar to hypertensive hemorrhages with location-specific findings and often an associated history of transient ischemic attacks.[50] Unlike hypertensive hemorrhages, CAA is more likely to be lobar than ganglionic, and recurrent hemorrhage is common. Confirmatory diagnosis is only possible via evaluation of brain tissue. No treatment is known.

Case Example

A 39-year-old woman presented with new-onset focal seizures of her right arm and no neurologic deficit. A CT scan of her head was performed and revealed a left parietal mass measuring 3 × 2 cm. MRI confirmed the lesion and showed minimal enhancement on contrasted study, little to no edema, and a 6 mm necrotic center. A stereotactic biopsy was scheduled and revealed a grade III astrocytoma. Postoperatively, the patient had elevated blood pressure with increased incision drainage. A repeat CT scan showed a 3 × 3 cm intracerebral hematoma at the end of the biopsy site. The patient was returned to the operating room for evacuation of the intracerebral hematoma. Upon recovery, the patient continues to have no neurologic deficit and is undergoing medical treatment of the tumor.

◆ Postprocedural Intracerebral Hemorrhage

Factors contributing to delayed postprocedural hemorrhages include multiple passes through the brain, specifics of the clotting status of the patient, and the type of procedure performed. Bleeding often contributes to erosion of surface veins or disruption of superficial blood vessels during the procedure. Routine postprocedural imaging is the best source of detection of hemorrhaging. This entity is frequently underdiagnosed because of the lack of routine repeat imaging and because small hemorrhages tend not to cause any additional symptoms or deficits. After stereotactic biopsy, 0.8 to 59.2% of patients will have a postoperative hemorrhage, the wide range depending on the postprocedural scanning schedule.[42,46,51] Only 10% of those with hemorrhage will have suspicious symptoms or deficits. A review of the literature reveals the incidence of postventriculoperitoneal shunt placement hemorrhages to be 0.4 to 4.0%.[52] Even major surgeries have the possibility of rebleeding. A study of 230 patients revealed an incidence of rebleeding after aneurysm clipping to be as high as 2.6%.[53]

Case Management

The patient was taken immediately to the operating room for evacuation of the hematoma. He improved slowly after surgery and was discharged to an acute rehabilitation facility.

References

1. von Bollinger O. Ueber traumatische spat-Apoplexie: ein Beitrag zur Lehre von der Hirnerschutterung. In: Internationale Beiträge zur wissenschaftlichen Medizin: festschrift, Rudolf Virchow gewidmet zur vollendung seines 70. Vol 2. Berlin, Germany: Hirchwald; 1891:459–470
2. Duret H. Traumatismes craniocérébraux: accidents primitifs, leurs grandes syndromes. Paris: Felix Alcan; 1922:833–851
3. Cohen TI, Gudeman SK. Delayed traumatic intracranial hematoma. In: Narayan RK, Wilberger JE, Povlishock JT, eds. Neurotrauma. New York: McGraw-Hill Health; 1996:689–702
4. Rockswold GL, Leonard PR. Analysis of management in thirty-three closed head injury patients who "talked and deteriorated." Neurosurg 1987;21-1:51–55
5. Bucci MN, Phillips TW. Delayed epidural hemorrhage in hypotensive multiple trauma patients. Neurosurg 1986;19-1:65–68
6. Borovich B, Braun J. Delayed onset of traumatic extradural hematoma. J Neurosurg 1985;63:30–34
7. Teasdale G, Galbraith S. Acute traumatic intracranial hematomas. In: Krayenbuhl H, Maspes PE, Sweet WH, eds. Progress in Neurosurgery. Vol 10. Basel: Karger; 1980:14–42
8. Poon WS, Rehman SU. Traumatic extradural hematoma of delayed onset is not a rarity. Neurosurg 1992;30(5):681–686
9. Youmans JR, ed. Diagnosis and treatment of moderate to severe head injury in adults. In: Neurological Surgery. Philadelphia: WB Saunders; 1996:1618–1718
10. Rivas J, Lobato R. Extradural hematoma: analysis of factors influencing the courses of 161 patients. Neurosurg 1988;23(1):44–51
11. Diaz F, Yock DH. Early diagnosis of delayed posttraumatic intracerebral hematomas. J Neurosurg 1979;50:217–223
12. Young HA, Gleave JR. Delayed traumatic intracerebral hematoma: report of 15 cases operatively treated. Neurosurg 1984;14(1):22–25
13. Alvarez-Sabin J, Turon A, Lozano-Sanchez M, Vasquez J, Codina A. Delayed posttraumatic hemorrhage "Spat-Apoplexie." Stroke 1995;26(9):1531–1535
14. Elsner H, Rigamonti D. Delayed traumatic intracerebral hematomas: "Spat-Apoplexie." Report of two cases. J Neurosurg 1990;72:813–815
15. Mendelow AD, Teasdale GD, Russell T, et al. Effect of mannitol on cerebral blood flow and cerebral perfusion pressure in human head injury. J Neurosurg 1985;63:43–48
16. Ashkenazi E, Constantini S, Pomeranz S, et al. Delayed epidural hematoma without neurologic deficit. J Trauma 1990;30:613–615
17. Piepmeier JM, Wagner F. Delayed post-traumatic extracerebral hematomas. J Trauma 1982;22(6):455–460
18. Aoki N, Sakai T. Traumatic aneurysm of the middle meningeal artery presenting as delayed onset of acute subdural hematoma. Surg Neurol 1992;37:59–62
19. Dowling JL, Brown AP, Dacey RG Cerebrovascular complications in the head-injured patient. In: Narayan RK, Wilberger JE, Povlishock JT, eds. Neurotrauma. New York: McGraw-Hill Health; 1996:655–672
20. Lipper MH, Kishore PR. Delayed intracranial hematoma in patients with severe head injury. Radiology 1979;133:645–649
21. Fukamachi A, Nagaseki Y. The incidence and development process of delayed traumatic intracerebral haematomas. Acta Neurochir (Wien) 1985;74:35–39
22. Young H, Gleave J. Delayed traumatic intracerbral hematoma: report of 15 cases operatively treated. Neurosurg 1984;14:22–25
23. Huneidi AH, Afshar F. Delayed intracerebral haematomas in moderate to severe head injuries in young adults. Ann Royal Coll Surg Eng 1992;74:345–350
24. Jaimovich R. Delayed posttraumatic intracranial lesions in children. Ped Neurosurg 1991;92(17):25–29
25. Gudeman S, Kishore P. The genesis and significance of delayed traumatic intracerebral hematoma. Neurosurg 1979;5:309–313
26. Riesgo P, Piquer J. Delayed extradural hematoma after mild head injury: report of three cases. Surg Neurol 1997;48:226–231

27. Pretorius ME, Kaufman HH. Rapid onset of delayed traumatic intracerebral haematoma with diffuse intravascular coagulation and fibrinolysis. Acta Neurochir (Wien) 1982;65:103–109

28. Kaufman HH, Moake JL. Delayed and recurrent intracranial hematomas related to disseminated intravascular clotting and fibrinolysis in head injury. Neurosurg 1980 7(5):445–449

29. Juvela S, Heiskanen O. The treatment of spontaneous intracerebral hemorrhage. J Neurosurg 1989;70:755–758

30. Magladery JW. The natural course of cerebrovascular hemorrhage. Clin Neurosurg 1963;9:106–113

31. Kase CS. Intracerebral hemorrhage: non-hypertensive crisis. Stroke 1986;17(4): 590–595

32. Bae HG, Lee KS. Rapid expansion of hypertensive intracerebral hemorrhage. Neurosurg 1992;31(1):35–41

33. Radberg JA, Olsson JE. Prognostic parameter in spontaneous intracerebral hematomas with special reference to anticoagulant treatment. Stroke 1991; 22(5):571–576

34. Snyder M, Renaudin J. Intracranial hemorrhage associated with anticoagulation therapy. Surg Neurol 1977;7:31–34

35. Franke CL, deJonge J. Intracerebral hematomas during anticoagulant treatment. Stroke 1990;21(5):726–730

36. Fredriksson K, Norrving B. Emergency reversal of anticoagulation after intracerebral hemorrhage. Stroke 1992;23(7):972–977

37. Winn HR, Richardson AE. The long-term prognosis in untreated cerebral aneurysms: the incidence of late hemorrhage in cerebral aneurysm. A 10-year evaluation of 364 patients. Ann Neurol 1977;1:358–370

37a. Hunt WE, Hess RM. Surgical risk as related to time of Intervention in the repair of intracranial aneuryms. J Neurosurg 1968;28:14–20

38. Jane JA, Kassell NF. The natural history of aneurysms and AVM's. J Neurosurg 1985;62:321–323

39. Hornig CR, Bauer T. Hemorrhagic transformation in cardioembolic cerebral infarction. Stroke 1993;24(3):465–468

40. Garcia JH. Pathology. In: Barnett HJ, Mohr JP, eds. Stroke. New York: Churchill Livingstone; 1992:125–135

41. Lee KS, Bae HG. Recurrent intracerebral hemorrhage due to hypertension. Neurosurg 1990;26(4):586–590

42. Field M, Witham TF. Comprehensive assessment of hemorrhage risks and outcomes after stereotactic brain biopsy. J Neurosurg 2001;94:545–551

43. Park YC. Clinical diagnosis of cerebrovascular accidents. J Kor Med Assoc 1973;28:303–308

44. Herbstein DJ, Schaumburg HH. Hypertensive intracerebral hematoma. Arch Neurol 1974;30:412–414

45. Kase CS. Intracerebral hemorrhage. In: Barnett HJ, Mohr JP, eds. Stroke. New York: Churchill Livingstone; 1992:561–616

46. Kalfas IH, Little JR. Postoperative hemorrhage: a survey of 4992 intracranial procedures. Neurosurg 1988;23(3):343–347

47. Little JR, Dial B. Brain hemorrhage from intracranial tumor. Stroke 1979;10(3): 283–288

48. Cole AJ, Aube MA. Migraine with vasospasm and delayed intracerebral hemorrhage. Arch Neurol 1990;47:53–56

49. Vinters HV, Gilbert JJ. Cerebral amyloid angiopathy: incidence and complications in the aging brain, I: Cerebral hemorrhage. Stroke 1983;14(6):915–923

50. Greenberg SM, Rebeck GW. Apolipoprotein and cerebral hemorrhage associated with amyloid angiopathy. Ann Neurol 1995;38:254–259

51. Kulkarni AV, Guha A. Incidence of silent hemorrhage and delayed deterioration after sterotactic brain biopsy. J Neurosurg 1998;89:31–35

52. Savitz MH, Bobroff LM. Low incidence of delayed intracerebral hemorrhage secondary to ventriculoperitoneal shunt insertion. J Neurosurg 1999;91: 32–34

53. Proust F, Hannequin D. Causes of morbidity and mortality after ruptured aneursym surgery in a series of 230 patients. Stroke 1995;26(9):1553–1557

12

Sedation and Pain Management in the Neurosurgical Intensive Care Unit Patient

Dan Miulli

Case Study

A 47-year-old female was involved in a rollover motor vehicle accident, with resultant severe closed head injury, consisting of mild cerebral edema, pneumothorax, and a fractured pelvis. The patient's pupils are 2 mm and reactive; she does not open her eyes, is intubated, and withdraws to painful stimuli, yielding a Glasgow Coma Scale (GCS) score of 6. The trauma team has placed a chest tube, and orthopedics decides to expectantly manage the pelvic fracture. The patient will remain on the ventilator while GCS is less than or equal to 8 and while the trauma team remains concerned about lung injuries. The vital signs demonstrate an increased heart rate and increased blood pressure anytime there is attempted movement of the patient; therefore, the patient is sedated and given pain medication.

See page 162 for Case Management.

◆ General Principles of Pain Management

Pain must be treated. Neglecting pain treatment results in undue suffering, anxiety expressed by the patient and the family, fear, anger, depression, slow recovery, decreased ability to participate in activities of daily living, weight loss, fever, increased heart and respiratory rates, increased blood pressure, chest pain, myocardial infarction (MI), atelectasis, constipation, and infection.[1–3] Overmedication results in the inability to perform a neurologic exam, which is the most important means of following a patient with neurologic disease or injuries. Overtreatment of pain and sedation leads to prolonged intubation, prolonged intensive care unit (ICU) stay, pneumonia, and deep venous thrombosis (**Table 12–1**).[4]

In a severe head injury or comatose patient who is intubated, only subtle changes may foretell drastic intracranial changes and problems such as contusions blossoming or other small abnormalities leading to midline shift and herniation. If the patient is overmedicated, a treatable lesion will be

Table 12–1   Results of Undertreatment and Overtreatment of Pain[4]

Undertreatment of pain	Overtreatment of pain
Suffering, anxiety, fear, anger, depression	Inability to perform neurologic exam
Slow recovery	Prolonged intubation
Decreased ability to participate in ADL	Prolonged ICU stay
Patient's family anxiety	Pneumonia
Weight loss, fever, increased heart and respiratory rates, increased blood pressure, chest pain, MI; atelectasis, constipation, infection	DVT

ADL, activities of daily living; DVT, deep venous thrombosis; ICU, intensive care unit; MI, myocardial infarction.

missed. Frequently, in patients with severe head injury or severe neurologic deficits, an intracranial pressure (ICP) monitor is inserted; however, the ICP, although rising and falling with movement, suctioning, and pain, will change exponentially as the brain has reached the ability to compensate. A gradual change in neurologic exam precedes large changes in ICP. Therefore, there must be a fine line that is maintained between pain and sedation, and under- and overmedication in the neurologic patient.

◆ What Is Pain?

Pain is "whatever the experiencing person says it is, existing whenever s/he says it does."[5] It is an unpleasant sensory and emotional experience associated with actual or potential tissue damage, or described in terms of such damage.[6] In biological terms, stimulus energy from any source is converted into nerve impulses and transferred from the site of transduction to the central nervous system (CNS) and brain, during which time the signal is modulated at multiple levels before being perceived at the highest centers of the brain.

Nociceptors are specific receptors that respond to tissue trauma or stimuli that may cause tissue trauma.[7] They are located in skin, connective tissue, muscle, tendon, muscle spindle, joint capsules, bone, and viscera, and around nerves and blood vessels. Thankfully, they are not located in the brain substance itself. The tissue changes from injury-released prostaglandins, substance P, bradykinins, cytokines, histamine, and serotonin. This is the first area where pain can be modulated. The impulses from the nociceptors responding to these substances or responding to simple mechanical deformation travel along slow conducting unmyelinated C fibers or faster conducting, small myelinated A delta fibers. Although both C fibers and large A delta fibers respond to pain, it is the ratio of response that determines the passage through the dorsal horns as pain; the response from C fibers must be greater than the response from A delta fibers. The impulses are mostly from the trunk and limbs, and therefore go to the dorsal horn of the spinal cord, usually activating N-methyl-D-aspartate (NMDA) receptors, the second site of pain modulation. NMDA receptor stimulation causes intraneuronal elevation of Ca^{2+}, which stimulates nitric oxide synthase (NOS) and the production of nitric oxide (NO).[8] Substances known to block NMDA receptors include d-methadone, dextromethorphan, ketamine, naloxone, and amantadine. It is at the NMDA receptors that inherent spinal cord nociceptor modulators such as γ-aminobutyric acid (GABA), serotonin, glutamate, substance P, norepinephrine, and endogenous opioids are released by spinal interneurons in laminae I, II, IV, and V of the dorsal horn, which are controlled by brain cortex centers, periaqueductal gray, or concurrent spinal cord input. The modified signal crosses in the spinal cord and ascends in multiple tracts, such as the spinoreticular, spinothalamic, spinomesencephalic, and spinohypothalamic, to the reticular formation, thalamus, mesencephalon, and hypothalamus, respectively, the third area of modulation. Sensations reaching the thalamus undergo complex modulation to determine if the sensation will be processed to reach the brain. From these intermediates, the signal passes to the frontal cortex, insular cortex, limbic structures, and sensory cortex to label the pain as good or bad, the fourth area of possible modulation.

A functioning brain is needed for the perception of pain. Each area through neurochemical release, such as GABA, norepinephrine, substance P, serotonin, and opioids, influences the pain. These same areas respond to memories, social influences, environmental influences, experiences, depression, and culture. Repeated stimuli at any location further change the characteristics of the pain and the threshold (**Table 12–2**).

Acute injury is mostly transmitted as nociceptive pain. This differs in treatment from neuropathic pain associated with chronic repeated stimuli and caused by aberrant signal processing in the peripheral or central nervous system. After repeated stimulation, the pathophysiological abnormalities of neuropathic pain become unrelated to the provocative event. This type of pain occurs infrequently in the ICU but may be seen in patients with multiple strokes, multiple fractures, or cancer pain.

◆ Assessment of Pain

Pain management depends on an appropriate assessment of the pain most often recorded on a pain scale. Outpatient and pain assessment in the awake cooperative patient requires obtaining a detailed history along with the examination. The history of the awake cooperative patient must include past medical and surgical history, medications, smoking and alcohol intake, family history, psychosocial history and review of symptoms, and physical examination. These areas will help identify physical and psychological modifiers of the pain, which is important when considering nonnarcotic

Table 12–2 Neurochemicals Released and Possible Modulators of Pain Pathway Areas[1-4]

Area in pain pathway	Neurochemical	Possible modulation
Nociceptor	Prostaglandins, substance P, bradykinins, cytokines, histamine, and serotonin	Local anesthetics, ASA, NSAIDs, opioids, acetaminophen, AEDs, and TCAs
Pain fiber C or A delta	Calcium and sodium channel	Channel blockers
Interneuron	NMDA, GABA, and endogenous opioids	Magnesium, PCP, GABA, and opioids
Reticular formation, thalamus, mesencephalon, and hypothalamus	GABA, norepinephrine, substance P, serotonin, and opioids	GABA, norepinephrine, β-blocker, capsaicin, serotonin, and opioids
Frontal cortex, insular cortex, limbic structures, and sensory cortex	GABA, norepinephrine, substance P, serotonin, and opioids	GABA, norepinephrine, β-blocker, capsaicin, serotonin, opioids, AEDs, TCAs, benzodiazepines, and barbiturates

AEDs, antiepileptics; ASA, acetylsalicylic acid (aspirin); GABA, γ-aminobutyric acid; NMDA, N-methyl-D-aspartate; NSAIDs, nonsteroidal anti-inflammatory drugs; PCP, phencyclidine hydrochloride; TCAs, tricyclic antidepressants.

and nonmedicinal treatments, such as ice, elevation, antidepressants, and environmental factors. The medical and surgical history is important when evaluating the patient for contraindications to types of therapy.

The characteristics of the pain also play a role in the treatment. It is important to obtain the following characteristics of the pain: its quality, location, intensity, duration, periodicity, exacerbating and relieving factors, present and past pain management, and associated signs and symptoms.

Pain is an unpleasant sensory and emotional experience associated with actual or potential tissue damage. Therefore, assessment of pain requires an examination of the area of pain referral and any other diagnostic tests that will assist in determining the appropriate treatment.

Often only pain intensity is considered in the pain history; by itself, however, it may lead to unnecessary treatments. When there are difficulties in communication such as may occur in the very young, the very old, the mildly confused, and patients of different language, culture, or background, a pain assessment rating scale may be the only information available. Most widely used "pain scales" are based on 10 divisions. Because it is necessary to follow pain trends over time and with treatment, often between varying health care workers and health facilities, only a 10-division scale should be used until other scales become universal.[9,10]

A numeric rating scale asks the patient or the health care worker to rate the pain on a scale of 0 to 10, with 0 being no pain at all and 10 being the worst possible pain the patient or health care worker could imagine. Often patients will state that they have a high pain threshold, much higher than others. However, it must be emphasized to patients that the worst possible pain that they could imagine is a 10, and the current pain is in relation to that level, not based on others' perception. It may be appropriate at times to ask women who have had children by vaginal delivery, as ascertained in the history, to compare the current pain to the pain experienced during labor, which may have been a 10 (**Fig. 12–1**).

The modified Visual Analog Scale is a 10 cm line marked from 0 to 10, with 0 being no pain at all and 10 being the worst possible pain the patient could imagine. When teamed with the commonly used scale such as the American Cancer Society, Facial Pain Scale or Wong-Baker Faces Rating Scale for Children, which consists of six or eight images of faces with varying expressions, from a smiling face (0) to a crying face (10), the Visual Analog Scale becomes the ultimate scale for the awake person (**Fig. 12–2**).

Severely debilitated patients and those with severe head injuries are physically not able to use these scales to indicate their level of pain. In these cases, health care workers are responsible for acting in the best interest of the individual patient to relieve suffering without causing untoward side effects. A behavioral pain scale is useful when patients cannot communicate. One of the most widely accepted behavioral pain scales is the 10-point FLACC scale. The patient is assessed in five categories and given 0, 1, or 2

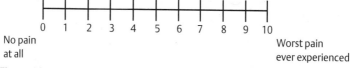

Figure 12–1 Commonly used pain scale. Patient points to number on scale after health-care worker describes "0" as no pain at all and "10" as worst pain ever experienced.

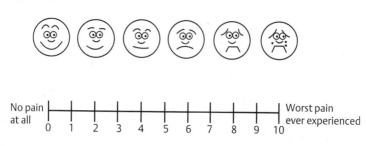

Figure 12–2 Visual Analog Scale (VAS) and Wong-Baker Faces Scale allows additional clues for patients to adequately assess their pain. The health-care worker describes "0" as no pain at all and "10" as worst pain ever experienced. The faces help the patient decide how he or she currently feels.

Table 12–3   FLACC Behavioral Pain Scale[1,2]

	Score		
	0	**1**	**2**
Facial expression	Smiles or no particular expression	Occasional grimace, frown; withdrawn	Frequent to constant frown, clenched jaw, quivering chin
Leg movement	Relaxed or normal posture	Uneasy, restless, tense	Kicking or legs drawn up
General activity	Normal position; lying quietly, moves easily	Squirming, shifting back and forth, tense	Arched, rigid, or jerking
Crying	No crying while awake or asleep	Moans, whimpers; occasional complaints	Crying steadily; screams or sobs; frequent complaints
Ability to be consoled	Content, relaxed	Reassured by occasional touching, hugging, or talking; distractible	Difficult to console or comfort

points depending on the behavior being demonstrated. The behaviors are facial expression, leg movement, general activity, crying, and ability to be consoled (**Table 12–3**). The FLACC scale can also be used with children ages 6 months to 3 years.

◆ Management of Pain

Nonsteroidal Anti-inflammatory Drugs

Once a patient's pain can be assessed using a pain scale, medication and other treatment can be quickly entertained. Pain that is rated as 4 or less can be managed with ice, acetaminophen, or nonsteroidal anti-inflammatory drugs (NSAIDs), with the last two inhibiting an isoform of the enzyme cyclo-oxygenase (COX 1–3) blocking prostaglandin synthesis.[11] The usual dose for acetaminophen (N-acetyl-p-aminophenol [APAP]) is 10 to 75 mg/kg/day in 4 to 6 divided doses. The maximum adult daily dose is 4000 mg. It is now believed that an initial large dose of 50 mg/kg can be given, yielding relief comparable to that of some narcotics while maintaining a high safety profile. The side effects of acetaminophen are seen with elevated multiple doses, although they can occur with a single dose. They are acute hepatic necrosis, or liver toxicity, nephrotoxicity, and, with chronic use, thrombocytopenia. The manufacturers of acetaminophen have voluntarily upgraded warnings that large doses can cause irreversible liver failure. Those with impaired liver function or regular alcohol use should take no more than 2 g daily. Anyone who takes more than three alcoholic drinks a day should be advised to avoid acetaminophen.

Analgesics, including aspirin (acetylsalicylic acid [ASA]) and APAP, inhibit cyclo-oxygenase, preventing the production of prostaglandins. COX receptors are found throughout the body, and a specific group's effect depends on which receptors are stimulated. COX-1 receptors are found in the CNS, kidneys, platelets, gastrointestinal (GI) system, skin, and other areas. COX-2 receptors are found in the brain and kidneys. COX-3 receptors are found in the CNS. Most NSAIDs are nonselective COX 1–3 receptor inhibitors. The location of the receptors in the CNS is the reason that APAP only lowers temperature and pain but does not inhibit platelet function or have any significant anti-inflammatory effect.

NSAIDs should be withheld for 4 to 10 days after mild bleeding and not given for at least 4 to 10 days after severe bleeding. NSAIDs inhibit platelet function only while at therapeutic dosage. They should be given with a stomach protectant and adequate hydration to help prevent side effects. The usual dose for ibuprofen is to 50 mg/kg divided into 4 to 6 doses per day.

Ketorolac is another anti-inflammatory drug that can be given intravenously or orally. The usual dose for ketorolac is 30 to 60 mg per dose and can be given every 6 to 8 hours. Ketorolac can be given immediately after such neurosurgical procedures as lumbar diskectomy and lumbar spinal fusion when bleeding has been controlled. During these procedures, ketorolac 30 mg IV may be given initially, followed by 120 mg in 500 cc saline at 10 cc/hour continuous drip until completed. This treatment modality, along with lidocaine patches or infusion, may greatly decrease or obviate the need for narcotics.

NSAIDs belong to multiple drug classes, with each class affecting individuals differently. Therefore, if one class of NSAID or even a drug in the same class does not work, consider treatment with another (**Table 12–4**).

NSAID Side Effects

None of the drugs in this group should be given if there is a known sensitivity to an NSAID. Salicylates should not be given to children with viral infections. In general, the nonselective COX inhibitor NSAIDs have similar side effects, such as dyspepsia; ulcers; GI perforation and bleeding (antiplatelet activity lasts for 2–3 days while therapeutic); kidney and liver dysfunction; hypersensitivity reaction, such as urticaria-angioedema; respiratory, attention, and memory deficits; headache; and tinnitus. Rofecoxib, a COX-2 inhibitor, was recently shown to have cardiac side effects, such as MI and stroke, and has been voluntarily removed from the market. Celecoxib, another COX-2 inhibitor, has not been removed from the market. Celecoxib side effects are thought to be less problematic than other NSAIDs.

There is no significant difference between the GI effects of nonselective COX NSAIDs and a proton pump inhibitor and selective COX-2 NSAIDs. ASA inhibits platelet function irreversibly, whereas NSAIDs inhibit platelet function only while at therapeutic dosage. Furthermore, certain nonselective COX inhibitors, such as ibuprofen, will block the antiplatelet of ASA, but others, such as naproxen, will not.

Table 12–4 Pain Medication for Pain Rated as 4 or Less on 0 to 10 Pain Scale[1-3,9-11,20]

Generic name	Average dose	Average frequency (hours)	Maximum daily dose	Class
Ice	Local area	Until it melts		
Acetaminophen	10–75 mg/kg/day	4–6	4000 mg	p-aminophenol, COX-3 inhibitor
Aspirin	5–100 mg/kg/day	4–6	8000 mg	Salicylate
Diflunisal	250–500 mg	8–12	1500 mg	Salicylate
Choline, magnesium, trisalicylate	30–60 mg/kg/day	8–12	4500 mg	Salicylate
Ibuprofen	5–50 mg/kg/day	4–6	3200 mg	Propionic acid
Naproxen	250–500 mg	6–8	1500 mg	Propionic acid
Ketoprofen	12.5–75.0 mg	6–8	300 mg	Propionic acid
Flubiprofen	50–100 mg	6–8	300 mg	Propionic acid
Oxaprozin	600–1200 mg	8–12	1800 mg	Propionic acid
Indomethacin	25–75 mg	8	200 mg	Indoleacetic acid
Piroxicam	10–20 mg	24	20 mg	Benzothiazine
Meloxicam	7.5–15.0 mg	24	15 mg	Benzothiazine
Diclofenac	25–75 mg	6–8	200 mg	Pyrroleacetic acid
Ketorolac	30–60 mg	IV, PO 6–8	150 mg	Pyrroleacetic acid
Celecoxib	200–400 mg	12–24 hour	800 mg	COX-2 inhibitor

COX, cyclo-oxygenase; IV, intravenously; PO, L, per os (orally).

Other Pain Treatment

There are numerous ways to administer effective pain treatment, and in the neurologic patient, these routes must be tried unless there is a contraindication. Initially, local pain should be treated with ice. Icing works by stimulating large A delta fibers in the peripheral nervous system, increasing output above C fibers, and inhibiting pain transmission. Longer lasting pain, such as that caused by muscle spasm, may be treated with ice, heat, or both, depending on the response. If there is severe extremity or axial pain epidural at the approximate dermatome or caudal, anesthetics and analgesics may be delivered. The elevated pain from the disruption or destruction of large muscle areas may be treated appropriately with the local continuous infusion of long- or short-acting lidocaine derivatives. When the pain is of less severity, or to augment delivery of other pain medication, topical solutions can be utilized. Although used for chronic and neuropathic pain, they can be used for acute pain. Compounds such as a 5% lidocaine patch can significantly reduce pain and improve the quality of life. Lidocaine is believed to block sodium channels in the damaged nerve endings. It can be applied to the newly traumatized or operated tissue. The 5% lidocaine patch should not be applied directly to the open tissue or freshly sutured tissue. In those cases, it can be applied on both sides of the wound for 12 continuous hours per day (**Table 12–5**).

Table 12–5   Initial Pain Medication and Delivery[1–3,9–11,20]

Treatment	Dosage	Delivery	Injury
Ice	30 minutes on and off	Topical	Local soft tissue injury
Lidocaine 5% patch	12 hours on	Topical	Local soft tissue injury
EMLA cream (2.5% lidocaine, 2.5% prilocaine)	Apply q 2 hours	Topical	Local soft tissue injury
Capsaicin cream	Apply bid, tid	Topical	Neuropathic
NSAID cream (e.g., diclofenac, indomethacin)	Apply tid, qid	Topical	Nonacute tendon or ligament injury
Lidocaine intramuscular infusion	2 mg/min	Intratissue infusion	Local soft tissue injury
Bupivacaine epidural infusion	0.03–0.06%	Epidural	Soft tissue, bone
Bupivacaine epidural infusion with opioid	0.030–0.125% and 0.5–1.0 mg morphine or 1 μg fentanyl	Epidural	Soft tissue, bone

bid, twice a day; EMLA, eutectic mixture of local anesthetics; NSAID, nonsteroidal anti-inflammatory drug; qid, 4 times a day; tid, 3 times a day.

Nonopioid Pain Treatment

For pain greater than 4 on a 0 to 10 pain scale, acetaminophen and NSAID, as well as other nonconventional, nonnarcotic complementary drugs, can be used (**Table 12–6**). Each may be used with narcotics, potentiating the effects of a smaller narcotic dosage, resulting in less sedation and other deleterious side effects. The nonconventional medications can be benefited from, especially if the history can provide clues as to environmental, physiologic, or psychological factors influencing the current pain. The nonconventional medications include antiepileptic drugs (AEDs), tricyclic antidepressants (TCAs), GABA, norepinephrine, α- and β-blockers, capsaicin, serotonin, benzodiazepines, caffeine, and barbiturates. These nonconventional medications are particularly beneficial in neuropathic and chronic pain.

Nonconventional pain medications work in multiple areas and by a variety of mechanisms, as listed here.

♦ *TCAs* inhibit neuronal discharge, decrease sensitivity of adrenergic receptors, block reuptake of norepinephrine and serotonin, and bind to histaminergic, cholinergic, and adrenergic receptors.

♦ *Selective serotonin reuptake inhibitors (SSRIs)* potentiate serotonin and norepinephrine pathways, inhibit cytochrome P-450, and assist in treating patients with depression and anxiety. Side effects include tremor, fever, diarrhea, delirium, and increased muscle tone.

♦ *AEDs* suppress abnormal neuronal discharges by blocking sodium channels, whereas others increase the inhibiting GABA transmission.

♦ *Benzodiazepines* potentiate inhibitory GABA transmission while also having antianxiety and antispasticity properties.

♦ *Alpha-adrenergic blockers* decrease hyperarousal symptoms by activating autoinhibitory presynaptic receptors of the locus cerulus.

Common potentiating adjuvant nonnarcotic pain medications are listed in **Table 12–6**. The medication should be carefully chosen and reflect the clinical situation associated with the drug's major use. For example, if depression exacerbates the pain, consider the addition of amitriptyline.

Opioid Pain Treatment

The most commonly prescribed medications for severe pain are opioids. Theophrastus first referenced opium in the third century BC; now there are four classes of opioids, representing the particular receptor they stimulate: mu, kappa, delta, and the newest, nociceptin/orphanin FG (N/OFQ).[7] Mu was named for the prototype agonist morphine. It is stimulated by endogenous enkephalins and β-endorphins. Known drugs are morphine, buprenorphine, fentanyl, meperidine, and methadone. Kappa was named for the prototype ketocyclazocine. It is stimulated by endogenous dynorphins. Known drugs are butorphanol, nalbuphine, and pentazocine. Delta was discovered in the mouse vas deferens. It is stimulated by endogenous enkephalins and

Table 12-6 Nonopioid Medication for Pain Rated as 4 or Greater on the 0 to 10 Pain Scale[1-3,9-11,20]

Generic name	Average dosage	Average frequency (hours)	Major use	Maximum daily dose
Caffeine	65–325 mg	8	Stimulant	
Methysergide	2–8 mg	8–12	Headache	6–8 mg
Gabapentin	100–1200 mg	8	Neuralgia	3600 mg
Carbamazepine	5–35 mg/kg/day	6–12	Neuralgia	1600 mg
Divalproex sodium	15–60 mg/kg/day	24	Migraine	4000 mg
Phenytoin	4–8 mg/kg/day	6–8	Trigeminal neuralgia	600 mg
Amitriptyline	0.5–2.0 mg/kg/day	6–12	Depression	300 mg
Nortriptyline	20–150 mg	6–12	Depression	150 mg
Dexamethasone	0.0233–0.333 mg/kg/day	4–8	Inflammation	16 mg
Tramadol (opioid and SSRI)	50–100 mg	4–6	Pain	400 mg
Zolmitriptan	1.25–5 mg	2	Headache	10 mg
Propranolol	0.5–16 mg/kg/day		Migraine	640 mg
Baclofen	10–20 mg	6–8	Spasm	80 mg
Ketamine	5 µg/kg/min		Pain	
Benzodiazepines (e.g., alprazolam)	0.25–1.00 mg	8	Anxiety	10 mg
Calcium channel blocker	Multiple			

SSRI, selective serotonin reuptake inhibitor.

β-endorphins, which also bind to the mu receptor. There are no known clinical drugs, although experimental drugs exist.

Clinically, the effect of opioids is to raise the pain threshold, increasing the minimal intensity needed to feel pain. At the anatomical level, opioids act by inhibiting nociceptive transmission to the spinal cord, activating descending inhibitory pathways, and altering the higher center activity of pain perception. The opiates may have a purely stimulatory effect on opiate receptors (agonists) or stimulate at low doses and block at higher concentrations (agonists/antagonists). At the cellular physiology level, all opioids decrease cyclic adenosine monophosphate (cAMP); increase K^+ efflux, especially mu and delta; decrease calcium entry into the neuron, especially kappa; cause cellular hyperpolarization; and decrease the release of neurotransmitters, providing a neuroprotective mechanism. Opioids are beneficial in treating patients with pain and neurologic injury. Specific opioid families are more beneficial than others and have fewer neurologic side effects. Kappa opioids provide the most benefits and should be used in patients with severe neurologic injury and disease.

Multiple investigators believe in the beneficial role of opioids. Faden[12] suggests that by utilizing selective opioids, novel approaches to the treatment of CNS injury can be developed. Among the subtypes of opioid receptors, mu and delta receptors either inhibit or potentiate NMDA receptor-mediated events, whereas kappa opioids antagonize NMDA receptor-mediated activity, providing more neurotoxic protection. To assist healing during times of nervous system injury, the body's opioid systems have both a neurodestructive and a neuroprotective role. Mu and kappa-1 subtype receptors appear to mediate neuroprotective actions, and kappa-2 receptors are involved in secondary injury responses. Dynorphin, an endogenous kappa receptor stimulator, has marked neurotoxic effects when given intrathecally at subinjury doses to rats, exacerbating the response to brain or spinal cord trauma,[12] probably by stimulating a kappa receptor subtype.

Using animal models, other selective opiate receptor antagonists, such as naloxone, and the endogenous opiate antagonist thyrotropin-releasing hormone (TRH) have improved outcome and physiological variables following hypovolemia, spinal cord trauma, and head injury. High-dose naloxone in the mg/kg range improves blood pressure, neurologic motor function, outcome, and survival.[13,14] To take full advantage of the effects opioids have on individual receptor stimulators and because humans experience the clinical effects of opioids differently, specific receptor stimulators and inhibitors must continue to be investigated and understood.

Kappa Opioid Receptor Stimulators

Opioid receptors are classified into four types: mu, delta, kappa, and N/OFQ. Among these types, the kappa receptor system has become most attractive. According to Ikeda and Matsumoto,[15] by targeting the kappa receptor, novel therapeutic agents beyond pain and its relief can potentially be developed. Endogenous opioid systems have been proposed as secondary or delayed brain injury factors, largely on the basis of the therapeutic efficacy of opioid receptor antagonists or agonists. Ikeda and Matsumoto[15] demonstrated that the novel kappa opioid agonist RU51599 has a neuroprotective effect on traumatic and ischemic brain edema, while also having an analgesic effect. Hudson et al[16] demonstrated the neuroprotective effects of the kappa opioid–related anticonvulsants U-50488H and U-54494A in a neurotoxic model of NMDA-induced brain injury in the neonatal rat. Tortella and DeCoster[17] found that kappa receptor opioids, specifically the arylacetamide series of kappa opioid analgesics, are novel pharmacotherapeutic treatments for epilepsy, stroke, or trauma-related brain or spinal cord injury. The kappa opioid shares common properties with all opioids, being neuroprotective but, unlike mu receptors, acting directly in the brain to reduce ICP by inhibiting antidiuretic hormone (arginine vasopressin [AVP]) secretion and promoting water excretion in humans.[18] AVP regulates brain water content and is elevated in the cerebrospinal fluid of patients with ischemia and traumatic brain injuries. Ikeda et al[19] demonstrated the protective effect of RU51599, a selective kappa opioid agonist and AVP release inhibitor, thereby improving brain edema. Kappa receptor stimulation increases diuresis, reducing edema and increasing ICP, leading to increases in cerebral perfusion pressure. Kappa receptor stimulators cause respiratory depression but less than mu receptor stimulation. They also cause dysphoria, which can be problematic.

Nalbuphine is a potent kappa agonist and mu antagonist analgesic with a low side effect profile and low abuse potential, possibly because it inhibits midbrain dopamine release. Because it is a mu antagonist, it should be used with caution in those individuals who are addicted to mu receptor stimulators, such as morphine, because it can cause a withdrawal problem.

Mu Opioid Receptor Stimulators

The prototypical mu receptor stimulator is morphine, which has many benefits. In neurologic disease, it is neuroprotective to the cell. Morphine may also be used for preoperative sedation and dyspnea associated with acute left ventricular failure and pulmonary edema. Camphorated tincture of opium, another mu receptor stimulator, can treat severe diarrhea and intestinal cramping, and codeine is helpful with severe persistent cough. At times when very mild hyperventilation may be used, such as after head injury, morphine blunts the reflex vasoconstriction caused by decreased pCO_2 and decreases peripheral vascular resistance.[20]

The potential adverse effects of ketamine in neurosurgical anesthesia have been well established. The side effects of this mu receptor stimulator are increased ICP and cerebral blood flow (CBF). De Nadal et al[21,22] demonstrated in human brain trauma subjects that when carbon dioxide reactivity was preserved, 56.7% of the patients showed impaired or abolished autoregulation to hypertensive challenge. In both groups after mu receptor stimulation with either morphine or fentanyl, there was a significant increase in ICP and a decrease in mean arterial blood pressure and cerebral perfusion pressure, but arterial-venous difference of oxygen ($AVDO_2$) estimated CBF remain unchanged. In patients with preserved carbon dioxide reactivity, the opioid-induced ICP increase was even greater. This demonstrated the vasodilating effects of fentanyl. In additional studies, de Nadal and others came to the conclusion that potent opioids cause greater increases of ICP, due to methods other than activation of the vasodilator cascade. Sperry et al[23] showed that mu receptor stimulators are associated with a statistically significant ICP increase of 8.2 mm Hg for fentanyl, and an increase of 6.1 mm Hg for sufentanil. Both drugs caused statistically significant decreases in mean arterial blood pressure (MAP): fentanyl, 11.6 mm Hg; sufentanil, 10.5 mm Hg. No significant changes in heart rate occurred. Their results indicate that modest doses of potent opioids can significantly increase ICP in patients with severe head trauma.[23] Other investigators proved the same, that sufentanil, fentanyl, and alfentanil infusions cause a significant but transient increase in ICP accompanied by a significant decrease in MAP.[24] Hydromorphone, a mu receptor agonist, also significantly increased regional CBF in the anterior cingulate cortex, both amygdalae, and the thalamus, all structures belonging to the limbic system. Not all mu receptor stimulators cause cerebral vasodilation.

Mixed Receptor Stimulators

Butorphanol, a kappa agonist/mu antagonist, causes a less distinct picture of regional CBF increases, mainly in the area of both temporal lobes. The same mu receptor antagonist shows improvement in outcome after experimental brain trauma by the actions of kappa-opioid receptor agonists, affecting cellular bioenergetics.[25]

In addition to vasodilation, mu receptor stimulators produce mainly euphoria, whereas kappa agonists are more likely to produce dysphoria. The administrations of morphine and pentazocine increased dopamine turnover in the striatum and hypothalamus in a drug dose–dependent manner. The stimulative effects of butorphanol on the dopamine system were weaker than those of morphine and pentazocine, and there were no dose dependencies in the effects of butorphanol. Butorphanol, morphine, and pentazocine increased 5-hydroxytryptamine (5-HT, serotonin) turnover. It has been hypothesized that the nucleus paragigantocellularis (PGi) plays an important role in the development of physical dependence on opioids, including the prototype mu-opioid receptor agonist morphine and the mixed agonist/antagonist butorphanol, which shows selective kappa-opioid receptor agonist activity.

Opioids and Their Side Effects

Just as NSAIDs belong to different groups, with considerable variability in efficacy, opioid groups vary in their ability to treat pain, even in the same individual. *If one opioid does not work, consider treatment with another one.* The first and most widely used opioid is the group that stimulates the mu receptor; these include morphine, Demerol, Dilaudid, and fentanyl. The side effects of this group share some commonality with most opioid receptor stimulators and, as expected, demonstrate unique risks. Mu receptor stimulators cause increased ICP, both directly and indirectly, by vasodilatory and nonvasodilatory ways;[7,9,10,20,26] respiratory depression; bronchoconstriction; chest wall rigidity; hypotension; increased edema by increasing antidiuretic hormone (ADH) release; stimulated dopamine release; constipation; reduced body temperature; sedation; nausea with or without vomiting;

itching; somnolence; confusion and disorientation; hallucinations; and seizures at high doses. The mu acting drug also stimulates dopamine release, leading to addiction.

Therefore, when prescribing a high-dose intravenous opioid or opioid infusion, vital signs must be closely monitored. There should be continuous pulse oximetry, and the physician should be notified for decreased oxygenation. Blood pressure and respirations should be recorded every 15 minutes for 2 hours, then every 1 hour for 4 hours, then every 4 hours thereafter. With each increase in dosage, the vital sequence should restart. The medication should be stopped and the physician notified if the respiratory rate is less than 10 per minute or the systolic blood pressure (SBP) is less than 90 mm Hg. Antidotes for opioids must be immediately available. Naloxone 1 mg ampule should be on the patient's floor. If the respiratory rate is less than 8 per minute, give naloxone 0.2 mg intravenous push (IVP) and call the attending physician; the dose may be repeated in 5 minutes. For itching, have available diphenhydramine 25 mg IV/PO every 6 hours. For initial nausea and vomiting, which usually resolve with the second dose, have available an antiemetic such as granisetron 10 µg/kg IV over 5 minutes every 4 hours or comparable agent. Furthermore, when discontinuing patient-controlled analgesia (PCA) if greater than 3 days of continuous infusion, wean the medication (**Table 12–7**).

Table 12–7   Opioid Receptors and Side Effects[1–3,9–11,15,16,18–20]

Receptor	Drug	Side effects	Contraindications or cautions
Mu	Morphine, fentanyl, hydromorphone, buprenorphine	Raises ICP, respiratory depression, bronchoconstriction, chest wall rigidity, hypotension; increases edema by increasing ADH release; stimulates dopamine release, pupil constriction (miosis); reduces body temperature; depresses cough reflex; constipation, sedation, and nausea with or without vomiting; itching; somnolence, confusion, and disorientation	Head injury, asthma, respiratory conditions, paralytic ileus, cholelytiasis
Kappa	Nalbuphine	Respiratory depression, euphoria, sedation, nausea, vomiting, sweating, headache, vertigo, confusion, dry mouth	
Delta	Experimental BW373U86, SB235863		

ADH, antidiuretic hormone; ICP, intracranial pressure.

Opioid medication should be prescribed only after understanding the risks and benefits of the medication. Additional resources for prescribing dosage and administration should be checked before giving the medication. Below are some of the commonly prescribed opiates with some general considerations. For each, the exact dose should be tailored to the patient and clinical circumstance.

♦ Ten percent of the population lacks the enzyme needed to activate codeine. As a desired treatment, codeine may cause nausea and constipation.

♦ Tramodol lowers the seizure threshold.

♦ Fentanyl transdermal takes 12 to 16 hours to produce a therapeutic effect and 48 hours to reach steady state.

♦ Seriously consider the use of meperidine in the neurosurgical intensive care unit (NICU) patient because of neurotoxic risks of anxiety, tremors, myoclonus, and seizures.

♦ Give a loading dose of the narcotic, then an hourly dose of approximately $\frac{1}{6}$ the loading dose.

♦ Most opiates are cleared by renal and hepatic means (**Table 12–8**).

♦ General Considerations in Treating Pain

Treat pain early, when it begins; do not wait until pain is out of control. When pain becomes severe, it will require a much greater dosage. Consider providing medication around the clock when there is an initial injury, as opposed to giving medication only when asked for by the patient or only when the patient appears symptomatic. There will also be times when there is breakthrough pain. This pain is usually of moderate to severe intensity, occurs rapidly, usually in less than 3 minutes, is of relatively short duration, and occurs 1 to 4 times per day. Therefore, different medications should be prescribed for initial treatment and recurring pain. It is even beneficial to prescribe patient-controlled analgesia or continuous intravenous infusion of pain medication (**Table 12–9**).

In addition to cautiously looking for reasons to decrease or discontinue the medication, NICU personnel must document the medication's efficacy. The attending physician must be notified if the pain remains greater than 4 on a 1–10 pain scale for 3 consecutive hours. If there is breakthrough pain, acetaminophen, 650 mg or more, can be given every 4 to 6 hours. Consider additional treatment should a pain pump or medication stop being available.

Table 12–8 Opioid Pain Medication for Pain of 5 or 6 Greater on the 0 to 10 Pain Scale[1-3,9-11,15,16,18-20]

Drug	Receptor agonist or antagonist	Route	Dosage	Frequency (hours)	Half-life (hours)
Morphine	Mu	IV	0.1 mg/kg	3–4	2.1–2.6
		IM	0.2 mg/kg	3–4	
		PO	0.3 mg/kg	3–4	
Ketamine	Mu	IV	5 μg/kg/min	3–4	
Hydromorphone	Mu	IV, IM	0.015 mg/kg	3–6	2.6–3.2
			0.5–1.0 mg/hr		
		PO	0.06 mg/kg	3–6	
Fentanyl	Mu	IV	25–50 μg/hr		3.7
		TC	25–100 μg/hr	72 hour patch	3.7
			600–7200 μg		
Oxycodone	Mu	PO	0.2 mg/kg	3–4	
Hydrocodone	Mu	PO	0.2 mg/kg	3–4	
Meperidine	Mu	IV	0.75 mg/kg	2–3	3
		IM	75 mg		3
		PO	Not given PO	Not given PO	3
Levorphanol	Mu	IM	0.02 mg/kg	6–8	11
		PO	0.04 mg/kg	6–8	11
Buprenorphine	Mu	IV	0.4 mg/kg	6–8	5
		SL	2–24 mg	6–8	5
Codeine	Mu	IV	1 mg/kg	6–8	3
		IM	1 mg/kg	6–8	3
		PO	1 mg/kg	3–4	3

Tramadol	Mu	PO	50–100 mg	6	5
Nalbuphine	Kappa agonist, mu antagonist	IV	0.15–2.5 mg/kg	3–6	
Butorphanol	Kappa agonist, mu agonist and antagonist	IV, IM	2 mg 0.5–4.0 mg 0.25–32 mg/day max	3–4	3
Thyroid-releasing hormone		IN IV	1 mg spray, 1–4 mg/day	3–6	
Naloxone	Binds mu receptor without stimulation; also binds kappa and delta	IV	0.4 mg every 2–3 minutes		1
Pentazocine	Kappa; mu agonist and antagonist	PO	50 mg	4–6	4
Propoxyphene HCl	Mu	PO	65 mg	4–6	9

HCl, hydrochloric; IM, intramuscularly; IN, intranasally; IV, intravenously; PO, L. per os (orally); SL, sublingual; TC, transdermal transcutaneous.

Table 12–9   Treatment of Pain

Scale score	Treatment
0–4	Ice + APAP; possibly low-dose NSAIDs, possibly topical
5–9	Ice + APAP + ketorolac; possibly high-dose NSAIDs, low-dose opioids
10	Ice + APAP + ketorolac; possibly high-dose NSAIDs, high-dose opioids

APAP, acetaminophen; NSAIDs, nonsteroidal anti-inflammatory drugs.

Case Management

The 47-year-old female involved in a rollover motor vehicle accident with resultant severe closed head injury, consisting of mild cerebral edema, a pneumothorax, and fractured pelvis, has GCS 6, a chest tube, increased heart rate, and increased blood pressure anytime there is attempted movement. She does require pain medication. The patient should be assessed initially using the FLACC scale and given an initial dose of nalbuphine, which should be repeated until a FLACC score <4 is achieved. A dosage should be given every 3 to 6 hours based on the FLACC score at the time of assessment. The pain therapy should also be augmented with acetaminophen 10 to 75 mg/kg/day in 4 to 6 divided doses unless contraindications exist. An alternative to a single intravenous nalbuphine dosage every 3 to 6 hours would be a continuous drip (see the algorithm in **Table 12–10**).

◆ Pain and Sedation Control in the Unconscious Patient

At times sedation may be required in patients with multiple injuries either to prevent further injury or in an attempt to temporarily assist with the management of increased intracranial pressure. It must be remembered that sedation and paralytics have not been shown to increase outcome in patients with severe head injury. Sedation and paralytics, however, have been shown to increase the possibility of pneumonia, ventilator dependency, and ICU length of stay.[4] Notwithstanding, sedation is sometimes required. During these times the initial agitation scale must be assessed, and the level of sedation required must also be recorded. Any sedation decreases the most sensitive and important means to assess neurologic injury: the neurologic exam. The favored assessment scale is the Ramsey or Modified Ramsey based on wakefulness (**Table 12–11**).

Table 12–10   Patient-Controlled or Continuous IV Analgesia Algorithm[1-3,9-11,15,16,18-20]

Document allergies:

Weight in kilograms:

Use continuous pulse oximeter; notify physician if less than _____%.

Record blood pressure and respirations every 15 minutes for 2 hours, then every 1 hour for 4 hours, then every 4 hours thereafter. With each increase in dosage, begin sequence of vital signs again. Stop infusion and notify attending physician if respiratory rate < 10/minute or systolic blood pressure < 90 mm Hg.

Keep pain ≤ 4 on 1–10 VAS or 1–10 FLACC pain scale. Assess and record pain every hour while awake.

Choose one medication to use:

_____morphine 1 mg/mL

_____hydromorphone (Dilaudid) 0.5 mg/mL

_____fentanyl 10 μg/mL

_____butorphanol (Stadol) 0.1 mg/mL (for increased ICP)

_____nalbuphine (Nubain) 1 mg/mL (for increased ICP)

Give initial bolus of the medication being used above:

_____ mg morphine sulfate (range: 1–5 mg)

_____ mg hydromorphone (Dilaudid) (range: 0.1–1.0 mg)

_____ mg fentanyl (range: 10–20 μg)

_____ mg butorphanol (Stadol) (range: 0.5–2.0 mg)

_____ mg nalbuphine (Nubain) (range: 10–20 mg)

PCA pump settings of the medication chosen above (continuous basal rate):

_____ mg/hr morphine sulfate (range: 1–4 mg)

_____ mg/hr hydromorphone (Dilaudid) (range: 0.5–1.0 mg)

_____ μg/hr fentanyl (range: 10–20 μg)

_____ mg/hr butorphanol (Stadol) (range: 0.1–1.0 mg)

_____ mg/hr nalbuphine (Nubain) (range: 5–10 mg)

PCA dose of the medication chosen above:

_____ mg morphine sulfate (range: 0.5–2.0 mg)

_____ mg hydromorphone (Dilaudid) (range: 0.1–0.2 mg)

_____ μg fentanyl (range: 10–20 μg)

_____ mg butorphanol (Stadol) (range: 0.1–0.5 mg)

_____ mg nalbuphine (Nubain) (range: 5–10 mg)

Lockout interval: _____ 5–30 minutes

Maximum dose per 4 hours of the medication chosen above:

_____ mg morphine (range: 10–40 mg)

_____ mg hydromorphone (Dilaudid) (range: 2–6 mg)

(Continued)

Table 12–10   Patient-Controlled or Continuous IV Analgesia Algorithm (*Continued*)

_____ µg fentanyl (range: 100–300 µg)
_____ mg butorphanol (Stadol) (range: 2–4 mg)
_____ mg nalbuphine (Nubain) (range: 40 mg)

Notify attending physician if pain > 4 for more than 1 hour.

Have available on the floor naloxone (Narcan) 1 mg ampule. Give 0.2 mg IVP if respiratory rate is < 8/min and call physician; may repeat dose in 5 minutes.

When discontinuing PCA if > 3 days of continuous infusion, wean:

_____ decrease morphine 1 mg/hr until < 2 mg/hr, then decrease 0.5 mg/hr

_____ decrease hydromorphone (Dilaudid) 0.5 mg/hr until < 1 mg/hr, then decrease 0.2 mg/hr

_____ decrease fentanyl 10 µg/hr until < 20 µg/hr, then decrease 5 µg/hr

_____ decrease butorphanol (Stadol) 0.5 mg/hr until less < 1 mg/hr, then decrease 0.2 mg/hr

_____ decrease nalbuphine (Nubain) 5 mg/hr until < 10 mg/hr, then decrease 1 mg/hr

Primary IV line to run at a rate of at least _____ to be piggybacked into the PCA line.

Have available diphenhydramine (Benedryl) 25 mg IV/PO every 6 hours prn pruritus.

Have available an antiemetic such as granisetron (Kytril) 10 µg/kg IV over 5 minutes every 4 hours prn nausea and vomiting.

For breakthrough pain, may give acetaminophen (Tylenol) 650 mg every 6 hours.

If pump is interrupted for > 1 hour, not due to respiratory changes or blood pressure changes, may give hydrocodone 5 mg PO every 4 hours.

IV, intravenously; IVP, intravenous push; PCA, patient-controlled analgesia; PO, L. per os (orally); prn, L. pro re nata (according as circumstances may require); VAS, Visual Analog Scale.

Table 12–11   Modified Ramsey Scale Score[1,5,9,10,20]

Score	Description
1	Anxious, agitated
2	Cooperative, oriented, tranquil
3	Responds to commands
4	Responds to shaking
5	Responds to noxious stimuli only
6	Unresponsive

Just as pain must be assessed and scored prior to treatment, so sedation needs must be considered. Based on the assessed needs, a sedation medication is then chosen. The drug of choice should provide the clinician with an opportunity to examine the patient closely on a regular basis. Thus the medication should be short acting and with controllable significant side-effects (e.g., propofol or midazolam). The patient must be monitored closely while on the sedative. Consider drugs other than propofol for sedation in children. The patient also should be intubated. Longer acting drugs may be necessary for nonneurological patients or when burst suppression is required, although propofol or midazolam can also be used. If propofol is used, it can be reversed with Romazicon (flumazenil); 0.2 mg can be given IVP. If systolic blood pressure becomes <90 mm Hg or heart rate <50, the attending physician should be notified. The dose may be repeated in 5 minutes.

Burst Suppression

Sometimes for status epilepticus, severe cerebral edema, or increased ICP refractory to other methods, cerebral burst suppression is indicated. There are many methods to induce burst suppression. The preferred drug of choice is pentobarbital; as with other drugs, one must watch for hypotension and cardiac depression. If ICP is uncontrolled and results in low cerebral perfusion pressure (CPP), if no surgical lesion is present, and if patient is viable, consider pentobarbital coma. Do not use pentobarbital coma prophylactically; it has not been shown to improve outcome.[27] Patient must be in a monitored bed and intubated (**Table 12–12**).

To initiate pentobarbital therapy:

1. Give pentobarbital 2.5 mg/kg every 15 minutes for 4 doses. *Follow blood pressure closely.*
2. Over the next 3 hours, give pentobarbital 10 mg/kg/hr continuous infusion.
3. Then initiate maintenance pentobarbital 1.5 mg/kg/hr infusion.
4. Maintain burst suppression 1–2 bursts/page.
5. Check daily levels; maintain pentobarbital level 5 mg% (a lab value, e.g., mg, μg/mL) or 50 μg/mL.

   a. Remember that this is not a phenobarbital level.
   b. Some people may not have burst suppression at higher levels.
   c. If ICP is controlled for >48 hours, then start to wean drug.
   d. If ICP is not controlled in 24 hours, this procedure is unlikely to work.

It is often difficult to adequately sedate the patient while providing proper analgesia. However, the same delivery of analgesia and sedation according to predefined and measurable criteria is possible using the FLACC and Ramsey/Modified Ramsey scores, as stated earlier (**Tables 12–13** and **12–14**).

Table 12–12 Patient Sedation Continuous Intravenous Schedule Algorithm[1–3,9–11,15,16,18–20]

Document allergies:

Document weight in kilograms:

Continuous EKG for burst suppression.

Use continuous pulse oximeter; notify physician if less than _____ %.

Patient must be intubated.

Record blood pressure and heart rate every 5 minutes for initiation of drug, then every 1 hour thereafter. With each increase in dosage, begin sequence of vital signs again. Stop infusion and notify physician if SBP < 90 mm Hg or heart rate < 50.

RAMSEY SCALE SCORE: 1 = anxious, agitated, 2 = cooperative, oriented, tranquil; 3 = responds to commands; 4 = responds to shaking; 5 = responds to noxious stimuli only; 6 = unresponsive

Check below patient's initial agitation category based on the above Ramsey Scale score where:

1 = severe agitation; 2 and 3 = moderate agitation; 4, 5, and 6 = mild agitation

☐ severe   ☐ moderate   ☐ mild

STANDARD ASSUMED SEDATION GOAL: Ramsey score 2–3 on 1–6 scale. Assess and record Ramsey score every hour.

SEDATION GOAL OPTION: Must check for different goal option.

_____ Keep sedation Ramsey Scale score 4, 5, or 6

_____ Use for burst suppression to achieve maximum of 2 bursts per continuous EEG page

Must assess neurologic exam and GCS at least every 8 hours by reducing or holding infusion rate to bring patient to Ramsey Scale score of 2 or 1, unless burst suppression.

OPTION:_____ Assess neurologic exam and GCS every _____ hours (range 1–24 hours)

Medication ordered (only one of these drugs can be used):

_____propofol (Diprivan)

_____midazolam (Versed) 1 mg/mL

_____lorazepam (Ativan) 1 mg/mL

Initial loading dose for agitation checked above:

propofol (Diprivan) ♦ severe 15 µg/kg/min ♦ moderate 10 µg/kg/min ♦ mild 5 µg/kg/min

midazolam (Versed) ♦ severe 0.06 mg/kg ♦ moderate 0.04 mg/kg ♦ mild 0.02 mg/kg

lorazepam (Ativan) ♦ severe 0.06 mg/kg ♦ moderate 0.04 mg/kg ♦ mild 0.02 mg/kg

(Continued)

Table 12–12   Patient Sedation Continuous Intravenous Schedule Algorithm *(Continued)*

Automatic increase/decrease rate for the following amount every 10 minutes until sedation goal of Ramsey Scale score indicated above is obtained

Maximum dose:

   propofol (Diprivan) 80 µg/kg/min, or for burst suppression 150 µg/kg/min
   midazolam (Versed) 0.2 mg/kg/hr
   lorazepam (Ativan) 0.06 mg/kg/hr

Notify physician if Ramsey Score < 2 for > 1 hour.

The reversal agent flumazenil (Romazicon) 1 mg ampule must be available on floor. Give 0.2 mg IVP; if SBP < 90 mm Hg or heart rate < 50, call physician. May repeat dose in 5 minutes.

For propofol (Diprivan): Change tubing and solution every 12 hours during continuous infusion using strict aseptic technique.

EEG, electroencephalogram; EKG, electrocardiogram; GCS, Glasgow Coma Scale; IVP, intravenous push; SBP, systolic blood pressure.

Note

All medications and dosages listed in this chapter are taken from *AHFS Drug Information*[9] and *Drug Facts and Comparisons*, 2004 edition.[10] This information is intended as a supplement to, and not a substitute for, the actual information from the sources. It is not meant to substitute for the knowledge, expertise, skill, and judgment of physicians, pharmacists, or other health care professionals in patient care. The absence of a warning for any medication should not be interpreted to indicate that the medication is safe, appropriate, or effective in any given patient.

Table 12–13   Medication for Sedation per Desired Ramsey Score[1,5,9,10,20]

Medication	Desired sedation goal of burst suppression	Desired Ramsey score (4–6)	Desired Ramsey score (2–3)
Propofol (Diprivan)	15 µ/kg/min	10 µg/kg/min	5 µg/kg/min
Midazolam (Versed)	0.06 mg/kg/hr	0.04 mg/kg/hr	0.02 mg/kg/hr
Lorazepam (Ativan)	0.06 mg/kg/hr	0.04 mg/kg/hr	0.02 mg/kg/hr

Table 12–14   Patient Sedation and Analgesia Intravenous Schedule Algorithm[1–3,9–11,15,16,18–20]

Initially, the patient is loaded with the appropriate analgesic and sedation. Further medication can be based on the following protocol being adjusted for patient characteristics.

Must fill out Patient Sedation Schedule

Select single Pain Analgesia to be given:

_____ morphine sulfate 1 mg/mL
_____ hydromorphone (Dilaudid) 0.5 mg/mL
_____ fentanyl 10 µg/mL
_____ butorphanol (Stadol) 0.1 mg/mL (for increased ICP)
_____ nalbuphine (Nubain) 1 mg/mL (for increased ICP)

For propofol (Diprivan) dose of 5–19 µg/kg/min, or midazolam (Versed) dose of 0.02–0.06 mg/kg/hr, or lorazepam (Ativan) dose of 0.02–0.04 mg/hr, administer:

morphine sulfate 1 mg/hr by continuous IV infusion *or*
hydromorphone (Dilaudid) 0.2 mg/hr by continuous IV infusion *or*
fentanyl 10 µg/hr by continuous IV infusion *or*
butorphanol (Stadol) 0.2 mg/hr by continuous IV infusion *or*
nalbuphine (Nubain) 5 mg/hr by continuous IV infusion

For propofol (Diprivan) dose of 20 to 39 µg/kg/min, or midazolam (Versed) dose of 5 to 7 mg/hr, or lorazepam (Ativan) dose of 3 mg/hr, administer:

morphine sulfate 3 mg/hr by continuous IV infusion *or*
hydromorphone (Dilaudid) 1 mg/hr by continuous IV infusion *or*
fentanyl 40 µg/hr by continuous IV infusion *or*
butorphanol (Stadol) 1 mg/hr by continuous IV infusion *or*
nalbuphine (Nubain) 10 mg/hr by continuous IV infusion

For propofol (Diprivan) dose above 40 µg/kg/min, or midazolam (Versed) dose above 7 mg/hr, or lorazepam (Ativan) dose above 3 mg/hr, administer:

morphine sulfate 5 mg/hr to a maximum of _____ by continuous IV infusion *or*
hydromorphone (Dilaudid) 1.5 mg/hr to a maximum of _____ by continuous IV infusion *or*
fentanyl 50 µg/hr to a maximum of _____ by continuous IV infusion *or*
butorphanol (Stadol) 2 mg/hr to a maximum of _____ by continuous IV infusion *or*
nalbuphine (Nubain) 15 mg/hr to a maximum of _____ by continuous IV infusion

Naloxone 1 mg ampule must be available on floor. Give 0.2 mg IVP, if SBP < 90 mm Hg, call physician. May repeat dose in 5 minutes.

When discontinuing the chosen analgesia if > 3 days of continuous infusion, wean:

_____ decrease morphine 1 mg/hr until < 2 mg/hr, then decrease 0.5 mg/hr

(Continued)

Table 12–14   Patient Sedation and Analgesia Intravenous Schedule Algorithm *(Continued)*

_____ decrease hydromorphone (Dilaudid) 0.5 mg/hr until < 1 mg/hr, then decrease 0.2 mg/hr

_____ decrease fentanyl 10 μg/hr until < 20 μg/hr, then decrease 5 μg/hr

_____ decrease butorphanol (Stadol) 0.5 mg/hr until < 1 mg/hr, then decrease 0.2 mg/hr

_____ decrease nalbuphine (Nubain) 5 mg/hr until < 10 mg/hr, then decrease 1 mg/hr

Primary IV line to run at a rate of at least _____ to be piggybacked into the PCA line.

Have available diphenhydramine (Benedryl) 25 mg IV/PO every 6 hours prn pruritus.

Have available granisetron (Kytril) 10 μg/kg IV over 5 minutes every 4 hours prn nausea and vomiting.

If pain pump is interrupted for > 1 hour, not due to respiratory changes or blood pressure changes, may give hydrocodone 5 mg NG tube every 4 hours.

ICP, intracranial pressure; IV, intravenously; NG, nasogastric; PCA, patient-controlled analgesia; PO, L. per os (orally); SBP, systolic blood pressure.

References

1. Joint Commission on Accreditation of Healthcare Organizations National Pharmaceutical Council, Inc. (JCAHO). Pain: current understanding of assessment, management, and treatment. Oakbrook Terrace, IL: JCAHO; 2001
2. Jacox AK, Carr DB, Chapman CR. Acute pain management: operative or medical procedures and trauma (Clinical Practice Guidelines No 1, AHCPR 92–0032). Rockville, MD: U.S. Department of Health and Human Services, Agency for Health Care Policy and Research; 1992
3. Pasero C, Paice JA, McCaffery M. Basic mechanisms underlying the causes and effects of pain. In: McCaffery M, Pasero C, eds. Pain Clinical Manual. 2nd ed. St. Louis, MO: Mosby; 1999:15–34
4. Guidelines for the Management of Severe Head Injury. New York: The Brain Trauma Foundation; 2000
5. McCaffery M. Nursing practice theories related to cognition, bodily pain and man–environmental interactions. Los Angeles: UCLA Student Store; 1968
6. Merskey H, Bugduk N. Classification of Chronic Pain Syndromes and Definitions of Pain Terms. 2nd ed. Seattle: IASP Press; 1994
7. Brody TM, Larner J, Minneman KP. Human Pharmacology: Molecular to Clinical. 3rd ed. St. Louis, MO: Mosby; 1998
8. Riedel W, Neeck GZ. Nociception, pain, and antinociception: current concepts. Z Rheumatol 2001;60(6):404–415
9. McEvoy GK, ed. AHFS Drug Information. Bethesda, MD: American Society of Health-System Pharmacists; 2004
10. Drug Facts and Comparisons 2004. 58th ed. St. Louis, MO: Facts and Comparisons; 2004
11. Chandrasekharan NV, Dai H, Roos KL, et al. COX-3, a cyclooxygenase-1 variant inhibited by acetaminophen and other analgesic/antipyretic drugs: cloning, structure, and expression. Proc Natl Acad Sci U S A 2002;99(21):13926–13931

12. Faden AI. Neurotoxic versus neuroprotective actions of endogenous opioid peptides: implications for treatment of CNS injury. NIDA Res Monogr 1996;163: 318–330
13. McIntosh TK, Faden AI. Opiate antagonist in traumatic shock. Ann Emerg Med 1986;15(12):1462–1465
14. McIntosh TK, Fernyak S, Hayes RL, Faden AI. Beneficial effect of non-selective opiate antagonist naloxone hydrochloride and the thyrotropin releasing hormone (TRH) analog YM-14673 on long-term neurobehavioral outcome following experimental brain injury in the rat. J Neurotrauma 1993;10:373–384
15. Ikeda Y, Matsumoto K. Analgesic effect of kappa-opioid receptor agonist. Nippon Rinsho 2001;59(9):1681–1687
16. Hudson CJ, Von Voigtlander PF, Althaus JS, Scherch HM, Means ED. The kappa opioid-related anticonvulsants U-50488H and U-54494A attenuate N-methyl-D-aspartate induced brain injury in the neonatal rat. Brain Res 1991;564(2):261–267
17. Tortella FC, DeCoster MA. Kappa opioids: therapeutic considerations in epilepsy and CNS injury. Clin Neuropharmacol 1994;17(5):403–416
18. Bemana I, Nagao S. Effects of niravoline (RU 51599), a selective kappa-opioid receptor agonist on intracranial pressure in gradually expanding extradural mass lesion. J Neurotrauma 1998;15(2):117–124
19. Ikeda Y, Teramoto A, Nakagawa Y, Ishibashi Y, Yoshii T. Attenuation of cryogenic induced brain oedema by arginine vasopressin release inhibitor RU51599. Acta Neurochir (Wien) 1997;139(12):1173–1179; discussion 1179–1180
20. Hardmann JG, Limbird LE. Goodman and Gillman's The Pharmacological Basis of Therapeutics. 10th ed. New York: McGraw-Hill; 2001
21. de Nadal M, Munar F, Poca MA, Sahuquillo J, Garnacho A, Rossello J. Cerebral hemodynamic effects of morphine and fentanyl in patients with severe head injury: absence of correlation to cerebral autoregulation. Anesthesiology 2000;92(1):11–19
22. de Nadal M, Ausina A, Sahuquillo J, Pedraza S, Garnacho A, Gancedo VA. Effects on intracranial pressure of fentanyl in severe head injured patients. Acta Neurochir Suppl (Wien) 1998;71:10–12
23. Sperry RJ, Bailey PL, Reichman MV, Peterson JC, Petersen PB, Pace NL. Fentanyl and sufentanil increase intracranial pressure in head trauma patients. Anesthesiology 1992;77(3):416–420
24. Albanese J, Viviand X, Potie F, Rey M, Alliez B, Martin C. Sufentanil, fentanyl, and alfentanil in head trauma patients: a study on cerebral hemodynamics. Crit Care Med 1999;27(2):407–411
25. Vink R, Portoghese PS, Faden AI. Kappa-opioid antagonist improves cellular bioenergetics and recovery after traumatic brain injury. Am J Physiol 1991;261 (6 Pt 2):R1527–R1532
26. Cottrell JE, Turndorf H. Anesthesia and Neurosurgery. 2nd ed. St. Louis, MO: Mosby; 1986
27. Schwartz M, Tator C, Towed D. The University of Toronto head injury treatment study: a prospective randomized comparison of pentobarbital and mannitol. Can J Neurol Sci 1984;11:434–440

Section III

Pathophysiology

13

Homeostatic Mechanisms in the Neurosurgical Intensive Care Unit Patient

Gayatri Sonti, Dan Miulli, and Javed Siddiqi

Case Study

A 28-year-old right-handed Caucasian male had a pituitary macroadenoma resection. Postoperatively, the patient's Glasgow Coma Scale (GCS) score decreased from 15 to 6. The patient started to have seizures. His temperature was 37.3°C (99.2°F), heart rate 80, respirations 16, and blood pressure 160/90. He was intubated and was transferred to the neurosurgical intensive care unit (NICU), where he had intracranial pressure (ICP) consistently above 30 and cerebral perfusion pressure (CPP) 70 to 80. Arterial blood gas showed pH 7.53, pCO$_2$ 20, and PaO$_2$ 98%. Electrolytes showed serum sodium 129, potassium 3.2, chloride 105, bicarbonate 30, blood urea nitrogen (BUN) 5, creatinine 0.3, and serum osmolality 282.

See page 178 for Case Management.

◆ Homeostasis of the Brain

The skull is a solid box within which the volume of all the components—the brain, cerebrospinal fluid (CSF), and blood—should remain constant. Alteration in pressure in one compartment of the skull is compensated by volume changes in the other. The energy requirements of the brain are met from oxygenation of glucose. In addition, the autoregulation of the cerebral vasculature attempts to maintain adequate perfusion to the brain.[1,2] The homeostasis of the brain results from a balance of the above mechanisms.

In the neurologically injured patient, this homeostasis is altered and must be understood. The treatment of patients in the NICU includes a thorough understanding of cerebral metabolism, intracranial pressure, cerebral perfusion pressure, management of fluids and electrolytes, and the correction of these parameters to achieve homeostasis after brain injury (**Table 13–1**).

Table 13–1   Therapeutic Targets for NICU Patients[2,7,9]

CPP	>70–95 or >60–95 if concerns about secondary injury from treatment
ICP	5–15 mm Hg
Hemoglobin	10
Hematocrit	30–35%
Core temperature	35–37.2°C, 95–99°F
PaO_2	>97%
pO_2	>115 mm Hg for 72 hours, then >100 mm Hg
Serum osmolality	<320 mOsm/L
pCO_2	35–40 mm Hg
Sodium	140–145 mmol/L
Glucose	80–110 mg/dL
PCWP	10–14
PAD	12–16
CVP	6–8

CVP, central venous pressure; ICP, intracranial pressure; NICU, neurosurgical intensive care unit; PAD, pulmonary artery diastolic pressure, PCWP; pulmonary capillary wedge pressure.

◆ Cerebral Blood Flow and Perfusion

Cerebral blood flow (50–75 mL/100 g/min) is affected by regional cerebral metabolism, cerebral perfusion pressure, and oxygen and carbon dioxide tension.[1] The neurointensivists must prevent ischemia. Without blood flow, glucose and glycogen are depleted in 4 minutes. In the ischemic penumbra, there is an increased metabolism attempting to deliver more substrate that results in increased brain temperature.[3] If brain tissue oxygen drops below 20 mm Hg, there is anaerobic respiration, followed by glucose storage dependent lactic acid accumulation, mitochondrial damage, decreased pH, vasodilation, failure of Na–K adenosinetriphosphatase (ATPase) pump, and Na and Cl influx followed by water, all which lead to cytotoxic edema.[1,2] Failure in the blood–brain barrier leads to vasogenic edema. Hydrogen ions accumulate and pH drops to 6.0 from 6.4, causing inhibition of mitochondrial respiration and failure to sequester calcium, and, in turn, leading to further cell activation in the face of no substrate. The cell dies. Cerebral autoregulation attempts to maintain blood flow according to this or any other change in cerebral metabolism.

Cerebral perfusion is the blood pressure gradient across the cerebral vasculature and usually is equal to the mean arterial pressure minus the intracranial pressure (MAP – ICP). The ability to maintain cerebral autoregulation is affected by pathological conditions such as hyperventilation, edema, and hypoxia. ICP is controlled through regulation of the intracranial

Table 13–2   Management of Elevated ICP and CPP[1]

- Surgical evacuation of mass lesion
- HOB elevated to 30 degrees
- Mild hyperventilation to $PaCO_2$ of 32–35 mm Hg
- Diuretics (e.g., mannitol 0.25–1 g/kg) if signs of herniation
- Ventricular drainage if GCS ≤ 8
- Vasopressors such as norepinephrine (0.2–0.4 µg/kg/min), low-dose dopamine (1.5–0 µg/kg/min), and phenylephrine (max 4 µg/kg/min)
- Sedation and paralytics using short-acting agent
- Pain control

Note: Initiate hypothermia and barbiturate coma if the above measures fail and if ICP is consistently above 25 mm Hg.
CPP, cerebral perfusion pressure; GCS, Glasgow Coma Scale; HOB, head of bed; ICP, intracranial pressure.

constituents of CSF, blood, and brain volume.[1,2] The pressure volume index (PVI) is the ability of the brain to compensate for increased intracranial volume. ICP slowly raises up to a point where a slight increase in intracranial volume causes a big change in ICP. When ICP is consistently increased to greater than 20 mm Hg, it may lead to ischemia and herniation, which eventually lead to brain death. The goal in the management of high ICP is to reduce the CSF, blood, and brain volume. This may be accomplished by CSF drainage, prevention of vasodilation, and surgery to remove a portion of the skull, allowing the brain to expand. A decompressive craniectomy may have some benefit in salvageable patients with consistently elevated ICP. **Table 13–2** outlines the basic approach to managing elevated ICP and CPP.

◆ Control of Blood Pressure

The CPP should be maintained >70 mm Hg and below 100. If there is a concern about secondary injury from therapy, consider maintaining CPP above 60 mm Hg. Significant decreases in blood pressure are a direct effect of ICP treatments using sedation, paralytics, or diuretics. In these hypotensive situations, moderate intravenous (IV) fluids followed by vasopressors can elevate blood pressure. In brain injury, the autoregulation of cerebral blood flow is altered; if CPP increases above 95 to 125, there can be an increase in blood volume and an increase in ICP. The first-line antihypertensive medication should be β-blockers or angiotensin-converting enzyme (ACE) inhibitors. Other medications such as nitrogen-containing compounds act quickly, but because they cause a direct vasodilator effect, they increase ICP.[2]

◆ Control of Serum Glucose

Tight control of glucose concentration is essential in head injury patients. Hypoglycemia of 50 mg/dL causes neuronal injury by changing cerebral blood flow and cerebral metabolism. In addition, glucose levels >110 to 150 mg/dL in nondiabetics and >200 to 250 mg/dL in diabetics also have deleterious effects. IV regular insulin infusion and frequent blood glucose checks are essential to maintain glucose levels between 80 and 110 mg/dL.[4]

◆ Fluids and Electrolyte Balance

The principles of homeostasis of body water are as follows: $^2/_3$ of total fluid resides inside cells, and $^1/_3$ of total fluid resides in the extracellular space. The extracellular space is composed of $^1/_3$ plasma and $^2/_3$ interstitial fluid. The osmotic forces created by solutes determine the movement of water across membranes. An estimate of serum osmolality is determined by the equation

$$2Na + BUN/2.8 + glucose/18,$$

where BUN is the blood urea nitrogen level.

Sodium is the main determinant of osmotic force because it does not easily cross the membrane. Therefore, an imbalance in sodium concentration and volume status results in disturbance in homeostasis.[1] The most common conditions seen are diabetes insipidus, syndrome of inappropriate antidiuretic hormone (SIADH), and cerebral salt wasting (CSW) (**Table 13–3**).[1,5]

Table 13–3   Common Conditions Leading to Sodium Concentration Imbalance[7,9]

Condition	Vascular volume	Serum sodium	Urine sodium	Urine osmolality
DI	Decrease	Increase	No change	Decrease
SIADH	Increase	Decrease	Increase	Increase
CSW	Decrease	Decrease	Increase	

CSW, cerebral salt wasting; DI, diabetes insipidus; SIADH, syndrome of inappropriate antidiuretic hormone.

Hypernatremia

Hypernatremia is usually caused by hypovolemia due to free water loss. It is often related to defective antidiuretic hormone (ADH) release or due to osmotic diuresis. When sodium levels are >160 mmol/L, decreased level of consciousness and confusion set in. Hypernatremia should be treated first with crystalloids, 0.45 or 0.9% NaCl; if needed, colloids such as 5% albumin can be used. Patients with diabetes insipidus should be carefully monitored for fluid balance, body weight, serum and urine sodium, and urine specific gravity. If urine output exceeds the input by 250 mL/hr for 2 consecutive hours, hormonal replacement with IV 1-deamino-8-D-arginine vasopressin (DDAVP, or desmopressin) 0.5 to 2 µg may be administered with caution.[5]

Hyponatremia

In NICU patients, hyponatremia results primarily from SIADH and CSW. In SIADH, the extracellular volume is increased, and CSW is decreased. If sodium is less than 135 mmol/L, due to excessive water retention or sodium excretion, serum osmolality should be measured immediately. An increase in glucose concentration by 100 mg/dL also accounts for a fall in sodium by 1.6 mmol/L and a rise in serum osmolality by 2 mOsm/kg. Patients usually become symptomatic after a drop of sodium below 120 mOsm/L, although mentation changes can be seen with levels below 130 mmol/L in the acutely injured patient. Some of the common symptoms are headache, nausea, and vomiting. Patients may also become lethargic or develop tonicoclonic seizures at low levels. Hyponatremia should be corrected slowly to prevent central pontine myelinolysis.[1,2]

◆ Hypothermia and Brain Injury

Brain temperature is higher than the core body temperature by 1°C. Several studies demonstrate that in head-injured patients, there are moderate to severe elevations in brain temperature. Hyperthermia is neurotoxic, and hypothermia attenuates these effects. Mild hypothermia is between 32 and 35°C and moderate hypothermia, 30 and 33°C.[6,7] Although spontaneous hypothermia and hyperthermia result from damage to the hypothalamus, several studies demonstrate the neuroprotective effects of iatrogenic-induced hypothermia.[3] Hypothermia can be induced by antipyretic medication, surface cooling using hypothermia blankets, gastric lavage with ice-cold water, or saline. However, the most efficient way is by an endovascular cooling device placed in the inferior vena cava via the femoral vein.[8] The duration, speed of cooling, and rate of rewarming are likely factors in determining whether hypothermia will be effective. **Tables 13–4** and **13–5** outline the advantages and disadvantages of hypothermia for brain-injured patients.[9–13]

Table 13–4   Advantages of Hypothermia for Brain-Injured Patients[9-13]

- Attenuation of release of excitatory amino acids such as glutamate and other chemicals, such as pyruvate and glycerol
- Decrease in reperfusion injury
- Decrease in ICP
- Improvement in CPP
- High temperatures increase brain metabolism; the adverse affects can be reduced by induced hypothermia.

CPP, cerebral perfusion pressure; ICP, intracranial pressure.

Table 13–5   Disadvantages of Hypothermia for Brain-Injured Patients[9-13]

- Temperature below 35°C may impair brain tissue oxygenation
- Hypokalemia and hyperglycemia
- Infections

Case Management

The described patient had a seizure and was hyperventilating. He is subsequently post-ictal. The seizures should be treated and an emergent head CT is obtained to rule out a mass lesion such as a fresh hematoma.

The patient is also hypervolemic as suggested by the low sodium, potassium, BUN, and creatinine. The glucose is presumably high because the serum osmolality does not correlate with the sodium level. A rising glucose is expected after falling sodium but also can occur with steroid administration after pituitary surgery. Although patients become lethargic or develop tonic-clonic seizures at sodium levels around 120, this can occur with higher levels of sodium when there is a rapid drop such as >0.5 mmol/hr.

When correcting hyponatremia, do not increase serum sodium more than 10 mEq/L in 24 hours or more than 1.3 mEq/L/hr. The patient may benefit from furosemide intravenously to decrease fluid overload, and a fluid restriction to 1 liter per day.

References

1. Bernard SA, Buist M. Induced hypothermia in critical care medicine: a review. Crit Care Med 2003;31:2041–2051
2. Broderick JP. Werner Hacke. Treatment of acute ischemic stroke, II: Neuroprotection and medical management. Circulation 2002;106:1736–1745

3. Ginsberg MD, Busto R. Combating hyperthermia in acute stroke: a significant clinical concern. Stroke 1998;29:529–534

4. Gordon CJ. The therapeutic potential of regulated hypothermia. Emerg Med J 2001;18:81–89

5. Gupta AK, Al-Rawi PG, Hutchinson PJ, Kirkpatrick PJ. Effect of hypothermia on brain tissue oxygenation in patients with severe head injury. Br J Anaesth 2002;88:188–192

6. Hammer MD, Kreiger DW. Hypothermia for acute ischemic stroke. Neurologist 2003;9:280–289

7. Layon AJ, Gabrielli A, Friedman WA. Textbook of Neurointensive Care. Philadelphia: Saunders; 2004:26–51

8. Berger C, Schabitz ER, Georgiadis D, Steiner T, Achoff A, Schwab S. Effects of hypothermia on exictatory amino acids and metabolism in stroke patients. Stroke 2002;33:519–529

9. Militsa B. Nutrition in neurologic and neurosurgical critical care. Neurol India 2001;49(Suppl 1):S75–S79

10. Schaller B, Graf R. Hypothermia and stroke: the pathophysiological background. Pathophysiology 2003;10:7–35

11. Steinberg GK, Ogilvy CS, Shuer LM, et al. Comparison of endovascular and surface cooling during unruptured cerebral aneurysm repair. Neurosurgery 2004;55:307–314

12. Yasui N, Kawamura S, Suzuki A, Hadeishi H, Hatazawa J. Role of hypothermia in the management of severe cases of subarachnoid hemorrhage. Acta Neurochir Suppl (Wien) 2002;82:93–98

13. Zauner A, Doppenberg EM, Menzel M, Gilman C, Young HF, Bullock R. The importance of brain temperature in patients after severe head injury: relationship to intracranial pressure, cerebral perfusion pressure, cerebral blood flow, and outcome. J Neurotrauma 2002;19:559–571

14

Neurophysiology in the Neurosurgical Intensive Care Unit: Options, Indications, and Interpretations

Dennis Cramer, Dan Miulli, and Javed Siddiqi

Case Study

A 70-year-old male, who works as a musician in an orchestra, is undergoing resection of a right cerebello-pontine angle mass. Monitoring for the operation includes brainstem auditory evoked response (BAER) and somatosensory evoked potentials (SSEP). During the resection there is an increase in SSEP latency by 50% in the left upper extremity and left lower extremity. BAER detects a prolonged III-V inter-peak latency on the right.

See page 195 for Case Management.

◆ Electroencephalogram

The electroencephalogram (EEG) records the sum of neuronal activity within the pyramidal layer of the cerebral cortex.[1] The electrode system uses channels (two electrodes per channel) arranged in different combinations, termed montages. Each channel reflects the summation of both excitatory and inhibitory potentials produced by the cell membranes between the two electrodes. EEG monitoring can be effectively used in[2]

◆ Seizure monitoring and differentiation
◆ Intracranial pressure (ICP) monitoring
◆ Hydrocephalus
◆ Postoperative monitoring
◆ Cerebral perfusion alterations
◆ Monitoring effectiveness of ischemia therapy

The four basic frequency patterns generated by the brain are referred to as beta, alpha, theta, and delta. Beta is associated with acts of mental concentration, alpha can be found in relaxed patients who have their eyes closed, theta waveforms are often seen during general anesthesia and rapid eye movement (REM) sleep, and delta is most often pathologic or representative of deep sleep (**Fig. 14–1**).

The EEG electrodes are attached in a standardized fashion, termed the International 10–20 system (**Fig. 14–2**). Even-numbered electrodes are on

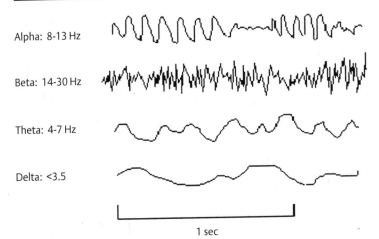

Alpha: 8-13 Hz

Beta: 14-30 Hz

Theta: 4-7 Hz

Delta: <3.5

1 sec

Figure 14–1 The four basic frequency patterns generated by the brain, as seen in electroencephalogram (EEG) readings.

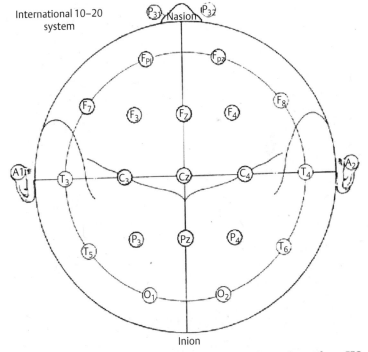

Figure 14–2 The international 10–20 system of electrode attachment for an EEG.

the patient's right and odd-numbered electrodes on the left, while electrodes with a *z* are midline. The letters used are *P* for parietal attachment, *T* for temporal, *O* for occipital, *F* for frontal, and *A* for auricular.

The signal processing in an EEG machine converts the voltage versus time plot to one of frequency plus power versus time. An EEG can filter out extraneous electrical input (i.e., 60 Hz interference) but not physiological "noise" (i.e., cardiac activity). This should be taken into account during analysis. When examining an EEG tracing, the key considerations are the patient's degree of alertness during the recording and any increased or decreased waveform, particularly if localized to specific channels, which can then be correlated to specific cerebral locations. A normal adult tracing is shown in **Fig. 14–3**, and common pathological tracings are depicted in **Fig. 14–4 (A–D)**.

Burst Suppression

Burst suppression is an abnormal pattern characterized by bursts of higher voltage sharp wave (8–12 Hz) and slow wave (1–4 Hz) activity appearing out of a background of relatively suppressed voltage. A flurry of activity is seen, followed by a period of electrical silence on the tracing. This can be seen during high-dose anesthesia administration. A common use of burst suppression monitoring is the titration of neuroprotective medications. The end point of titration is the induction of the burst suppression

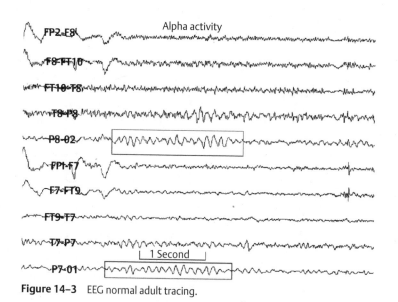

Figure 14–3   EEG normal adult tracing.

pattern on the EEG (**Fig. 14–5**). Common burst suppression doses are listed here:[3]

- *Pentobarbital:* 10 mg/kg load, then 1 to 3 mg/kg/hour
- *Midazolam:* 200 µg/kg as a slow intravenous (IV) bolus, followed by 0.75 to 10.0 µg/kg/minute
- *Etomidate:* 0.4 to 0.5 mg/kg
- *Propofol:* 1 mg/kg loading dose, titrate down rapidly starting at 20 mg/kg/hour

◆ Somatosensory Evoked Potentials

Somatosensory evoked potentials (SSEPs) allow for the monitoring of the spinal cord and peripheral nerves, as well as both cortical and subcortical structures. The evoked potential is generated when repetitive stimuli are applied to a peripheral nerve. Responses are then recorded centrally. Common nerves used are the median, ulnar, common peroneal, and posterior tibial. SSEPs are less affected by anesthesia than EEG and are more sensitive indicators of ischemia than EEG monitoring. SSEP waveforms move in parallel to regional blood flow and reflect changes when blood flow falls to near critical levels. It is notable to point out that SSEPs can be affected by medical equipment generating strong electrical fields (i.e., if a computed tomography [CT] scanner is next door to the neurosurgical intensive care unit [NICU]). A finding requiring investigating in SSEPs is an amplitude reduction by more than 50% or increase in latency by 1 msec.[4,5]

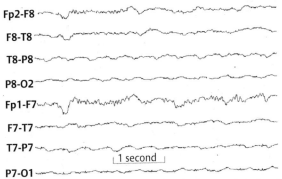

Figure 14–4   EEG pathological tracings: **(A)** alpha coma, (*Continued on pages 184 to 186*)

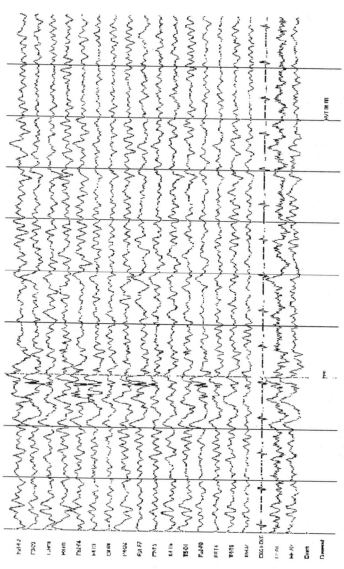

Figure 14–4 *(Continued)* **(B)** bifrontal partial epilepsy, and

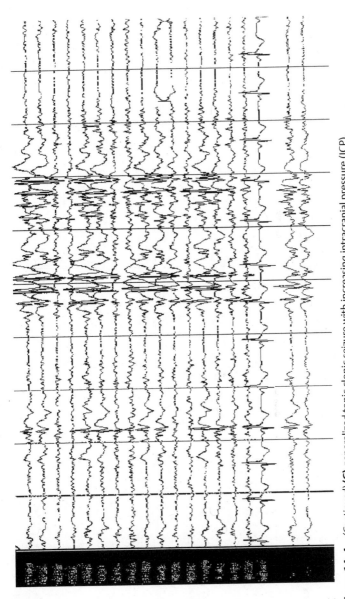

Figure 14–4 *(Continued)* **(C)** generalized tonic-clonic seizure with increasing intracranial pressure (ICP).

C

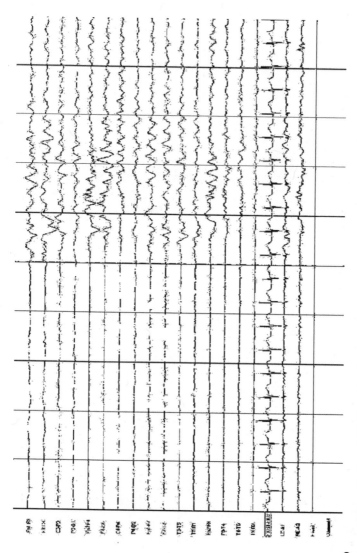

Figure 14–4 *(Continued)* **(D)** Closed head injury with increased intracranial pressure.

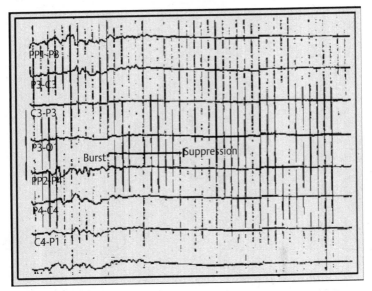

Figure 14–5   EEG burst suppression pattern.

SSEPs have the following NICU applications:[4]

- Differentiating preganglionic versus postganglionic injury
- Evaluating peripheral nerve trauma and postoperative progress
- Evaluating postsurgical premotor and motor strip operations
- Investigating postoperative paraplegia after posterior spinal fusion
- Evaluating the comatose patient

Limitations of SSEPs

SSEPs can be poor in predicting function in areas of the brain not involved with the somatosensory pathways.

Predictive Value of SSEPs

SSEPs have been used in evaluating the predicted prognosis of spinal cord injured (SCI) patients in many studies. The tibial or common peroneal nerves are used, and the latency times are compared to those of normal subjects (**Fig. 14–6A**). Further delineation between ischemic and traumatic SCI patients allows for more specifically tailored outcome. The outcome after rehabilitation can also be predicted using SSEPs (**Fig. 14–6B**).[6]

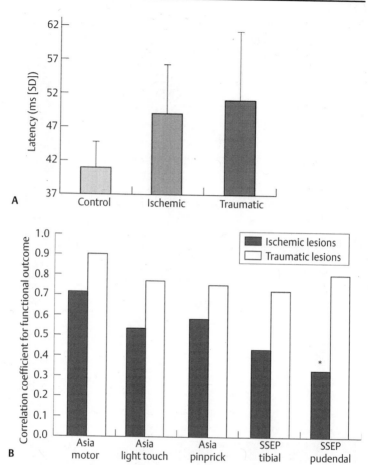

Figure 14–6   Predictive value of somatosensory evoked potentials (SSEPs) from tibial or common peroneal nerve latency in groups of patients. (**A**) Comparison of SSEPs for normal (control) subjects with those from ischemic or traumatic spinal cord–injured (SCI) subjects. (**B**) SSEPs can help predict outcomes for ischemic versus traumatic SCI subjects.

Fig. 14–7 shows a normal median nerve SSEP. The labels used stand for Erb's point (EP), a negative dorsal cervical spine potential (N13), a negative potential recorded from the contralateral scalp (N20), and a positive scalp potential (P22). The overlapping of tracings occurs as the previous tracing is retained while a new evoked potential is written over it for comparison. Each nerve has its own physiologic limits on the SSEP. The criteria for an abnormal study are prolonged central conduction time,[1] abnormal internerve (right-left) central

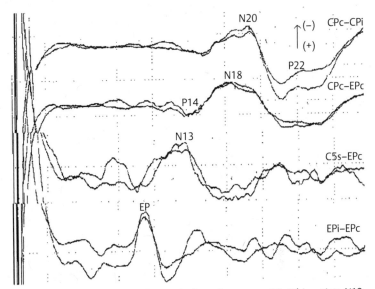

Figure 14–7 SSEP tracing of a normal median nerve. EP, Erb's point; N13, negative dorsal cervical spine potential; N20, negative potential recorded from the contralateral scalp; P22, positive scalp potential.

conduction time difference,[2] and absent EP, N13, N18, or N20 waves.[3] A typical value for the upper limit of normal for an EP-N20 is ~11 msec.

◆ Electromyelogram

The electromyelogram (EMG) captures electrical activity produced by the depolarization of muscle membrane. Most data regarding EMG usage are derived from the large number of studies that have been done on the facial nerve during acoustic neuroma removal. EMGs may be used to monitor[7]

- ◆ Cranial nerve functioning
- ◆ Spinal nerve roots

Interpretation of EMG Results

When a nerve is electrically excited using EMG, the signal is displayed visually, and the output can be coupled to a speaker for auditory feedback during a procedure. **Fig. 14–8** shows the spectrum of EMG discharge types that are encountered during passive nerve monitoring.

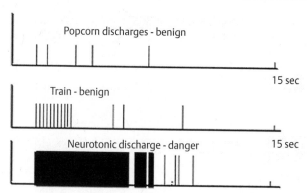

Figure 14–8 Spectrum of EMG discharge types that are encountered during passive nerve monitoring.

No activity in an intact nerve is the best situation. The "popcorn" discharge is commonly caused by mechanical stimulation of the nerve. Sustained muscle activity indicates serious nerve irritation. The neurotonic discharge is indicative of serious nerve trauma. The amplitude of the EMG potentials shows how many nerve fibers are activated; accordingly, a reduction in amplitude indicates a conduction block. Anesthesia can induce spontaneous nerve discharge, which can mimic neurotonic discharge.[8]

◆ Transcranial Doppler Ultrasound

Transcranial Doppler ultrasound has been regarded as the earliest detector of impending damage because it detects blood flow abnormalities prior to ischemic injury. This noninvasive monitor is used in the early postoperative period to evaluate middle cerebral artery (MCA) flow for signs of velocity increases and pulsatile changes.[9] These early changes are predictive of an intracerebral hemorrhage (ICH) before the symptoms of headache or hypertension. Cerebral vasospasm can be assessed by comparing the ratio of blood flow in the MCA and the ICA (the Lindegaard ratio). This differentiates hyperemia from true vasospasm.

Table 14–1 outlines the interpretation of values for the Lindegaard ratio.[4,10] **Table 14–2** lists the clinical applications of transcranial Doppler ultrasound.[11]

Recommendations for patients with subarachnoid hemorrhage (SAH) are as follows: if no vasospasm is detected by day 7–8 in patients with grade I SAH, transcranial Doppler ultrasound is usually discontinued. Transcranial Doppler ultrasound is performed every other day after days 8 through 10 in patients with higher SAH grades and no spasm.

Table 14–1   Lindegaard Ratio Interpretation[9–11]

0–3 Normal
3–6 Mild vasospasm
>6 Severe vasospasm

Table 14–2   Clinical Applications of Trancranial Doppler Ultrasound[9–11]

Applications	Rating	Evidence	
		Quality	Strength
Sickle cell disease	Effective	Class I	Type A
Ischemic cerebrovascular disease	Established	Class II	Type B
Subarachnoid hemorrhage	Established	Class II	Type B
Arteriovenous malformations	Established	Class III	Type C
Cerebral circulatory arrest	Established	Class III	Type C
Perioperative monitoring	Possibly useful	Class III	Type C
Meningeal infection	Possibly useful	Class III	Type C
Periprocedural monitoring	Investigational	Class III	Type C
Migraine	Doubtful	Class II	Type D
Cerebral venous thrombosis	Doubtful	Class III	Type D

◆ Brainstem Auditory Evoked Response

The brainstem pathway for the auditory system includes the cochlea, spiral ganglion, eighth cranial nerve (CN VIII), cochlear nucleus (lower pons), superior olivary nucleus (lower $^3/_5$ of pons), lateral lemniscus (upper pons), inferior colliculus (midbrain), and medial geniculate body (thalamus). Input from CN VIII ascends both ipsilateral and contralateral, and there are crossing fibers at each level.

Small ear inserts placed in the external auditory canal (EAC) apply a stimulus in which the patient hears a clicking noise or tone bursts. These bursts are recorded from electrodes placed on the scalp along the vertex and on each earlobe. The brainstem auditory evoked response (BAER; also known as the auditory brainstem response, evoked auditory potential, brainstem auditory evoked potential, and evoked response audiometry) consists of five waves (I, II, III, IV, and V). Waves I, III, and V are the most robust of the waveforms. The absolute and interpeak latencies, amplitude, and overall morphology of the waves are measured and evaluated. The auditory brainstem values have a normal range, which varies among patients and instruments used. It may be difficult to differentiate the origins of waves II to V because of the relatively small area of the auditory structures. The localization errors are ~1 cm at worst.[12]

Indications for BAER in the NICU

Indications for the use of BAER in the NICU are

- Lateralization of pathology
- Hearing loss (including Meniere's disease)
- Neoplasms of the brainstem (including the cerebellopontine angle)
- Multiple sclerosis
- Central pontine myelinolysis
- Leukodystrophies and other degenerative diseases of the central nervous system
- Infarctions and ischemia
- Pontine hemorrhages
- Screening for ototoxic drugs
- Coma and brain death

Abnormal auditory brainstem response findings may consist of delays in the absolute latency times of the individual waves, or an increased latency time between waves I to V, or waves I to III, or waves III to V. Poor wave morphology is also considered to be abnormal (**Tables 14–3, 14–4, 14–5,** and **14–6; Figs. 14–9** and **14–10**).

Table 14–3 Anatomical Correlations to BAER[12]

Wave	Location
I	Auditory nerve
II	Cochlear nucleus
III	Superior olive
IV	Lateral lemnisci
V	Inferior colliculus

BAER, brainstem auditory evoked response.

Table 14–4 BAER Montage[12]

BAER channel	Recorded waveform location
Channel 1	Ai-CZ
Channel 2	Ac-CZ
Channel 3	Ai-Ac
Channel 4	Inion-CZ

Ai and Ac refer to earlobe ipsilateral and earlobe contralateral, respectively, to the ear being stimulated.
CZ, center, midline, midplane between earlobes.

Table 14–5   BAER Reference Values[12]

Wave	Mean latency (ms)	Range (ms)
Wave I	1.62	1.26–1.98
Wave II	2.80	2.23–3.37
Wave III	3.75	3.24–4.26
Wave IV	4.84	4.15–5.53
Wave IV/V	5.27	4.61–5.93
Wave V	5.62	4.93–6.31
	Female	**Male**
I–V (age ≤ 60 years)	<4.60	<4.65
I–V (age > 60 years)	<4.70	<4.75
I–III	2.63	
I–IV/V	4.32	
III–V	2.31	

Table 14–6   Interpretation of BAER Results[12]

Wave finding	Interpretation
Abnormal I–III IPL	This abnormality suggests the presence of a conduction defect in the brainstem auditory system between the CN VIII close to the cochlea and the lower pons.
Abnormal III–V IPL	This abnormality suggests the presence of a conduction defect in the brainstem auditory system between the lower pons and the midbrain.
I absent and III–V is normal	Wave I (CN VIII activation potential) could not be recorded. This is usually due to a peripheral hearing disorder. Because of this, the state of conduction in the brainstem auditory pathway between peripheral CN VIII and lower pons could not be determined. Lower pons to midbrain conduction was normal.
IV or V absent or of abnormally low amplitude	This abnormality suggests the presence of a conduction defect in the brainstem auditory system rostral to the lower pons.
Absent II, III, IV, and V with normal I	This abnormality indicates a significant lack of function in brainstem auditory tracts.

BAER, brainstem auditory evoked response; CN, cranial nerve; IPL, interpeak latency.

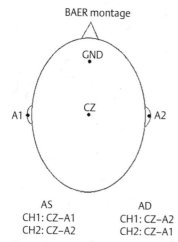

AS
CH1: CZ–A1
CH2: CZ–A2

AD
CH1: CZ–A2
CH2: CZ–A1

Figure 14–9 Brainsterm auditory evoked response (BAER) montage.

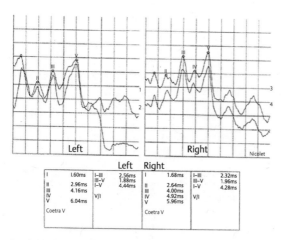

Left			Right		
I	1.60ms	I–III 2.56ms	I	1.68ms	I–III 2.32ms
		III–V 1.88ms			III–V 1.96ms
II	2.96ms	I–V 4.44ms	II	2.64ms	I–V 4.28ms
III	4.16ms		III	4.00ms	
IV			IV	4.92ms	
V	6.04ms	V/I	V	5.96ms	V/I
Coetra V			Coetra V		

Normal adult ABR waveform response. I–V absolute latencies and interpeak intervals (I–III, III–V, I–V) are within normal limits bilaterally. Interaural differences for the I–V interpeak intervals (.16ms) and wave V absolute latencies (.08ms) are within normal limits.

Figure 14–10 Normal adult auditory brainstem response (ABR) waveforms.

Case Management

In this patient, the change in BAER reflects an abnormality between the midbrain and lower pons. The SSEP localizes the change to an area above the pyramidal decussation, possibly due to ischemia. Possible etiologies for the monitoring changes include vascular injury, increased edema from venous damage compression, retractor injury, increased iatrogenic compression, use of cold water irrigation, or decreased blood flow. First blood pressure and oxygenation should be addressed through the anesthesiologist; then, the temperature of the irrigation must be checked. Ideally, the surgeon may need to stop till an explanation for the changes is available.

References

1. Youman JR. Neurological Surgery: A Comprehensive Reference Guide to the Diagnosis and Management of Neurosurgical Problems. 4th ed. Philadelphia: WB Sanders; 1996:402–430
2. Vespa PM, Nenov V, Nuwer MR. Continuous EEG monitoring in the intensive care unit. J Clin Neurophysiol 1999;16:1–13
3. Jordan KG. Continuous EEG monitoring in the neurosciences intensive care unit and emergency department. J Clin Neurophysiol 1999;16:14–39
4. Greenberg MS. Handbook of Neurosurgery. 5th ed. New York: Thieme; 2001: 549–552
5. Czosnyka M, Kirkpatrick PJ, Pickard JD. Multimodal monitoring and assessment of cerebral haemodynamic reserve after severe head injury. Cerebrovasc Brain Metab Rev 1996;8:273–295
6. Iseli E, Cavigelli A, Dietz V, Curt A. Prognosis and recovery in ischaemic and traumatic spinal cord injury: clinical and electrophysiological evaluation. J Neurol Neurosurg Psychiatry 1999;67:567–571
7. Houlden DA, Schwartz ML, Klettke KA. Neurophysiologic diagnosis in uncooperative trauma patients: confounding factors. J Trauma 1992;33:244–251
8. Murthy JM. Somatosensory evoked potentials by paraspinal stimulation in acute transverse myelitis. Neurol India 1999;47:108–111
9. Wilterdink JL, Feldmann E, Furie KL, et al. Transcranial Doppler ultrasound battery reliably identifies severe internal carotid artery stenosis. Stroke 1997;28:133–136
10. Report of the American Academy of Neurology, Therapeutics and Technology Assessment Subcommittee. Assessment: transcranial Doppler. Neurology 1990;40:680–681
11. Aaslid R, Huber P, Nornes H. Evaluation of cerebrovascular spasm with transcranial Doppler ultrasound. J Neurosurg 1984;60(1):37–41
12. Chiappa KH. Evoked Potentials in Clinical Medicine. 3rd ed. Philadelphia: Lippincott-Raven; 1997:199–268

15

Cerebral Perfusion

Dan Miulli and Javed Siddiqi

Case Study

A 20-year-old male presents after a fall from a second-story window with obvious contusions to his chest, abdomen, and head. At the scene of the accident, he does not open his eyes or talk, and he exhibits extensor/decerebrate posturing. His pupils are equal and sluggishly reactive. There is no obvious distension or rigidity of the abdomen. His blood pressure is 90/50.

See page 207 for Case Management.

◆ Blood–Brain Barrier

The brain capillary varies from the systemic capillary by several unique features; these establish the blood–brain barrier. The brain capillary endothelial cells are the distinguishing elements of the blood–brain barrier. The brain capillary endothelial cells are not fenestrated, lack intracellular clefts, and are closed by intercellular tight gap junctions. The tight gap junctions of the brain capillary endothelial cells assist in keeping substances out of the brain interstitial space. The body systemic capillary endothelial cells are not in contact with one another; they do not make a circumferential ring barrier but instead have multiple fenestrations that allow fluid to pass freely.

The circumferential ring of brain capillary endothelial cells regulates which substances reach the brain's interstitial space, the supporting astrocytes, and the neurons. In an intact blood–brain barrier, all substances pass through the capillary endothelial cell and the other regulator, the choroid plexus epithelial cell. The blood–brain barrier regulates the biochemical, immunological, and electrical passage of material into the brain. The tight gap junctions, the strong intercellular connections, have a high electrical impedance, preventing ions from passing. The capillary endothelial cells exclude plasma proteins from the brain interstitial space because the endothelial cells have very little pinocytic vesicles to transport the proteins and contain unique cerebral enzymes, cellular channels, and transport systems. The brain capillary endothelial cells require large amounts of energy to serve as the complex regulatory interface between the brain and the blood circulation. The brain capillary endothelial cell energy dependent transport organizations have 3 to 5 times the amount of mitochondria as the systemic capillary cells. Maintaining the blood–brain barrier's unique functions, the brain capillary membrane has a different structural surface, and its lack of permeability is assisted by pericytes and astrocytic foot process.

The pericyte or perivascular cells are not unique to the brain; they are found partially wrapping systemic capillaries and venules in endothelial cells. The selective permissiveness into the brain interstitial space is not present in the neural hypophysis, subfornicele organ, median eminence, area postrema, and pineal gland (**Table 15–1**).[1,2]

Brain Interstitial Circulation

In the normal state, for substances to pass from the blood to the brain interstitial space, they must pass through the capillary endothelial cell. The brain capillary endothelial cell allows certain compounds to pass with relative ease into the brain interstitial space via transcellular diffusion or ubiquitous transport mechanisms. These substances are lipid soluble, low molecular weight of ~500 daltons or less, nonpolarized, and not bound to proteins. Such substances include glucose, low-density lipoproteins, transferrin, bromide, morphine, and bile salts. These substances when not actively transported must still diffuse down a concentration gradient from blood to capillary endothelial cell to brain interstitial space. The blood–brain barrier is not permeable to ions and amino acids, and the exact type of permeability to water is controversial. Water does not enter through a lipid membrane but must pass through selective water channels regulated by aquaporins. The blood–brain barrier excludes water-soluble molecules with a molecular weight greater than 180 daltons. It is not permeable to vital dyes, epinephrine, curare, bile pigments, and fluorescein. Substances that enter the brain interstitial space fluid could alter nervous system function. These substances pass from the blood–brain capillary to the interstitial space, where they may be absorbed by neurons, glial cells,

Table 15–1   Blood–Brain Barrier Characteristics: The Brain Capillary Endothelial Cell[1-3]

Tight gap junction	Different membrane structure
Basement membrane	Neuronal enzymes
Minimal pinocytic activity	Transport mechanisms
High mitochondrial content	Pericytes (also seen in systemic circulation)
High electrical impedance	Astrocytic foot process

or others; they then pass through, but sometimes around, subependymal glial cells and ependymal gap junctions into the cerebrospinal fluid (CSF) of the ventricles, cisterns, and Virchow-Robin spaces, where they eventually circulate back into the blood via the arachnoid villi.[1–3]

Blood–Cerebrospinal Fluid Barrier

The choroid plexus epithelial circumferential junction actively secretes substances into the CSF. The blood–CSF barrier is similar to the blood–brain barrier of the capillary endothelial cell. Substances dissolved in the choroid capillary blood pass more easily through the choroid endothelium, are selectively passed by the connective tissue of the choroid plexus, and then are regulated by the choroid epithelium. The choroid epithelial cells contain circumferential junctions, which must secrete CSF into the ventricle. The CSF acts as a sink for the brain interstitial fluid, with a gradient of substances carrying components away from the interstitial space.

Blood–Brain Barrier Disruption

Diseases of the nervous system disrupt the blood–brain barrier, resulting in most of the devastation. The barrier is disrupted by hypertension, hypercapnia, hypocapnia, trauma, hyperthermia, chemicals such as intra-arterial lactated Ringer's, mannitol, leukotriene C_4, nitric oxide synthetase, arabinose, and lactamide, as well as in the center of tumors, but necessarily in the periphery. The disrupted blood–brain barrier leads to brain edema, accumulation of fluids and electrolytes, increased cerebral volume, increased intracranial pressure (ICP), cellular swelling, and cell death. There are many studies of brain edema in a variety of pathologies. However, there is a clinical situation that, when thoroughly understood, will clarify most questions about the blood–brain barrier and cerebral edema. That situation is head trauma.

Vasogenic Edema

At the moment of impact, the blood–brain barrier's tight gap junctions are stretched, which essentially turns the brain capillary for ~30 to 60 minutes into a sieve, leading to vasogenic edema. There is accumulation of serum, albumin, and proteins. The opening is also prolonged for an unknown duration by hypoxia and for a single time of 6 hours by a hypertension surge. The mechanical disruption traumatizes microvessels, cells, and cellular organelles, releasing calcium, ornithine decarboxylase, and free radicals. Sustained increases of free radicals meant to oxidize toxins will disrupt the cellular membrane. An increase in intracellular and extracellular stores of calcium will be sustained by hypoxia.

The activity of ornithine decarboxylase is increased 2000% due to up-regulation of its messenger ribonucleic acid (mRNA).[4] It acts to decarboxylate ornithine forming putrescine, which is then converted into spermidine, then finally into spermine. All three are released immediately after cellular injury because of the necessity for regeneration, development, cell growth, and neuronal survival. Putrescine accumulation induces shrinkage in cerebral microvessels after trauma, opening the blood–brain barrier and increasing vasogenic edema. Putrescine can be increased by isoflurane and decreased by ketamine.

Bradykinins are released, which, with other pathway products, increase calcium at the time of mechanical disruption. This calcium increases calcium-calmodulin and calcium protein kinase C and opens the blood–brain barrier.

The disrupted blood–brain barrier is stabilized by dexamethasone, copper, zinc, superoxide dismutase, serotonin antibodies, and progesterone.

Cytotoxic Edema

The most common type of edema after head injury, cytotoxic edema, occurs in the cell 30 to 60 minutes after insult as a response to the intracellular accumulation of the toxic levels of lactate, hydrogen-ion acidosis, potassium, oxygen free radicals, and glutamate, among others. The sodium potassium adenosinetriphosphatase (ATPase) pump fails secondary to depletion of cellular energy, allowing sodium to build up intracellularly and drawing in water. Hydrogen accumulation is the most common reason for buffering the cell by increasing the water content. The cell osmotically swells, reacting to the increasing glycogen granules that are sequestered to provide more substrate to the tricarboxylic acid (TCA) cycle. The additional energy is required to supply cellular active transport mechanisms, which include

- Sodium potassium ATPase
- Sodium potassium chloride cotransporter
- Calcium-activated potassium channels
- Sodium hydrogen antiporter
- Chloride bicarbonate exchanger
- Carrier-mediated transport of nutrients
- Receptor-mediated transport of peptides

As the cellular membrane starts to fail, glutamate is released, increasing cellular metabolism, which, under its current anaerobic conditions, leads to further lactate production and, without utilization, accumulation and then to failure of energy metabolism and cell death.[3]

Interstitial Edema

Interstitial fluid drains down the gradient into the CSF sink. That sink begins to get clogged with toxins and proteins. CSF production is increased to buffer the brain interstitial fluid acidosis run off by up-regulation of the chloride bicarbonate exchanger. One method to decrease interstitial edema and the major contributor to traumatic brain injury cytotoxic edema is by decreasing the sink into which brain fluid drains. Decreasing the CSF in the

Table 15–2 Means to Decrease Brain Edema[1-3,6]

Type of edema	Means to decrease
Cytotoxic (the most common type in head injury)	Alpha-difluoromethylornithine, α-trinositol, amiloride, THAM
Vasogenic	CuZn SOD, 5HT1B, progesterone, indomethacin, naloxone, dexamethasone, CSF drainage
Interstitial	CSF drainage, acetazolamide

CSF, cerebrospinal fluid; CuZn SOD, copper-zinc superoxide dismutase; THAM, tris-(hydroxymethyl)-aminomethane.

ventricles does this; decreasing the pressure of the intracranial contents does not.

There is no silver bullet to treat brain injury. Fortunately, the brain can adapt and recover from multiple insults. Brain injury occurs because several innate brain systems fail to compensate for the overwhelming insult. Currently, there are experimental chemicals that are available to ameliorate different types of edema (**Table 15–2**).[5]

The aim of aggressive early treatment is to prevent ischemia. Glucose and glycogen are depleted in 4 minutes; there is increased metabolism in the layer surrounding the ischemic penumbra, the brain temperature increases, metabolism increases, and brain tissue pO_2 drops to less than 20 mm Hg, favoring anaerobic respiration. Anaerobic respiration causes lactic acidosis and brings hydrogen into the cell. Lactate accumulation approximates glucose stores at the time of ischemia. The cell swells in response to increasing levels of hydrogen. Multiple neuromodulators stimulate cyclic adenosine monophsphate (cAMP)–dependent ion transport, bringing more hydrogen into the cell. The ischemia leads to the cellular pH dropping to 6.0 to 6.4, inhibiting mitochondrial respiration and the ability to sequester calcium. When the cell is deprived of energy and oxygen, calcium stores are released, stimulating phosphorylation of protein kinase C and further increasing intracellular hydrogen in a vicious cycle, leading to degradation of cell membranes. Therefore, increasing cerebral blood flow in excess of edema is necessary to increase oxygen delivery.

◆ Cerebral Blood Flow

Cerebral blood flow (CBF) averages 45 to 65 mL/100 g/minute (55 mL/100 g/minute used by most references), being higher in gray matter (75–80 mL/100 g/minute) and somewhat less in white matter (20–30 mL/100 g/minute). Changes occur sooner when the entire CBF is affected compared to changes in regional CBF. Protein synthesis declines at 40 to 50 mL/100 g/minute, and anaerobic glycolysis at 35 mL/100 g/minute. Drastic elec-troencephalography (EEG) changes of absent activity are seen as early as 25 mL/100 g/minute; however, brainstem auditory evoked responses (BAERs) occur at 12 mL/100 g/minute, and loss of transcellular function begins at 10 to 20 mL/100 g/minute and anoxic depolarization at 8 to 15 mL/100 g/minute. Brain tissue tolerates slightly lower regional CBF changes before similar effects. Of course, the duration of decreased perfusion also differen-tiates ischemia from infarction.[6]

Cerebral Vascular Resistance

The physiology of cerebral vascular resistance (CVR) differs from the sys-temic circulation. One half of the systemic mean arterial pressure (MAP) is lost just distal to the cerebral arteries and arterioles. CVR is complex and neither always proportional nor linear to cerebral perfusion pressure (CPP). Therefore, knowing CPP does not allow direct calculation of CBF. CVR varies with edema, $PaCO_2$, and a host of other conditions. Under normal steady state conditions, autoregulation occurs as CVR varies with CPP to maintain a constant CBF. However, during extremes of pathological states, or extremes of autoregulation, CVR cannot vary enough. Between a CPP of 50 and 125 mm Hg, the blood vessel dilates and constricts to maintain constant CBF. At CPP of 50 to 60 mm Hg, the blood vessel is maximally dilated, and further decrease in CPP only results in decreased CBF. Likewise, at a CPP of 125 mm Hg, the blood vessel is maximally constricted. Any further increase in CPP is similar to increasing the flow through a rigid tube. This will cause vasogenic edema as the tight gap junctions are split apart. The amount of autoregulation or the amount of CVR changes daily, hourly, and by the minute. During head trauma, unless secondary injury occurs, or hypoten-sion, ischemia, or hyperventilation, autoregulation is maintained but shift-ed to the left.[7] To date there is no direct way to continuously measure CVR. Criteria are being developed utilizing transcranial Doppler ultrasound, its pulsatile index and resistance, in an attempt to quantify CVR and CBF, as given here:

$$CBF = CPP/CVR = MAP - ICP/CVR$$

Hypotension

After severe head injury around contusions, in punctate hemorrhages CBF cannot be maintained. CBF drops to less than 20 mL/100 g/minute and remains less than 30 mL/100 g/minute during the first 8 to 24 hours. It remains lowest under subdural hematomas and diffuse axonal injuries and, as expected, with hypotension. However, it is not only low around the area of injury; globally, it can be decreased to half the normal level after injury. A single episode of hypotension doubles the morbidity and mortality associat-ed with severe head injury. Hypotension leads to vasodilation 165% above baseline, increasing cerebral blood volume and ICP. Hypotension is not used initially to treat severe head injury. Although hypertension to maintain CPP in the normal range is beneficial,[8] if CPP exceeds the upper limit of autoregulation, whether artificially changed or not, it too will increase cerebral blood volume and ICP. *Guidelines for the Management of Severe Head Injury,*[7] published by The Brain Trauma Foundation, recommends the following:

> **Guideline:** Hypotension (SBP < 90 mm Hg) or hypoxia (apnea or cyanosis in the field, PaO$_2$ < 60 mm Hg, saturation < 90%) must be scrupulously avoided, if possible, or corrected immediately

> **Option:** Mean arterial pressures should be maintained above 90 mm Hg through the infusion of fluids throughout the patient's course to attempt to maintain cerebral perfusion pressure greater than 70 mm Hg.

Systolic blood pressure and mean arterial pressure can be treated in the field. However, if there is severe head injury, the patient must be taken to a trauma center where a neurosurgeon is present. The neurosurgeon will insert an external ventricular drain (EVD) and ICP monitor.

Cerebral Perfusion Pressure

Older studies compared the CPP to mortality in the adult mostly male population and found that if the CPP was greater than 80 mm Hg the mortality at that time in history was only 35 to 40%. If the CPP was less than 80 mm Hg mortality increased for each 10 mm Hg decrease CPP yielding a mortality of 95% for a CPP less than 60 mm Hg. Other investigators also found that the single most important therapy was to keep the CPP greater than 60 mm Hg.[9] Similarly, *Guidelines for the Management of Severe Head Injury* recommends that CPP should be maintained at a minimum of 70 mm Hg.[7]

Several caveats must be made. This is the recommendation for the average adult male, not for children and not for some adult females who have a normal systolic blood pressure (SBP), let alone MAP lower than 90 mm Hg. A CPP greater than 70 mm Hg should not be maintained at the expense of causing other injuries, such as pulmonary edema and acute respiratory distress syndrome (ARDS). Hlatky et al[10] demonstrated that for maximum CPP treatment in patients with difficult-to-manage increased ICP, more fluids were used, more vasopressors were utilized, and there was a 5-fold increase in ARDS. If secondary injury is becoming apparent, and that secondary injury may decrease outcome in the management of severe head injury, then CPP should be kept above a minimum of 60 mm Hg.

When attempting to manage the patient with severe head injury, orders must be written to maintain the CPP above a certain level, such as 70 mm Hg, or a minimum of 60 mm Hg, and must be written to maintain the CPP below an upper limit. The upper limit is variable from 90 to 120 mm Hg.

Blood Pressure Management in Infarction

There is considerable debate regarding the appropriate blood pressure to maintain in a patient who has suffered ischemia or who has suffered an intracerebral hemorrhage (ICH). Lowering blood pressure extensively during cerebral ischemia can lead to infarction. Blood pressure usually increases during the first few hours after ischemia in an attempt to correct the underlying physiological problem; but once the injury has equilibrated, the blood pressure decreases within 24 hours, returning to the patient's normal level in 4 to 7 days. The rise in blood pressure does not change CBF in areas of the brain where autoregulation is intact. However, in areas of ischemia where there is decreased blood flow, it is a requirement; coupled with dysfunctional autoregulation, there is a dramatic decrease in blood flow. There are no large randomized clinical studies in humans to support this theory. Current theories for treating elevated blood pressure in acute ischemic stroke are based largely on expert opinion and vary with regard to treatment thresholds. One 16-patient randomized study demonstrated no difference in outcome in patients who underwent antihypertensive treatment versus placebo. Several reports observed and recorded data from patients who presented with ischemia and attempted to correlate the data without experimental protocol. The researchers observed that for every 20 mm Hg drop in SBP, the relative risk of worsening within 36 hours of stroke onset increased by a factor of 0.66.[11] There are several management schemes; one is to lower blood pressure by 15% over 24 hours. However, the current guidelines for management of acute post-stroke hypertension have not changed prescribing patterns. There still remains considerable disparity due to uncertainty caused by lack of evidence from randomized controlled trials.[12]

For patients with SBP >220 mm Hg or diastolic blood pressure (DBP) >120 to 140 mm Hg on two readings 5 to 10 minutes apart,

◆ Give labetalol 10 mg intravenously (IV) every 10 minutes up to 150 mg. If no response, use nitroprusside 0.5 to 10.0 µg/kg/minute.

Patients who have had a stroke and are hypertensive are at high risk for an additional stroke. Those patients should receive blood pressure treatment when elevated to 140/90 mm Hg or higher. However, the decision to treat blood pressure at these levels should be made 4 to 7 days after the return to baseline blood pressure was to be expected. Blood pressure should be gradually reduced to 120/80, the optimal level for reducing cardiovascular risk.[11]

Blood Pressure Management in Hemorrhage

Management of hemorrhagic stroke is controversial, and there is no standardized system for treatment. Some advocate lowering blood pressure to reduce the risk of bleeding, edema formation, and systemic hypertensive complications, whereas others advocate allowing blood pressure to run its natural course as a protective measure against cerebral ischemia. Current American Heart Association guidelines[13,14] recommend maintaining MAP <130 mm Hg, SBP <180 mm Hg, and CPP >70 mm Hg. Lowering SBP to <160 mm Hg in the first hours after ICH may prevent additional bleeding. Ohwaki et al[15] studied patients with ICH and hypertension. They lowered SBP to targets of 140, 150, or 160 mm Hg and followed hematoma enlargement, defined as an increase in volume of ≥140% or 12.5 cm.[3] Hematoma enlargement occurred in 16 patients. Maximum SBP was significantly associated with hematoma enlargement ($p = .0074$). Maximum SBP was independently associated with hematoma enlargement (odds ratio per mm Hg: 1.04; 95% CI, 1.01–1.07). Target SBPs of ≥160 mm Hg were significantly associated with hematoma enlargement compared to those of ≤150 mm Hg ($p = .025$).

For hypertension treatment in acute ICH,

- For patients with a history of hypertension, maintain SBP <160 mm Hg.
- For patients with no history of hypertension, maintain SBP <150 mm Hg.
- Give labetalol 10 mg IV every 10 minutes up to 150 mg.
- If no response, give enalapril 0.625 mg IV q 6 hours; may repeat 0.625 mg q 16 minutes to a total of 2.5 mg q 6 hours.

There remains some debate in treating patients with ICH on whether surgery improves perfusion and thus outcome. The STICH trial randomized 1033 patients from 83 centers and reported that patients with spontaneous supratentorial ICH in neurosurgical units show no overall benefit from early surgery when compared to initial conservative treatment.[16]

There is new evidence that ICH progression can be minimized with recombinant activated factor VII (RFVII) and consequently reduce morbidity and mortality after ICH.[17] One to three doses of 40, 80, or 160 μg/kg given within the first 3 to 4 hours after symptom onset, or in patients at risk of additional bleeding, such as those with coagulopathy, demonstrated a 3 month mortality of 18% when compared to the placebo group mortality of 29%.[18]

However, there still remain subsets of patients that may benefit from surgical evacuation of ICH. The risk for rebleed is highest in the first 3 to 6 hours and lowest after 12 hours. Waiting until the patient is herniating before surgical intervention is no better than medical management alone.

Patients who may benefit from surgery for ICH include

- Patients who are symptomatic from a cerebellar hemorrhage >3 cm or >30 cc
- Patients who have a supratentorial ICH >20 to 30 cc and who present with a Glasgow Coma Scale (GCS) score of 13–5 or a decrease of 2 GCS points (carefully weigh the decision to take the patient to surgery if the bleed is in the left deep gray matter)
- Patients with lobar ICH
- Patients with amyloid ICH, on average, do not require surgery.

The goal of surgery is volume reduction to less than 20 cc.

Finally, the question of elevated blood pressure in aneurysmal subarachnoid hemorrhage (SAH) must be addressed. There is concern that the patient may rebleed if blood pressure is high and/or pulse pressure is large. However, lower GCS patients may require higher perfusion pressures to prevent infarction.

For hypertension treatment in acute SAH:

♦ If the patient has a GCS score of 3 to 6 (World Federation of Neurological Surgeons scale[18a] grade 5) or has a history of hypertension, maintain SBP <140 mm Hg.

♦ If the patient has a GCS score >6 and no history of hypertension, maintain SBP <120 mm Hg.

At times the patient's blood pressure or CPP is too low despite adequate fluid resuscitation. There is no consensus regarding which vasopressor to use. Small-dose IV vasopressin infusion may be beneficial in patients with acute brain injuries and with unstable hemodynamics who are refractory to fluid resuscitation and catecholamine vasopressors.[19] Biestro et al[20] commented that noradrenaline at a dose of 0.5 to 5.0 mg/hour is effective and safe and might be considered the drug of choice, whereas dopamine was not as effective at a high dose of 10.0 to 42.5 μg/kg/minute, and methoxamine given as a bolus controls sudden decreases in MAP. The use of vasoconstrictor drugs to increase CPP may impair oxygenation in the ischemic penumbra and to other tissues of the body, such as the intestinal mucosa and the kidneys. Several human and animal studies suggest that norepinephrine improves CBF better than dopamine at high doses (**Table 15–3**).[21]

Table 15–3   Vasopressors Used in Hypertension Treatment in SAH[21]

Agent	Receptor stimulus	Dosage	Effects
Dopamine	B2	1–3 μg/kg/min 5 μg/kg/min	Vasodilates Increases CO and SV.
	B1	+10 μg/kg/min; titrate up to 20 μg/kg/min	Vasoconstricts
	A		
Dobutamine	B1	5–20 μg/kg/min	Increases CO/HR/SV, vasodilates
	B2		
Phenylnephrine (Neosynephrine)	A	2–180 μg/min	Vasoconstricts, increases SVR
Epinephrine	A high and B low	1–8 μg/min	Increases HR/CO/SVR
Norepinephrine (Levophed)	A mostly and B little	8–12 μg/min	Increases CO/HR/SVR
Isuprel (Isoproterenol)	B	1–4 μg/min	Vasodilates, increases HR/CO

CO, cardiac output; HR, heart rate; SAH, subarachnoid hemorrhage; SVR, systemic vascular resistance.

◆ Cerebral Oxygenation

The brain cells need oxygen and need adenosine triphosphate (ATP). In an injured state, the brain does not respond well to blood pressure or volume that is excessively elevated. Blood pressure that is too high will cause cerebral edema, bleeding, and increased ICP. Therefore, a dilemma exists as to the exact titration of therapy; this dilemma has been answered with the introduction of technology that allows the monitoring of cerebral metabolism and brain oxygenation. The literature is replete with documentation that supernormal PaO_2 improves brain tissue oxygenation and outcome in hundreds of patients.[9,22–35] The hemoglobin molecule has the capacity to carry 17 to 21 mL O_2/100 mL blood when all four binding sites are saturated. PaO_2 reflects only free oxygen molecules dissolved in plasma and not those bound to hemoglobin. Neither PaO_2 nor SaO_2 reflects total oxygen in the blood. At 100% saturation, pO_2 can be as low as 80 mm Hg; at 75% saturation, pO_2 can be as low as 40 mm Hg; and at 50% saturation, pO_2 can be as low as 27 mm Hg. It must be remembered that blood cells plus plasma carry more oxygen than can be accounted for by the hemoglobin molecule. The red blood cells (RBCs) reach only 85% of the brain cells, with plasma supplying the remainder. Treating the patient must account for decreased affinity of hemoglobin from increased temperature, pCO_2, 2,3-diphospoglycerate, and a decrease in pH. A rightward shift, by definition, causes a decrease in the affinity of hemoglobin for oxygen. This makes it harder for the hemoglobin to bind to oxygen (requiring a higher partial pressure to achieve the same oxygen saturation), but it makes it easier for the hemoglobin to release bound oxygen. Physiologically, increasing FiO_2 past the maximal saturation of hemoglobin only increases the dissolved O_2 in plasma by 2 to 3%. Furthermore, FiO_2 levels higher than 60% may be harmful when used for longer than 24 hours in adults.

Increasing PO_2 to higher levels than necessary to saturate hemoglobin drives O_2 into the oxygen-starved brain tissue. With supernormal pO_2, during the early period after severe head injury, the lactate levels in brain tissue are reduced, and outcome is improved. Brain-injured patients may benefit from 100% O_2 during the first 8 to 24 hours, PaO_2 >150 mm Hg for 2 to 4 days during peak edema, and >100% thereafter, each in an attempt to maintain brain tissue oxygenation around 40 mm Hg and not below 20 mm Hg. Cerebral tissue monitoring systems measure four areas of brain metabolism, as well as physiological information about the progression of secondary injury at the cellular level, which may indicate the onset of ischemic injury. Experiments have demonstrated good recovery with mean brain partial oxygen pressure at 39±4 mm Hg, moderate to severe disability with mean brain partial oxygen pressure at 31±5 mm Hg, and dead or vegetative disability with a mean brain partial oxygen pressure at 19±8 mm Hg.[23–35]

Cerebral perfusion must be provided in a tightly regulated manner. The blood pressure must be maintained so that appropriate CPP and CBF continue without causing additional edema, increased ICP, or bleeding. Oxygen has to be supplied in supernormal levels to prevent the ischemic penumbra from infarcting.

Case Management

A 20-year-old male presents after a fall from a second-story window with obvious contusions to his chest, abdomen, and head. At the scene, he does not open his eyes or talk, and he exhibitis extensor/decerebrate posturing. His pupils are equal and sluggishly reactive. There is no obvious distension or rigidity of the abdomen. His blood pressure is 90/50.

The patient has a GCS = 4 and is hypotensive. The patient must first be resuscitated with fluids and his GCS reassessed. If he remains at GCS $\leq$ 8 or less, an ICP monitor and a cerebral metabolic monitor should be placed. FiO_2 and blood pressure should be adjusted to maintain a brain tissue oxygenation of 40 mm Hg. The CPP should be maintained >70 and <90 mm Hg. The patient should have augmentation of blood pressure with vasopressors such as norepinephrine or low-dose dopamine if CVP is in the desired range of 6 to 8 or pulmonary capillary wedge pressure is 10 to 14 mm Hg or pulmonary artery diastolic pressure is 12 to 16 mm Hg. The patient should be placed on 100% O_2 for 8 to 24 hours.

References

1. Kandel E, Schwartz J, Jessel TH, eds. Principles of Neural Science. 3rd ed. New York: Elsevier; 1991
2. Joynt R, Griggs R. Clinical Neurology. Baltimore, MD: Lippincott-Raven; 1996
3. Youmans JR, ed. Neurological Surgery. 5th ed. Philadelphia: WB Saunders; 2004
4. Henley CM, Muszynski C, Cherian L, Robertson CS. Activation of ornithine decarboxylase and accumulation of putrescine after traumatic brain injury. J Neurotrauma 1996;13:487–496
5. Edvinsson L, Krause DN. Cerebral Blood Flow and Metabolism. 2nd ed. Philadelphia: Lippincott Williams & Wilkins; 2002
6. Narayan RK, Wilberger JE, Povlishock JT. Neurotrauma. New York: McGraw-Hill; 1994
7. Guidelines for the Management of Severe Head Injury. New York: The Brain Trauma Foundation; 2000
8. Bouma GJ, Muizelaar JP. Relationship between cardiac output and cerebral blood flow in patients with intact and with impaired autoregulation. J Neurosurg 1990;73:368–374
9. Kiening K, Hartl R, Unterberg A, Schneider G, Bardt T, Lanksch W. Brain tissue pO_2 monitoring in comatose patients: implications for therapy. Neurol Res 1997;19:233–240
10. Hlatky R, Valadka AB, Robertson CS. Intracranial hypertension and cerebral ischemia after severe traumatic brain injury. Neurosurg Focus 2003;14:e2
11. Cohen S. Management of ischemic stroke. New York: McGraw-Hill; 2000
12. Kanji S, Corman C, Douen AG. Blood pressure management in acute stroke: comparison of current guidelines with prescribing patterns. Can J Neurol Sci 2002;29:125–131
13. Broderick J, Adams H, Barsan W, et al. Guidelines for the management of spontaneous intracerebral hemorrhage. Stroke 1999;30:905–915
14. Qureshi A, Tuhrim S, Broderick J, Batjer H, Hondo H, Hanley D. Spontaneous intracerebral hemorrhage. N Engl J Med 2001;344:1450–1460
15. Ohwaki K, Yano E, Nagashima H, Hirata M, Nakagomi T, Tamura A. Blood pressure management in acute intracerebral hemorrhage: relationship between elevated blood pressure and hematoma enlargement. Stroke 2004;35:1364–1367

16. Mendelow AD, Gregson BA, Fernandes HM, et al. STICH investigators; early surgery versus initial conservative treatment in patients with spontaneous supratentorial intracerebral haematomas in the International Surgical Trial in Intracerebral Haemorrhage (STICH): a randomised trial. Lancet 2005;365:387–397

17. Grotta JC. Management of primary hypertensive hemorrhage of the brain. Curr Treat Options Neurol 2004;6:435–442

18. Mayer SA, Brun NC, Begtrup K, et al. Recombinant activated factor VIIHTI: recombinant activated factor VII for acute intracerebral hemorrhage. N Engl J Med 2005;352:777–785

18a. Drake CG. Report of World Federation of Neurological Surgeons Committee on a universal subarachnoid hemorrhage grading scale. J Neurosurg 1988;68:985–986

19. Yeh CC, Wu CT, Lu CH, Yang CP, Wong CS. Early use of small-dose vasopressin for unstable hemodynamics in an acute brain injury patient refractory to catecholamine treatment: a case report. Anesth Analg 2003;97:577–579

20. Biestro A, Barrios E, Baraibar J, et al. Use of vasopressors to raise cerebral perfusion pressure in head injured patients. Acta Neurochir Suppl (Wien) 1998;71:5–9

21. Kroppenstedt SN, Sakowitz OW, Thomale UW, Unterberg AW, Stover JF. Influence of norepinephrine and dopamine on cortical perfusion, EEG activity, extracellular glutamate, and brain edema in rats after controlled cortical impact injury. J Neurotrauma 2002;19:1421–1432

22. Sheinberg M, Kanter M, Robertson C, et al. Continuous monitoring of jugular venous oxygen saturation in head injured patients. J Neurosurg 1992;76:212–217

23. Van Santbrink H, Maas A, Avezaat C. Continuous monitoring of partial pressure of brain tissue oxygen in patients with severe head injury. Neurosurg 1996;38:21–31

24. Zauner A, Doppenberg E, Woodward J, Choi S, Young H, Bullock R. Continuous monitoring of cerebral substrate delivery and clearance: initial experience in 24 patients with severe acute brain injuries. Neurosurg 1997;41:1082–1093

25. Kiening KL, Schneider GH, Bardt TF, Unterberg AW, Lanksch WR. Bifrontal measurements of brain tissue-pO_2 in comatose patients. Acta Neurochir (Wien) 1998;71:172–173

26. Zauner A, Doppenberg J, Soukup J, Menzel M, Young H, Bullock R. Extended neuromonitoring: new therapeutic opportunities. Neurol Res 1998;20:S85–S90

27. Menzel M, Doppenberg E, Zauner A, et al. Increased inspired oxygen concentration as a factor in improved brain tissue oxygenation and tissue lactate levels after severe human head injury. J Neurosurg 1999;91:1–10

28. Menzel M, Doppenberg E, Zauner A, et al. Cerebral oxygenation in patients after severe head injury monitoring the effects of arterial hyperoxia on cerebral blood flow, metabolism, and intracranial pressure. J Neurosurg Anesthesiol 1999;11:240–251

29. Manley G, Pitts L, Morabito D, et al. Brain tissue oxygenation during hemorrhagic shock, resuscitation, and alterations in ventilation. J Trauma 1999;46:261–267

30. Van den Brink W, van Santbrink H, Steyerberg E, et al. Brain oxygen tension in severe head injury. Neurosurg 2000;46:868–876

31. Rockswold SB, Rockswold GL, Vargo JM, et al. Effects of hyperbaric oxygenation therapy on cerebral metabolism and intracranial pressure in severely brain injured patients. J Neurosurg 2001;94:403–411

32. Longhi L, Valeriani V, Rossi S, De Marchi M, Egidi M, Stocchetti N. Effects of hyperoxia on brain tissue oxygen tension in cerebral focal lesions. Acta Neurochir Suppl (Wien) 2002;81:315–317

33. Reinert M, Alessandri B, Seiler R, Bullock R. Influence of inspired oxygen on glucose lactate dynamics after subdural hematoma in the rat. Neurol Res 2002; 24:601–606

34. Reinart M, Barth A, Rothen H, Schaller B, Takala J, Seiler R. effects of cerebral perfusion pressure and increased fraction of inspired oxygen on brain tissue oxygen, lactate and glucose in patients with severe head injury. Acto Neurochir 2003;145:341–350

35. Tolias C, Reinert M, Seiler R, Gilman C, Scharf A, Bullock R. Normobaric hyperoxia induced improvement in cerebral metabolism and reduction in intracranial pressure in patients with severe head injury: a prospective historical cohort matched study. J Neurosurg 2004;101:435–444

16

Cerebrospinal Fluid Dynamics and Pathology

Lynn M. Serrano, John D. Cantando, and Dan Miulli

Case Study

A 21-year-old female was struck in the head by falling objects resulting in a loss of consciousness. Her Glasgow Coma Scale (GCS) score was 7. Computed tomography (CT) scan revealed a small amount of epidural intracranial air. There were multiple facial fractures including those of the orbit and zygoma. An intraventricular drain and monitor were placed upon admission. During her hospital course the external ventricular drain was raised to 15 mm Hg after 5 days. She remained intubated. She developed fluid leakage from her nostrils.

See page 218 for Case Management.

Cerebrospinal fluid (CSF) is found within the four ventricles of the brain, the subarachnoid space, and the central canal of the spinal cord. It is also called liquor cerebrospinalis.[1] CSF circulates a variety of chemicals and nutrients necessary for normal brain function and metabolism; it also acts as a shock absorber, cushioning the brain from both day-to-day activity and traumatic events.

◆ Cerebrospinal Fluid Identification

Grossly, CSF should be a colorless, odorless, serous fluid. There is an estimated 70 to 160 cc of fluid in the central nervous system at any time (~50% intracranial, 50% spinal). Certain pathological conditions will change both the chemical and gross appearance of CSF. In the majority of cases, it is simple to ascertain whether fluid is CSF or not. However, at times, especially when contaminated with other fluids, it is necessary to analyze the fluid for its constituents to determine if an unknown fluid is CSF, contains CSF, or is another body fluid.[2–8] **Table 16–1** compares the composition of CSF with plasma. To determine if a fluid is CSF, the following tests can be done:

◆ *Glucose analysis* Analysis should be done immediately after collection to prevent fermentation. Nasal/lacrimal fluid or mucosal secretion will

Table 16–1   Chemical Constituents of Cerebrospinal Fluid and Plasma[2-8]

Constituent	Units	CSF	Plasma
Formation	mL/min	0.35	–
Osmolarity	mOsm/L	295	295
H_2O	%	99%	93%
Sodium	mEq/L	138–150	135–145
Potassium	mEq/L	2.2–3.3	4.1–4.5
Chloride	mEq/L	119–130	102–112
Calcium	mEq/L	2.1	4.8
Bicarbonate	mEq/L	22.0–23.3	24.0–26.8
Magnesium	mEq/L	2.3–2.7	1.7–1.9
Phosphorus	mg/dL	1.6	4.0
Ammonia	µg/dL	22–42	37–70
pCO_2	mm Hg	43–47	38–41
PH		7.33–7.35	7.41
pO_2	mm Hg	43	104
Glucose	mg/dL	45–80	90–110
Lactate	mEq/L	0.8–2.8	0.5–1.7
	mg/dL	10–20	6–13
Pyruvate	mEq/L	0.08	0.11
lactate: pyruvate		26	17.6
Glutamine	mg/dL	<20	>23
	µmol/L	552	641
Glutamate	µmol/L	26.1	61.3
GABA	µmol/L	3.5	29.8
Total protein	mg/dL	5–45, 5–15 ventricular, 10–25 cisternal, 15–45 lumbar	7000
Albumin	mg/L	155	36,600
Prealbumin	mg/L	17.3	238
Amino acids	% blood	30	3.6–7.2
	mEq/L	0.72–2.62	
IgG	mg/L	5–12	9870
RBCs	/mm³	0	3.6–5.4 M
WBCs	/mm³	<6/mm³; in children, up to 20/mm³	5000–10,000
Oligoclonal bands		<2	0
GOT	U	7–49	5–40
LDH	U	15–71	200–680
CPK	U	0–3	0–12
BUN	mg/dL	5–25	6–28
Bilirubin	mg/dL	0	0.2–0.9
Iron	µg/dL	1.5	15

BUN, blood urea nitrogen; CPK, creatine phosphokinase; CSF, cerebrospinal fluid; GABA, γ-aminobutyric acid; GOT, glutamic-oxaloacetic transaminase; IgG, immunoglobulin G; LDH, lactate dehydrogenase; RBC, red blood cell; WBC, white blood cell.

have <5 mg/dL of glucose. A negative test is more reliable, because even with meningitis, the glucose level is usually 5 to 20 mg/dL and associated with other changes. However, there is a 45 to 75% chance of a false-positive.[2,3,6,7,9,10]

♦ *Beta2-transferrin* This test can only be performed by electrophoresis of at least 0.5 cc of sample. Beta2-transferrin is only found in CSF and vitreous humor. (Note: This test is not reliable in patients with liver disease or in newborns.[11,12])

♦ *Ring sign* Also known as the "halo," this sign is particularly useful for blood-tinged samples. A drop of suspected fluid is placed on linen; as the fluid feathers out into the surrounding area, blood and mucus will stay centrally placed, and the CSF (which is less viscous) will continue spreading, creating a clear ring around the central colored area.

♦ Chemical Regulators of Cerebrospinal Fluid

Cerebrospinal fluid constituents are affected by secretion and absorption rates of CSF, hormones, and chemicals. The secretion rates and effects of hormones and chemicals on CSF vary from the vascular to the ventricular side of the choroid plexus.[13-15] These are described in **Table 16–2.**

♦ Flow Pattern of Cerebrospinal Fluid

CSF from blood plasma is actively transported by the choroid plexus (80%), or invaginations of the pia mater, into the ventricles, with the remaining 10 to 20% produced by ventricular ependymal cells, brain parenchyma, and indirect cellular fluid shifts. The approximate CSF secretion is 450 cc per day, which corresponds to a rate of 0.3 (0.35–0.37) mL/minute. The flow of CSF is in constant movement in a continuous pattern. Starting from the choroid plexus in the lateral ventricles, CSF continues through the foramen of Monro into the third ventricle and passes into the cerebral aqueduct prior to the fourth ventricle. From the fourth ventricle, fluid escapes into the cisterns and subarachnoid space via the foramen of Luschka and the foramen of Magendie. Some enters the central canal of the spinal cord, although most spinal fluid then circulates through the subarachnoid space and is reabsorbed in the venous system via the arachnoid villi. To keep the total spinal fluid in circulation throughout the ventricular system and subarachnoid space at ~150 cc, the absorption into the venous system is relatively constant at 450 cc/day, matching the daily production. There should be at least 3 to 5 mm Hg pressure of CSF for absorption to take place. Pathological states can alter the production, secretion, and/or circulatory flow of CSF.

Table 16–2 Hormone and Chemical Secretions in Cerebrospinal Fluid[13–15]

Vascular side of choroid plexus
Nonadrenergic sympathetic innervation (near CP epithelial cells and blood vessels) decreases CSF flow by 30%.
Cholinergic input primarily near the third ventricle stimulates CSF production up to 100%.
Endothelin binding sites are found in CP of lateral and third ventricles. Endothelin decreases blood flow and subsequently CSF production.
Antidiuretic hormone (ADH) regulates norepinephrine, dopamine, and endorphin release within the ventricle. ADH has been shown to indirectly decrease plasma Na^+.

Ventricular side of choroid plexus
5-hydroxytryptamine (5HT)   The CP contains 10 times the amount of 5HT receptors relative to other areas of the brain. It is released from the supraependymal nerve fibers into the CSF and interacts with the CP-5HT receptors. 5HT reduces the rate of CSF secretion.
Melatonin binding sites are located in the fourth ventricle and stimulate CSF secretion.
Carbonic anhydrase   High concentrations within the CP increase CSF production by facilitating Na^+ transport.
L-dopa is the most abundant monoamine in the CSF. The CP has D_1 receptors but lacks direct dopaminergic innervation. Dopamine effects on the CP are via the CSF, similar to 5HT.
Norepinephrine is secreted by noradrenergic periventricular neurons in contact with the ventricles and decreases CSF production. It follows circadian variations similar to systemic circulation.
Arginine vasopressin (AVP) is released by vasopressinergic neurons into the CSF, which stimulates CSF production. AVP in the CSF follows circadian variations, whereas plasma levels do not. The CP has V_1 receptors for AVP. AVP has been shown to indirectly lower plasma Na^+.
Arial natriuretic peptide (ANP) reduces CSF production. It is elevated in hydrocephalus cases. Evidence supports ANP involvement in the regulation of water and electrolyte passage across the blood–brain barrier. ANP has a direct negative effect on CSF production as substantiated by increased levels of ANP circulating within the CSF in hydrocephalic patients (both normal and high pressure). Systemically, ANP stimulates renal inhibition of Na^+ and water absorption, leading to hyponatremia. Within the brain, ANP reduces the net flux of Na^+ from the circulation by inhibiting the $Na^+/K+/Cl^-$ cotransport system that is known to decrease CSF production.[8,9]

CP, choroid plexus; CSF, cerebrospinal fluid.

◆ Pathology Involving Cerebrospinal Fluid

Table 16–3 notes changes in the gross appearance and the chemical composition of CSF due to certain diseases states.

Table 16-3 Cerebrospinal Fluid Findings in Pathological Conditions

Constituent	Color	Clarity	Pressure	Glucose mg/dL	Lactate mg/dL	Protein mg/dL	Cells/mm³	Oligoclonal bands
SAH bleed	Xanthochromic in <6–12 hours	Bloody, no clots	↑	Normal	Normal	↑	RBC to 5 days, PMN, then lymphocytes	
Multiple sclerosis	Colorless	Normal	Normal	Normal	Normal	Min. ↑25–50	Lymphocytes	≥2
Spinal obstruction	Colorless	Normal	Normal	Normal	Normal	>500	Normal	
Spinal tumor	SI xanthochromic	Cloudy	↓	Normal	Normal	↑, Froin's syndrome	Lymphocytes	
Bacterial infection	White, yellow	Cloudy	↑	↑, ½ or less serum glucose	>35 mg/dL	↑ 80–500	PMN > 500	
Viral infection	Colorless	Clear	SI ↑	Normal	Normal	Normal-SI ↑ 30–100	Lymphocytes < 500	
TB meningitis	Colorless	Cloudy	↑	↓	>35 mg/dL	↑ 50–300	Lymphocytes 200–500	
Fungal meningitis	Colorless	Cloudy, varies	↑	↓, varies	↑	↑ 50–300	PMN/lymphocytes 50–150	
Aseptic meningitis	Colorless	Clear	Normal	Normal	Normal, varies	Normal-SI ↑	Lymphocytes	
Abscess	Colorless	Clear	↑	Normal	Normal, varies	↑ 20–120	PMN	
Infarction	Colorless	Clear	SI ↑	Normal	Normal, varies	SI ↑	SI PMN < 50	
Traumatic LP	Not xanthochromic	Bloody, does clot	Normal	Normal	Normal	4 mg/dL increase/5000 RBCs	Same as peripheral	

LP, lumbar puncture; PMN, polymorphonuclear neutrophil leukocytes; RBC, red blood (cell) count; SAH, subarachnoid hemorrhage; SI, signal intensity; TB, tuberculosis.
Source: Adapted from Greenberg M. Handbook of Neurosurgery. 5th ed. New York: Thieme, 2001, with permission.

Disorders of Volume and Pressure

Normal pressure hydrocephalus (NPH) is associated with a classic triad of symptoms: dementia, gait disturbance, and urinary incontinence. The etiology is usually idiopathic but can be secondary to other intracranial pathology, such as Alzheimer's disease, carcinomatosis, infectious meningitis, and subarachnoid hemorrhage.[16] Diagnosis is primarily clinical, with documented normal pressure via lumbar puncture and a full workup of other causes of dementia. Some clinicians augment clinical symptoms by performing a quantitative lumbar puncture. Usually a cognitive assessment, such as a neuropsychological test, precedes the lumbar puncture. The lumbar puncture measures the opening pressure, allows 20 to 40 cc of fluid to drain off, then measures the closing pressure. If the brain is normally compliant when the change in volume divided by the change in pressure is ~0.62, the closing pressure may be reduced by 0.45 cm of CSF pressure for every 1 cc of CSF removed. Thus removing 30 cc of fluid should reduce closing pressure by ~13 cm CSF (10 mm Hg). This is the adult normal pressure-volume index (PVI; 25–30 mL change in volume causes a 10-fold change in pressure in mm Hg). No change in CSF pressure may indicate poor cerebral compliance, low PVI, and increased intracranial pressure; a large lowering in CSF pressure may indicate low intracranial pressure, herniation, or complete block of CSF pathways. Following the lumbar puncture, there should be a repeat cognitive assessment, such as a neuropsychological test, to determine if the quantitative lumbar puncture resulted in clinical improvement. Some clinicians do not rely on this test, whereas others will not shunt questionable cases of NPH without a positive improvement in cognitive assessment after a quantitative lumbar puncture. Treatment of NPH is shunting, either ventricular or, at rare times, lumbar-peritoneal.

Communicating and noncommunicating hydrocephalus symptoms include nausea, vomiting, gait disturbance, frontal headache (frequently worse in the morning), paresis of upward gaze, disorders of sodium, and papilledema. Temporizing measures for relief may include a ventricular catheter and/or diuretics (acetazolamide or furosemide). Permanent treatment should be directed at the offending pathology; however, frequently, a CSF-diverting procedure, such as a shunt or third ventriculostomy, is required.[16–20]

Obstructive (noncommunicative) hydrocephalus is blockage of the normal flow of CSF, causing dilatation of the ventricles proximal to the obstruction.

Triventricular hydrocephalus is specifically a stenosis occurring at the sylvian aqueduct, yielding dilatation of both lateral ventricles and the third ventricle. Common etiologies include edema, mass effect, mass lesion, and congenital abnormality.

Communicating (nonobstructive) hydrocephalus is a disruption of the equilibrium of secretion and absorption of CSF, yielding increased volume of CSF. It is most commonly caused by malabsorption of the CSF by the arachnoid granulations. Common etiologies include infection, hemorrhage, trauma, and noninfectious meningitis.

Table 16–4   Four Diagnostic Criteria for Pseudotumor Cerebri

CSF pressure > 20 cm H_2O
Normal CSF composition
Symptoms of elevated intracranial pressure without focal deficit
Normal imaging studies (occasionally slit ventricles may be seen)

CSF, cerebrospinal fluid.

Pseudotumor cerebri (idiopathic benign intracranial hypertension) symptoms may include nausea, vomiting, headache, retro-orbital pain, visual changes, including blindness (may be permanent) associated with increased intracranial pressure, possible optic atrophy, and, when progressive, papilledema (**Table 16–4**).

Treatment includes medical management with diuretics (acetazolamide or furosemide); if refractory, surgical management is warranted, with serial lumbar punctures, shunting, or optic nerve decompression.[21]

Leptomeningeal or Arachnoid Cysts

Leptomeningeal cysts are congenital fluid collections between two layers of the arachnoid. They are not related to post-traumatic leptomeningeal cysts due to growing skull fractures. There are two types of arachnoid cysts classified by histological findings: (1) simple, in which the lining of the cyst consists of cells capable of secreting CSF (this is the most common type of middle fossa arachnoid cyst); and (2) complex, in which the lining of the cyst is multicellular, often containing neuroglia and ependyma.

Classic presentation is in early childhood, when there is a sudden onset associated with hemorrhagic conversion or cyst rupture. Symptoms and presentation vary according to location and mass effect; asymptomatic lesions are usually identified incidentally (**Table 16–5**).

Diagnosis is via computed tomography (CT) scan or magnetic resonance imaging (MRI). Most cysts are static, however; repeat imaging can be used

Table 16–5   Arachnoid Cysts: Signs and Symptoms[2,4,5]

Location	Signs and symptoms
Middle fossa 50% of cysts in adults, 30% of cysts in children	Asymptomatic; unilateral headaches, nausea/vomiting, seizures, mild hemiparesis, present at younger age, male:female ratio 3:1, more in left hemisphere, hemorrhage
Suprasellar 9% of cysts	Increased ICP, hydrocephalus, craniomegaly, developmental delay, precocious puberty, bobbing head, visual loss

ICP, intracranial pressure.

to rule out cystic changes or enlargement. Treatment is indicated only when the patient is symptomatic and other etiologies have been ruled out. Most common treatments are shunting using a low-pressure valve, which has a low rate of reoccurrence, marsupialization, or a combination of both (**Table 16–6**).[4,5]

Infectious and Noninfectious Irritants Causing Meningitis

Post-traumatic meningitis is usually limited to head trauma with an associated skull fracture. Organisms are most commonly gram-positive cocci and gram-negative bacilli. Treatment should be directed at the offending agent (**Table 16–7**).[2,3,6,7,9,10]

Trauma-Related Cerebrospinal Fluid Abnormalities

Infectious

See Chapter 24, **Table 24–2**, cerebrospinal fluid analysis.

Cerebrospinal Leak

CSF leaks are associated with basal skull fractures and anterior fossa fractures resulting in otorrhea and/or rhinorrhea. Diagnosis is made by clinical exam; however, contrasted CT scans and radionuclide cisternograms can help identify the source of the leak. Analysis is required (see **Table 16–1**) to confirm the fluid as CSF. Treatment consists of general measures to lowering intracranial pressure, raising the head of the bed, acetazolamide to decrease CSF production, lumbar drain insertion, and/or surgical repair. Surgical repair is indicated in refractory and recurrent CSF leaks.

Pneumocephalus is evidence of air intracranially. Air can be intra-parenchymal, intraventricular, subdural, or epidural. It is associated with a skull defect or injury to the tegmen tympani (congenital/traumatic/related to pressure changes, e.g., deep-sea diving). The skull defect can be

Table 16–6 Treatment of Congenital Middle Fossa Arachnoid Cysts[2,4,5]

Cyst type	Description	Treatment
Type I	Communicates with subarachnoid space	No treatment, follow-up imaging every 6 months for 18 months
Type II	Large, quadrangular, mass effect; delayed uptake with cisternogram contrast	Surgery if symptoms severe; surgery either cystoperitoneal shunting or cyst marsupial fenestration
Type III	Large, round, mass effect; no communication with subarachnoid space; bone expansion of middle fossa	Surgery if symptoms severe; either cystoperitoneal shunting or cyst marsupial fenestration

Table 16–7   Treatment of Meningitis[2,3,6,7,9,10]

Patient population	Organism	Suggested antibiotics
Neonates (<1 month)	Group B/D *Streptococcus* Enterobacteriaceae *Listeria*	Ampicillin Gentamycin (alt. third-generation cephalosporin)
Newborns (1–3 months)	Pneumococci Meningococci *Haemophilus influenzae*	Ampicillin Third-generation cephalosporin +/– dexamethasone
Children (3 months–7 years)	Pneumococci Meningococci *H. influenzae*	Third-generation cephalosporin (alt. ampicillin)
Older children (>7 years) and Adults	*Streptococcus pneumoniae* *Neisseria* Meningococci	Third-generation cephalosporin Ampicillin (in combination with resistance, add rifampin +/– vancomycin
Alcoholics, immunocomprised, and elderly	Pneumococci Enterobacteriaceae *Pseudomonas* *Listeria*	Vancomycin Third-generation cephalosporin
Postprocedural	*Staphylococcus aureus* Enterobacteriaceae *Pseudomonas* Pneumococci	Vancomycin Ceftazidime +/– gentamycin

congenital, postprocedural, or post-traumatic. Pneumocephalus must be closely monitored with frequent CT scans to confirm resolution. Prophylactic antibiotic use is controversial. A tension pneumocephalus is the result of expanding trapped gas and can be associated with gas producing bacterial infection, room temperature air expanding due to increased body temperature after sealing the access, and the continued use of nitrous oxide anesthesia gas after the closure of the dura.

Traumatic Lumbar Puncture

Traumatic lumbar puncture can occur during a procedure to obtain CSF; local trauma or disruption of nearby vascular structures can produce a traumatic tap. The CSF analysis will still be accurate in most pathologies; however, its appearance can complicate the diagnosis of subarachnoid hemorrhage. When CT scan is negative for subarachnoid hemorrhage, yet the patient history and physical exam are highly suspicious, a lumbar puncture can be used to limit the differential diagnosis. **Table 16–8** itemizes the characteristics of a traumatic tap.

Table 16–8   Traumatic Punctures[2,4,5]

Decline in number of RBCs with succeeding tubes

WBCs proportional to blood RBCs.

Blood will clot.

No xanthochromia if first attempt within 2–12 hours, unless protein > 150 mg/dL or RBCs > 1.5 M/mm^3 or high lipid levels

Xanthochromia appears in the CSF within 2 hours in limited cases, 6 hours 70% of time, and 12 hours 90% of time.

Protein consistent with plasma or increased above-normal CSF levels by 1 mg/1000 RBCs.

CSF, cerebrospinal fluid; RBC, red blood cell; WBC, white blood cell.

Case Management

Initially, it is possible that the fluid coming out of her nose was CSF; however, this was less likely as there was no evidence of intradural air on the CT scan. The intracranial air was purely epidural. Furthermore, because of intubation, air sinus congestion can certainly develop. The fluid leak from the nose can be tested for glucose, but there is a 45–75% chance of false-positive finding. Any leakage of fluid onto the bed linen can also be observed for a "halo sign," which represents central blood and mucous surrounded by a ring of spreading CSF. The best test to determine if the fluid coming from the nose is CSF is beta2-transferrin. Since there was no globe damage, it is unlikely that the fluid is vitreous humor.

During external ventricular drain insertion, it is prudent to test the CSF for possibility of infection. These tests include: color, clarity, glucose, protein, and cell count. Any concerns of possible CSF leak could be initially treated with slightly lowering the drainage bag. The bag should not be dramatically lowered as this may allow air into the intracranial or intradural compartment.

References

1. Dorland's Illustrated Medical Dictionary. Philadelphia: WB Saunders; 1994
2. Greenberg MS. Handbook of Neurosurgery. 5th ed. New York: Thieme; 2001
3. Gilroy J. Basic Neurology. 3rd ed. New York: McGraw-Hill; 2000
4. Winn HR. Youman's Neurological Surgery. 5th ed. Philadelphia: WB Saunders; 2004
5. Wilkins RH, Regengachary SS. Neurosurgery. 2nd ed. New York: McGraw-Hill; 1996
6. Sacher RA, McPherson RA. Widmann's Clinical Interpretation of Laboratory Tests. 11th ed. Philadelphia: FA Davis; 2000

7. Ropper AH, Brown RH. Adams and Victor's Principles of Neurology. 8th ed. New York: McGraw-Hill; 2005

8. Kandel ER, Schwartz JH, Jessel TM. Principles of Neural Science. 4th ed. New York: McGraw-Hill; 2000

9. Layon AJ, Gabrielli A, Friedman WA. Textbook of Neurointensive Care. Philadelphia: WB Saunders; 2004

10. Rowland LP. Merritt's Neurology. 10th ed. Philadelphia: Lippincott Williams & Wilkins; 2000

11. Ryall RG, Peacock MK, Simpson DA, et al. Usefulness of B2-transferrin assay in the detection of cerebrospinal fluid leaks following head injury. J Neurosurg 1992;77:737–739

12. Fransen P, Sindic CJ, Thauvoy C, et al. Highly sensitive detection of beta-2 transferrin in rhinorrhea and otorrhea as a marker for cerebrospinal fluid (CSF) leakage. Acta Neurochir (Wien) 1991;109:98–101

13. Perez-Figares J, Jimenez AJ, Rodriguez EM. Subcommissural organ, cerebrospinal fluid circulation, and hydrocephalus. Microsc Res Tech 2001;52:591–607

14. Illowsky BP. Polydipsia and hyponatremia in psychiatric patients. Am J Psychiatry 1988;145:675–683

15. Migliore A, Paoletti P, Villani R. The rate of exchange of Na and other ions between plasma and cerebrospinal fluid in normal subjects and in hydrocephalic infants. Dev Med Child Neurol 1965;7:310–316

16. Mayberg MR. Neurosurgery Clinics of North America. Philadelphia: WB Saunders; 2001

17. Mori K, Tsutsumi K, Kurihara M, et al. Alteration of atrial natriuretic peptide receptors in the choroid plexus of rats with induced or congenital hydrocephalus. Childs Nerv Syst 1990;6:190–193

18. Tsutsumi K, Niwa M, Himeno A, Kurihara M, et al. Alpha-atrial natriuretic peptide binding sites in the rat choroid plexus are increased in the presence of hydrocephalus. Neurosci Lett 1988;87:93–98

19. Diringer M, Kirsch JR, Ladenson PW, Borel C, Hanley DF. Cerebrospinal fluid atrial natriuretic factor in intracranial disease. Stroke 1990;21:1550–1554

20. Milhorat T. The third circulation revisited. J Neurosurg 1975;42:628–645

21. McGirt MJ. Cerebrospinal fluid shunt placement for pseudotumor cerebri-associated intractable headache: predictors of treatment response and an analysis of long-term outcomes. J Neurosurg 2004;101:627–632

17

Intracranial Pressure Fundamentals

Daniel Hutton, Javed Siddiqi, and Dan Miulli

Case Study

A 42-year-old male is brought to the emergency department after rear-ending another vehicle at a high speed. He was an unrestrained driver and tested positive for ethanol and methamphetamines. His initial Glasgow Coma Scale (GCS) score was 12, but he was combative and was subsequently intubated. He has obvious signs of facial trauma and several scalp lacerations. His paralytics and sedatives have worn off, and he is localizing to central pain, but less on the left side, with no eye opening to verbal or painful stimulus. His pupils are 2 mm and reactive on the left, 4 mm and sluggish on the right. His noncontrast brain computed tomography (CT) scan shows an 8 mm right subdural hematoma with 11 mm of midline shift at the septum pellucidum. His basilar cistern is effaced. Traumatic subarachnoid hemorrhage is also noted bilaterally in the posterior frontal region, near the vertex.

See page 227 for Case Management.

◆ What Is Intracranial Pressure?

Elevated intracranial pressure (ICP) remains a frequently encountered dilemma in the neurosurgical intensive care unit (NICU). Few other pathologies challenge clinicians' insight and vigilance as does intracranial hypertension. In addition, treatment is limited because of a lack of true understanding and randomized trials for documentation of outcome. Intracranial hypertension is seen in 50% of those with intracranial mass lesions and 33% of those with diffuse injuries.[1]

ICP is a function of the contents of the cranial vault. The sum of the volumes of blood, brain, cerebrospinal fluid (CSF), and other elements (tumor, hematoma, abscess, edema) in an inelastic bony cranial vault together comprise the ICP. This is known as the Monro-Kellie hypothesis.[2] Therefore, an increase in any of the intracranial elements causes a concomitant decrease in the other elements. This principle does not apply to children with unfused sutures or to patients with comminuted skull fractures.

◆ Cerebral Blood Flow and Intracranial Pressure

The intracranial fluid model in a subject without head trauma has shown that adequate perfusion, or cerebral blood flow (CBF), is exquisitely autoregulated and relatively constant, with small amounts of flux. Numerous variables are available to monitor and manipulate in the NICU. Tenets are based on knowledge of the cardiopulmonary system, specifically, cardiac output. In this, adjustments of vasopressors, inotropes, chronotropes, and other medication are made to optimize cerebral perfusion. Though usually requiring invasive monitoring, cardiac output may be approximated with a simple calculation:

$$\text{Cardiac output} = \text{SV} \times \text{HR} = \frac{\text{VO}_2}{\text{AVDO}_2 \times 10}$$

where SV is stroke volume, HR is heart rate, VO_2 is oxygen consumption, and AVDO_2 is arteriovenous oxygen content difference. CBF is measurable with neuroimaging modalities, including xenon CT, positron emission tomography (PET) scanning, and functional magnetic resonance imaging (MRI). These techniques are quite expensive and usually unavailable on a continuous basis to most clinicians. CBF is dependent on cerebral perfusion pressure (CPP), which is the net driving hemodynamic force with consideration of ICP. Normal adult CPP is >50 mm Hg.

CBF is related to CPP via Poiseuille's law. Using this formula, CPP is directly proportional to CBF and also to vessel radius; it is inversely proportional to blood viscosity and vessel length. Shown mathematically, Poiseulle's law is

$$\text{CBF} = \frac{8(\text{CPP})r^4}{\pi(n)(l)},$$

where r is vessel radius, n is viscosity, and l is vessel length.

$$\text{CPP} = \text{MAP} - \text{ICP},$$

where MAP is mean arterial pressure.

$$\text{MAP} = \text{DBP} + \frac{(\text{SBP} - \text{DBP})}{3}$$

where DBP is diastolic blood pressure and SBP is systolic blood pressure.

Table 17–1   Normal Intracranial Pressure Levels[1–3,5,6]

cm CSF x 1.36 = mm Hg	
Dependent upon atmospheric pressure (varies with altitude), hydrostatic pressure, and filling pressure	
CSF pressure needs to be 3 to 5 mm Hg higher than venous pressure for absorption.	
Adults and older children	5 to 15 mm Hg
	6.5 to 19.5 cm CSF
Young children	<3 to 7.4 mm Hg
Term infants	<1.5 to 5.9 mm Hg
CSF pressure decreases 0.5 to 1.0 cm CSF for every milliliter of CSF removed. A minor decrease in pressure suggests hydrocephalus, whereas a large drop in pressure may signify tumor.	

CSF, cerebrospinal fluid.

Optimization of CPP at 60 to 70 mm Hg has been more reliably shown to be associated with an improved neurologic outcome. Normal ICP is age dependent (**Table 17–1**).

Although many definitions for a pathological threshold of ICP have been given, 20 to 25 mm Hg is generally accepted as truly pathological.[3]

◆ Etiology of and Findings Associated with Intracranial Hypertension

The causes of intracranial hypertension include the following:

- ◆ Cerebral edema
- ◆ Hyperemia (loss of autoregulation)
- ◆ Hematoma: epidural hematoma (EDH), subdural hematoma (SDH), intracerebral hemorrhage (ICH), foreign body, or combination with depressed skull fracture
- ◆ Hydrocephalus
    - ◇ Communicating from post-traumatic, secondary to aneurysmal subarachnoid hemorrhage (SAH) or arteriovenous malformation (AVM), meningitis
    - ◇ Obstruction from tumor and aqueductal stenosis
- ◆ Hypercarbia (minute ventilation is too low or impaired alveolar gas exchange)
    - ◇ Low minute ventilation
    - ◇ Impaired gas exchange: hemothorax, pneumothorax, and pulmonary contusions

◇ Pneumonia
◇ Acute respiratory distress syndrome (ARDS)
- Venous obstruction/thrombosis
- Agitation (increased intrathoracic and intra-abdominal pressures)
- Status epilepticus (may be without overt tonic-clonic activity)
- Vasospasm
- Hyponatremia

The following findings are associated with intracranial hypertension:

- Drowsiness → Somnolence → Obtundation
- Nausea/vomiting
- Blurred vision or diplopia
- Cushing's triad:
  ◇ Hypertension
  ◇ Bradycardia
  ◇ Respiratory irregularity
- Motor or sensory deficits
- Cranial nerve (CN) palsies: CN III for uncal herniation; CN VI for acute hydrocephalus; CN VI and VII for enlarging cerebellar hemorrhage[4]

◆ Monitoring Intracranial Pressure

Previously, much confusion existed regarding which patient populations would benefit from monitoring ICP. Indications for ICP monitoring were refined in 1995 by Bullock et al.[3] They include GCS ≤ 8 (postresuscitation) and abnormal noncontrast brain CT[5] or normal brain CT, but with at least two of the following: age > 40 years, SBP < 90, decerebrate or decorticate posturing on motor exam.

Relative contraindications to ICP monitoring include coagulopathy (International Normalized Ratio [INR] > 1.3), anoxic injury ("postcode"), and metabolic causes of coma, including intoxication (**Table 17–2**).

Types of Monitors

Various forms of monitoring have been used to assess ICP. Currently, intra-ventricular catheters are by far the most common. Their usefulness is twofold: proper assessment of ICP with less drift than other modalities, and the ability to treat intracranial hypertension by evacuation of CSF. Other methods include intraparenchymal, subarachnoid, subdural, and epidural bolts and, in infants, fontanometry.

Table 17–2   ICP Ventriculostomy Monitor

Indications	Contraindications
1. GCS ≤ 8	1. Coagulopathy
2. Unclear GCS; patient going to operating room for other reason	2. GCS > 9 (with certain exceptions)
3. Multisystem injury, making fluid management and neurologic exam difficult	3. Rapidly improving neurologic exam in patient with GCS < 8 (6 hour cutoff)
4. Anticipate prolonged sedation/ paralysis from other injuries (that appear more severe than head injury)	4. Patient known to be postictal (and without obvious intracerebral injury)
	5. ICP bolt harmful to patient (i.e., increases shift in patient with trapped ventricle)
	6. Appearance of "brain death"
	7. "Intoxication" (without good evidence of head injury)

GCS, Glasgow Coma Scale; ICP, intracranial pressure.

Intraventricular catheters are typically placed at Kocher's point in the frontal lobe. Other sites commonly used for ventriculoperitoneal shunts may be used, including Keen's point, Dandy's point, and Frazier's point. Landmarks exist for frontal lobe placement of intraventricular catheters. Generally, placement is performed on the nondominant side, 1 to 2 cm anterior to the coronal suture.

Procedure

Kocher's point is located 12.5 cm posterior to the nasion in the sagittal plane, then 2.5 cm lateral to midline. A small patch of hair is shaved, and the sterile site is prepped. After infusing lidocaine with epinephrine into the subcutaneous tissue and periosteum, a 1 to 2 cm linear incision is made. The hand drill is introduced in the trajectory of the opposite medial canthus of the eye and approximately 1 cm anterior to the tragus. After bone purchase is made through both tables of the skull, the drill is removed, and the dura is incised in a cruciate manner. A catheter is placed in the same trajectory as the drill, with the catheter advanced approximately 4 to 6 cm. A palpable "pop" through the ependymal surface is often felt, and retrieval of CSF is seen. Depending on the system used, the system is secured into place and attached for monitoring and drainage of CSF. Sterile dressings are then applied.

Intraparenchymal pressure monitors may also be placed with the above described procedure and placement of the parenchymal fiber 2 to 3 cm into the brain substance.

At many locations, triple lumen ventricular catheters are used and are supplemented with microdialysis catheters, temperature, pH, and oxygenation probes. This has provided advanced therapeutic models for optimization of multiple variables. With the exception of brain tissue oxygen sensors, improved outcome has yet to be determined.

Waveforms

Normal waveforms are rarely seen due to changes associated with the traumatic population. However, the tallest peak of the ICP wave corresponds to the atrial systolic wave. The smaller peak corresponds to the A wave on the central venous pressure (CVP) waveform.

Pathological waves are due to alterations of CPP, whether resulting from increased ICP or decreased MAP, or both. An increase in ICP is thought to be associated with a sharpened appearance of the waveforms. An increase in venous pressure, conversely, has a more rounded appearance (**Table 17–3**).

In 1960, Lundberg described several pathologies and associated changes in waveform characteristics.[6] Lundberg A waves (plateau waves) are usually seen with ICP >50 mm Hg. It has been postulated that there may be an associated increase in MAP. Lundberg B waves (pressure pulses) are described as an amplitude of 10 to 20 mm Hg and are associated with various types of breathing. Lundberg C waves have a frequency of 4 to 8/minute and have

Table 17–3   Normal and Abnormal Intracranial Pressure Waveforms[5,6]

Normal ICP waveform		
Peak	**Wave**	**Origin**
First large peak	Percussion wave W_1 (pulsatile)	Systolic pressure, large intracranial arteries and choroid plexus CBF
Second small peak	Tidal wave W_2 (pulsatile)	Central venous wave from right atrium, from brain increased elastance/ decreased compliance
Inverted	Inverted	Miscalibrated monitor
Third small peak	Dicrotic wave W_3	Arterial pulse
Expiration	Increases overall wave	Increasing central venous pressure
Inspiration	Decreases overall wave	Decreasing central venous pressure
Increased ICP waveform		
Peak	**Change with increased ICP**	
First large peak	Increases slightly	
Second small peak	Increases disproportionately to first wave	
Third small peak	Increases disproportionately to first wave	

ICP, intracranial pressure; CBF, cerebral blood flow.

Table 17–4   Abnormal Intracranial Pressure Waveform Analysis[5,6]

Lundberg A wave (plateau wave)

Mean wave > 50 mm Hg

Entire wave lasts 5 to 20 minutes, then returns to slightly elevated baseline.

Increased cerebral blood volume from low CPP, then vasodilation, increasing ICP, lowering CPP, causing ischemia, and resulting in brainstem response.

Occurs when ICP exceeds the limits of cerebral compliance; reflects ischemia

Lundberg B wave (pressure wave)

Mean wave > 20 to 50 mm Hg

Entire wave lasts over $1/2$ to 3 minutes.

Possibly not due to increased ICP; may be due to respiratory changes and variations in CBF

Can be seen in sleep

Suggests that Lundberg A (plateau) waves may form

Lundberg C wave (preterminal wave)

Mean wave < 20 mm Hg

Entire wave increased every 10 seconds

ICP transmission of cyclic variation in SBP

CBF, cerebral blood flow; CPP, cerebral perfusion pressure; ICP, intracranial pressure; SBP, systemic blood pressure.

been seen in normal pressures as well as with Lundberg A waves in the pre-morbid state (**Table 17–4**).

◆ Surgery to Relieve Intracranial Hypertension

Decompression of mass lesions is of critical value. Unfortunately, only guidelines exist to help govern surgical intervention. Surgery previously was performed on an exploratory basis. Exploratory bur holes were made ipsilateral to the pupillary abnormality or contralateral to the worst motor response. If blood was encountered, a full craniotomy was performed. Advances in imaging techniques have antiquated this technique.

Principle evacuation of the mass lesion is paramount. However, one should remain keen to the possibility of craniectomy. A large incision and flap should be turned for maximal exposure for visualization and the possibility of allowing for cerebral edema should bone flap be left off. The general size of an adult bone flap should be at least 11 × 15 cm.

Case Management

The patient had a GCS score of 7 upon reexamination after his sedatives and paralytics wore off. The patient has an intracranial hematoma on the right with mass effect, with a larger right pupil (which is observed to be sluggishly reactive to light). This is an acute emergency, and the patient should be taken to the OR immediately for evacuation of the hematoma. On the way to the OR, his head of bed should be raised to 30 degrees. He should be hyperventilated to PCO_2 of 30 and given intravenous mannitol. After the clot is evacuated, the patient should also have a ventriculostomy/ICP monitor inserted in the OR for diagnosis and treatment of ICP in the NICU postoperatively.

References

1. Winns R. Youman's Neurological Surgery. 5th ed. New York: WB Saunders; 2004
2. Greenberg MS. Handbook of Neurosurgery. 5th ed. New York: Thieme 2001
3. Bullock R, Chestnut RM, Clifton G, et al. Guidelines for the Management of Severe Head Injury. New York: The Brain Trauma Foundation, American Association of Neurological Surgeons, and Joint Section of Neurotrauma and Critical Care; 1995
4. Heros RC. Surgical treatment of cerebellar infarction. Stroke 1992;23:937–938
5. Narayan RK, Kishore PRS, Becker DP, et al. Intracranial pressure: to monitor or not to monitor? A review of our experience with severe head injury. J Neurosurg 1982;56:650–659
6. Lundberg N. Continuous recording and control of ventricular fluid pressure in neurosurgical practice. Acta Psychiatr Scand Suppl 1960;36:1–193

18

Cerebral Protection Measures

Dennis Cramer, Dan Miulli, and Javed Siddiqi

Case Study

A 32-year old male was an unrestrained driver involved in a head-on traffic collision at high speed. The patient was intubated in the field and Glasgow Coma Scale (GCS) score on arrival to the emergency room was 6T. Head computed tomography (CT) scan shows diffuse petechial hemorrhages and left frontal contusion, no midline shift or surgical hematoma demonstrated. The patient is transferred to the ICU where an intracranial pressure (ICP) monitor and cerebrospinal fluid (CSF) drainage device is promptly placed. Initial ICP is 20 mm Hg; however, 4 hours later the on-call physican is notified that the ICP has slowly been trending upward and is now at 35 mm Hg.

See page 234 for Case Management.

The ultimate result of a severe head injury primarily depends on the extent of injury at the time of incident. A primary brain injury from trauma includes contusions, epidural or subdural hematomas, intracerebral hemorrhage, and diffuse injuries. Initially, surgical intervention for a space-occupying mass should always be considered before proceeding to the management of secondary brain insults. These secondary brain injuries include edema, ischemia, and hypoxemia, which can result in infarction and/or herniation. Upon secondary injury, the brain undergoes numerous pathological and chemical changes that significantly impact the patient's neurologic outcome. The mainstay of treating a secondary brain insult is to ensure adequate cerebral blood flow (CBF) via control of intracranial and cerebral perfusion pressures.

Because CBF is difficult to measure, physicians can easily follow the mean arterial and intracranial pressures to estimate cerebral perfusion pressure (CPP). CBF is related to mean arterial pressure (MAP) and ICP, as shown in these equations:

$$CBF = CPP/CVR = (MAP - ICP)/CVR,$$

where CVR is cerebrovascular resistance.

The equations show the complex relationship between brain perfusion and blood pressure. The Monro-Kellie hypothesis, which helps to explain the significance of ICP, states that the sum of the intracranial volumes of blood, brain tissue, and cerebrospinal fluid (CSF) are constant and that any increase in one component will be counterbalanced by a decrease in another. The volume of brain tissue is 90%; blood and CSF are 5% each. All of these are contained within the rigid skull. The introduction of additional volume, such as from hemorrhage or edema, must be compensated by changes in the blood or CSF volumes. Failure to counterbalance these changes will result in increased ICP and possibly intracranial shifts (herniation). Increased ICP can be compensated by shifting CSF from the ventricles and subarachnoid space to the spinal canal or by decreasing the intracranial blood volume via collapsing veins and constricting cerebral arteries. Changes in vessel diameter can result in a reduction of cerebral intravascular volume by as much as 70 mL, easily buffering a new volume mass, such as a hemorrhage.[1]

After compensatory mechanisms for increased ICP are exhausted the patient begins suffering from secondary brain insults. Eighty to 90% of traumatic brain-injured patients who die are found to have histopathologic evidence of cerebral ischemia.[2] Studies show that approximately one third of patients with traumatic brain damage experience an "ultra-early" period of significantly decreased cerebral blood within 6 hours of injury.[3] The ischemia is characterized by focal reductions in CBF below the threshold of 18 mL/100 g/minute, resulting in ischemic neuronal cell death.[4] The hypoxic conditions perpetuate a hypermetabolic rate, resulting in an aerobic to anaerobic metabolism and leading to an increased concentration of lactic acid.[5] Ionic homeostasis is then compromised, leading to a complex process of calcium influx and cellular injury and death.[6]

◆ Pharmacologic Cerebral Metabolic Depressants

An estimated 15% of all head-injured patients suffer from refractory ICP.[7] When there is deteriorating CPP in the face of increasing ICP, hypertonic saline can be used to increase blood osmolarity, expand plasma volume, and reduce brain edema via the extraction of water from neurons and interstitial tissue. Hypertonic saline results in improved microvascular blood flow, thereby lowering ICP. Variable concentrations of hypertonic saline from 3 to 23.4% have been used. Although limited use of hypertonic saline is relatively safe, prolonged use can affect cellular homeostasis, and, in the alcoholic, rapid correction of hyponatremia can lead to central pontine myelinolysis. However, when this and all other medical and surgical modalities have failed to adequately control elevated ICP, the physician may attempt the use of pharmacologic agents to reduce cerebral metabolic rate (CMR) and hence ICP in a patient who is deemed salvageable. Many pharmacologic agents have been used to lower ICP, such as pentobarbital, thiopental, etomidate, propofol, isoflurane, and desflurane, but not enough data exist to recommend one drug over another. Most published information addresses the use of barbiturates, especially pentobarbital.

In 1974, Shapiro et al were the first to report the use of pentobarbital-augmented hypothermia in reducing CMR and ICP.[8] This therapy remains controversial mainly because of the potential side effects of myocardial hypotension, hypothermia, immunosuppression, hypokalemia, and hepatic and renal dysfunction.[9] Accordingly, the Brain Trauma Foundation, in cooperation with the American Association of Neurological Surgeons, has recommended a guideline using high-dose barbiturate therapy in hemodynamically stable head-injured patients with elevated ICP resistant to maximal medical and surgical treatment modalities.[9a]

Because of marked hypotension seen in ~50% of patients treated with barbiturates, many will require cardiac inotropes and/or vasopressors to maintain an MAP resulting in a CPP $\geq$ 70 mm Hg,[10] unless increased secondary risk concerns favor an acceptable lower CPP. Dopamine (primarily a vasoconstrictor) is commonly used starting at 3 μg/kg/minute and titrating to a maximum 20 μg/kg/minute to maintain CPP $\geq$ 70 mm Hg. Phenylephrine starting between 100 and 180 μg/minute, with a maintenance dosage of 40 to 60 μg/minute, or Levophed at 8 to 12 μg/minute is frequently used for progressively decreasing CPP and/or hypotension. Swan-Ganz catheterization and hemodynamic monitoring may be necessary to adjust cardiac medications and to ensure adequate volume status.

Many protocols have been used to administer barbiturate therapy. Eisenberg's protocol starts with a loading dose of pentobarbital at 10 mg/kg intravenous (IV) over 60 minutes, followed by 5 mg/kg every hour for 3 hours, with a maintenance dosage of 1 to 3 mg/kg/hour.[11] In a study by Cormio et al on 67 severely head-injured patients undergoing treatment for refractory intracranial hypertension, pentobarbital loading doses decreased ICP and MAPs on average by 12 and 9 mm Hg, respectively.[12] It can generally be considered that if the induced pentobarbital coma does not lower the ICP within 1 to 4 hours, it is unlikely to succeed without any other therapy.

Thiopental has been used when large doses of pentobarbital are not available or when a rapidly acting barbiturate is needed. It works by producing cerebral metabolic depression and cerebral vasoconstriction. The loading dose is 5 mg/kg IV over 10 minutes, with a continuous infusion of 5 mg/kg/hour (range: 3–5 mg) for 24 hours. After 24 hours, the infusion may be decreased to 2.5 mg/kg/hour because fat stores have now become saturated.

Propofol is a well-established sedative-hypnotic agent that has been used as an alternative to control elevated ICP, but questions remain regarding the pharmacodynamics of the drug. A study by Oertel et al has suggested a key mechanism responsible for the metabolic suppressive effect is a decrease in CO_2 production, resulting in a global "pharmacological hypocapnia."[13] The starting dose is 5 to 10 μg/kg/minute and increases by 5 to 10 μg/kg/minute every 5 to 10 minutes until ICP is controlled. Like the barbiturates, propofol exhibits hypotensive effects that may require cardiac medications or eventual discontinuation. In addition to the cardiotoxic effects, propofol may cause electrocardiogram changes and discoloration of urine.

A continuous electroencephalogram is recommended to monitor electrocerebral activity. Burst suppression of 1 to 3 bursts/page may not be necessary if control of ICP ≤ 20 to 25 mm Hg is achieved without the use of larger doses of the cerebral metabolic depressant agents.

Pharmacologically induced burst suppression is generally maintained 3 to 7 days; if computed tomography (CT) does not show any new findings, and ICP has been controlled, then therapy can be withdrawn slowly by reducing the infusion rate while monitoring ICP. Because of prolonged high-dose barbiturate therapy and the long half-lives of these drugs, it is difficult to distinguish the residual pharmacologic effects from the clinical condition. If a high index of suspicion for brain death is entertained, a nuclear cerebral metabolic test is warranted; if the test is negative, one should proceed with a cerebral angiogram before pronouncing brain death.

The prophylactic use of barbiturates for ICP treatment has shown no benefits in patients with intracranial mass lesions and was even found to be harmful in patients with diffuse injury (mortality of 77% vs 41% in the mannitol group).[14] A 2000 Cochrane Database review evaluating barbiturate therapy in acute traumatic brain injury concluded that there was no evidence that barbiturate therapy improves outcome for patients with acute severe brain injuries. The review also demonstrated that barbiturate therapy results in a decrease in blood pressure in 1 in 4 patients, and this hypotensive effect will offset any ICP-lowering effect on cerebral perfusion.[14]

Alternative agents to pentobarbital have not been well studied, but they have been used because of easier accessibility. A study comparing etomidate, isoflurane, and thiopental in animals undergoing 3 hours of middle cerebral artery occlusion found injured brain volume largest in the etomidate and isoflurane groups and smallest in the thiopental group.[15]

◆ Hypothermia

Control of temperature is of extreme importance in the head-injured patient. There have been many small studies on the effect of hypothermia causing reduced cerebral metabolism and ICP. In 1993, Clifton et al reported a 16% increase in favorable outcome in head-injured patients who underwent induced hypothermia (32–33°C).[16] A small study from 1999 showed mild hypothermia (34°C) to be an effective ICP control in patients with focal cerebral lesions.[17] Tokutomi and colleagues reported that lowering body temperatures to 35 to 36°C could reduce intracranial hypertension while maintaining CPP without significant cardiac dysfunction or oxygen delivery abnormalities.[18]

However, the results from a prospective, multicenter, randomized study consisting of 392 subjects demonstrated that traumatic brain-injured subjects who were randomly assigned to treatment with hypothermia (33°C) initiated within 6 hours of incident and maintained for 48 hours or normothermia showed no difference to normothermic patients at 6 months as measured by the Glasgow Outcome Score (GOS). Conversely, there were poorer outcomes in patients over 45 years old who were treated with hypothermia compared with the normothermia group. Also, the hypothermia group showed a higher cumulative fluid balance, greater use of vasopressors, and a higher percentage of days with complications.[19] This well-conducted study brings a renewed interest in the field of hypothermic treatment and the need for future trials to elucidate a clearer understanding and treatment guidelines.

◆ Blood Glucose Control

Traumatic brain injury leads to numerous neurochemical events and is associated with a catecholamine stress response, including hyperglycemia.[20] Many studies have shown hyperglycemia to correlate with the severity of brain injury and to be a predictor of neurologic outcome.[21-23] A study by Young et al showed that patients who had the highest peak admission 24 hour serum glucose level had the worst neurologic outcome at 18 days from injury.[21] The researchers also found that patients with a peak 24 hour serum glucose level >200 mg/dL had a 2 point decrease in their GOS and that those patients with a serum glucose level <200 mg/dL experienced a 4 point increase during the 18 day study period. Rovlias and Kotsou also found serum glucose levels >200 mg/dL in the first 24 hours to be highly predictive of an unfavorable outcome.[24]

Kushner et al found the median initial serum glucose level in acute ischemic cerebral infarction patients to be 155 mg/dL.[23] Additionally, clinical recovery was significantly poorer in patients with an initial glucose level greater than the median. The researchers reported that serum glucose admission levels correlated with the extent of metabolic brain abnormalities seen on acute positron emission tomography (PET) scanning.

During normal aerobic metabolism, energy in the brain is formed primarily when glucose is oxidized to CO_2 and water. The cellular metabolism of glucose begins with the process of glycolysis, resulting in the generation of pyruvate, the reduced form of nicotinamide-adenine dinucleotide (NADH), and adenosine triphosphate (ATP):

$$\text{Glucose} + 2 \text{ ADP} + 2 \text{ P}_i + 2 \text{ NAD}^+ \rightarrow 2 \text{ Pyruvate} + 2 \text{ ATP} + 2 \text{ NADH} + 2 \text{ H}^+ + 2 \text{ H}_2\text{O},$$

where ADP is adenosine diphosphate.

Pyruvate can be converted to lactate or to the amino acid alanine, or it can enter the citric acid, or Krebs, cycle (**Fig. 18–1**). The energy products derived from the citric acid, or Krebs, cycle (tricarboxyclic acid) are used in the final step of glucose metabolism as it enters the electron transport chain (ETC; **Fig. 18–2**). The end result of glucose breakdown is 38 moles of ATP, which is more efficient than the 6 moles of ATP produced via glycolysis alone. The detrimental effects of hypoxic or ischemic brain injury result from anaerobic

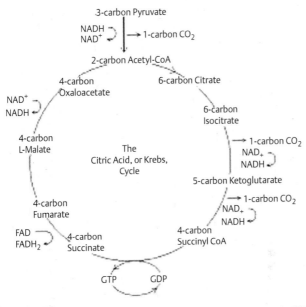

Figure 18–1   The citric acid, or Krebs, cycle. CoA, coenzyme A; GDP, guanosine diphosphate; GTP, guanosine triphosphate; COQ, coenzyme Q.

metabolism in which glucose is converted to lactate and hydrogen ions, rather than pyruvate. With increased levels of glucose available for lactate production, excessive lactate accumulation leads to greater tissue acidosis and subsequently neuronal damage.[25] There is considerable evidence of traumatic

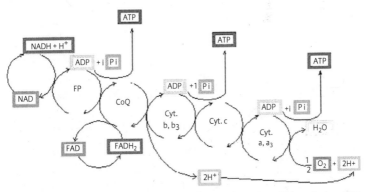

Figure 18–2   Electron transport chain. ADP, adenosine diphosphate; ATP, adenosine triphosphate; COQ, coenzyme Q; FP, flavoprotein.

brain-injured patients with serum glucose levels correlated with neurologic outcome. However, further clinical trials are needed to address neurologic outcome with strict glucose control in the acute brain injury.

Case Management

In the case of the 32-year-old male, a repeat CT scan should be repeated to identify any surgical hematomas. Efforts to decrease the ICP and increase the CPP should be done. Initially, the physician should ensure that the head-injured patient is well sedated and that his pain is being treated. If elevated ICP issues continue, the physican may consider mannitol and/or hypertonic saline, and possibly starting a vassopressor and/or inotrope to maintain the CPP at the desired goal. If the patient's elevated ICP remains refractory to the previous medications, one may consider placing him into a pharmacologically induced coma.

References

1. Wijdicks E. The Clinical Practice of Critical Care Neurology. New York:Lippincott-Raven; 1997
2. Graham DI. The pathology of brain ischemia and possibilities for therapeutical intervention. Br J Anaesth 1985;57:3–25
3. Bouma GIJ, Muizelaar JP, Stringer WA, Choi SC, Fatouros PP, Young HF. Ultra-early evaluation of regional cerebral blood flow in severely head injured patients using xenon-enhanced computerized tomography. J Neurosurg 1992;77:360–368
4. Schroder ML, Muizelaar JP, Bullock R, Povlishock JT, Salvant JB. Focal ischemia due to traumatic contusion documented by stable xenon CT and ultrastructural studies. J Neurosurg 1994;82:966–971
5. Kraig RP, Petito CK, Plum F. Hydrogen ions kill brain at concentrations reached in ischemia. J Cereb Blood Flow Metab 1987;7:379–386
6. Bullock R, Zauner A, Woodward JJ, Myseros J, Choi SC, Kaura SC, Ward JD, Marmarou A, Young HF. Factors affecting excitatory amino acid release following severe human head injury. J Neurosurg 1998;89:507–518
7. Gudeman SK, Miller JD, Becker DP. Failure of high-dose steroid therapy to influence intracranial pressure in patients with severe brain injury. J Neurosurg 1979;51:301–306
8. Shapiro HM, Wyte SR, Loeser J. Barbiturate-augmented hypothermia for reduction of persistent intracranial hypertension. J Neurosurg 1974;40:90–100
9. Schalen W, Messeter K, Nordstrom CH. Complications and side effects during thiopentone therapy in patients with severe head injuries. Acta Anaesthesiol Scand 1992;36:369–377
9a. Brain Trauma Foundation (U.S.). Management and Prognosis of Severe Traumatic Brain Injury. New York:Brain Trauma Foundation;2000
10. Rea GL, Rockswold GL. Barbiturate therapy in uncontrolled intracranial hypertension. Neurosurgery 1983;12:401–404
11. Eisenbeurg HM, Frankowski RF, Contant CF, et al. High-dose barbiturate control of elevated intracranial pressure with severe head injury. J Neurosurg 1988;69:15–23
12. Cormio M, Gopinath SP, Valadka A, Robertson CS. Cerebral hemodynamic effects of pentobarbital coma in head-injured patients. J Neurotrauma 1999;16:927–936

13. Oertel E, Kelly DF, Lee JH, et al. Metabolic suppressive therapy as a treatment if intracranial hypertension: why it works and when it fails. Acta Neurochir 2002;81:69–70

14. Roberts I. Barbiturates for acute traumatic brain injury. Cochrane Database Syst Rev 2000;(2):CD000033

15. Drummond JC, Cole DJ, Piyush PM, Lowell W, Reynolds. Focal cerebral ischemia during anesthesia with etomidate, isoflurane, or thiopental: a comparison of the extent of cerebral injury. Neurosurgery 1995;37:742–749

16. Clifton GL, Allen S, Barrodale P, et al. A phase 2 study of moderate hypothermia in severe brain injury. J Neurotrauma 1993;10:263–271

17. Shiozaki T. Selection of severely head-injured patients for mild hypothermia therapy. J Neurosurg 1999;89:206–211

18. Tokutomi T, Morimoto K, Miyagi T, Yamaguchi S, Ishikawa K, Shigemori M. Optimal temperature for the management of severe traumatic brain injury: effect of hypothermia on intracranial pressure, systemic and intracranial hemodynamics, and metabolism. Neurosurgery 2003;52:102–111

19. Clifton GL. Lack of effect of induction of hypothermia after acute brain injury. N Engl J Med 2001;344:556–563

20. Rosner MJ, Newsome HH, Becker DP. Mechanical brain injury: the sympathoadrenal response. J Neurosurg 1984;61:76–86

21. Young B, Ott L, Dempsey R, Haack D, Tibbs P. Relationship between admission hyperglycemia and neurological outcome of severely brain-injured patients. Ann Surg 1989;210:466–473

22. Feibel JH, Hardy PM, Campbell RG, et al. Prognostic value of the stress following stroke. JAMA 1977;238:1374–1376

23. Kushner E, Nencini P, Reivich M, et al. Relation of hyperglycemia early in ischemic brain infarction to cerebral anatomy, metabolism, and clinical outcome. Ann Neurol 1990;8:129–135

24. Rovlias A, Kotsou S. The influence of hyperglycemia on neurological outcome in patients with severe head injury. Neurosurgery 2000;46:335–343

25. Marsh WR, Anderson RE, Sundt TM. Effect of hyperglycemia on brain pH levels in areas of focal incomplete cerebral ischemia in monkeys. J Neurosurg 1986;65:693–696

Section IV

Care of the Patient

19

Neuropharmacology

Nicholas Qandah, Evan A. Houck, and Dan Miulli

Case Study

A 45-year-old male was an unrestrained driver of a motorcycle that was involved in an accident. He is taken to the trauma center with a Glasgow Coma Scale (GCS) of 8; his pupils are sluggish and reactive. He is intubated. He has multiple fractures and an elevated intracranial pressure (ICP) of 30, cerebral perfusion pressure (CPP) of 55.

See page 266 for Case Management.

As with other medical conditions, neurosurgical conditions can be treated or ameliorated with medications. The foremost consideration when initiating care in the neurosurgical intensive care unit is to restore cerebral blood flow, thus delivering essential oxygen and substrates that would allow the brain to heal. The brain needs an adequate cardiac output and ample pulmonary function to survive. Blood pressure must be restored to a range that is not so low it leads to neuronal death or so high that it leads to hyperemia, increased edema, and even hemorrhage. This chapter examines the medications used in conjunction with neurosurgical procedures.

We discuss hemodynamic medications for lowering and raising blood pressure, electrolyte solutions to assist the body in dealing with all manner of insult, blood products to replace losses, antiepileptics to control seizures, steroids to treat tumors or as an adjunct in certain types of spinal cord injuries, anticoagulants, sedatives to calm patients or decrease the cerebral metabolic rate of oxygen consumption, pain medications, and antiemetics; and when too much medication is given the agents to reverse the effects.

◆ Hemodynamic Agents

Hypertension

Before treating increased blood pressure, it is important to rule out intracranial causes, such as Cushing's reflex. Before choosing an agent, evaluate the effects of the drug on CPP and ICP. Always remember to order blood pressure and heart rate parameters when writing for a drug.[1,2]

Sodium Nitroprusside (Nipride)

Action: Reacts with oxyhemoglobin to form cyanide and nitric oxide (NO). NO stimulates cyclic guanosine monophosphate (cGMP) production, causing potent vasodilation (arterial > venous), hepatic and renal metabolism.[1,3]

Contraindications: Increased ICP, intracranial mass lesion (raises ICP), pregnancy[1]

Rx: Intravenous (IV) drip 0.25 to 8 μg/kg/minute. To prepare: 50 mg in 500 mL dextrose 5% in water (D5W) = 100 μg/mL; can be double concentrated to reduce fluid or glucose load[1,4]

Side effects: "Cerebral and coronary steal" phenomenon due to preferential peripheral vasodilation before cerebral vasodilation. Thiocyanate/cyanide toxicity causes neurologic deterioration and hypotension (cover bottle with foil: light sensitive). Nausea, diuresis, platelet inhibition; may increase ICP.[1,3]

Nitroglycerin (Tridil)

Action: Releases NO, resulting in guanylyl cyclase stimulation of cGMP synthesis. Acts predominantly on venous capacitance vessels, affecting arterial vascular smooth muscle at higher concentrations. Primarily venodilation without reflex tachycardia[1,3]

Contraindication: Increased ICP or decreased cerebral perfusion[1,2]

Rx: IV drip 10 to 20 μg/minute (increase by 5–10 μg/minute q 5–10 minute)[1,3,4]

Side effects: Does not cause "coronary steal"; can cause transient increase in ICP, headache, hypotension, rebound hypertension, and methemoglobinemia[1–4]

Labetalol (Normondyne)

Action: Blocks α-1 selective, β nonselective; hepatic glucuronide conjugation; may lower ICP[1,3]

Contraindications: Asthma, pregnancy[1]

Rx: Give each dose slow intravenous push (IVP) (over 2 minutes) q 10 minutes until desired blood pressure (BP) achieved; dose sequence: 20, 40, 80, 80, then 80 mg (300 mg total). Once controlled, use = same total dose IVP q 8 hours. Alternative: IV drip: add 40 mL (200 mg) to 160 mL of intravenous fluids (IVF) (result 1 mg/mL). Run at 2 mL/minute (2 mg/minute) until desired BP (usual effective dose 50–200 mg) or until 300 mg given, then titrate rate.

Bradycardia limits dose; increase slowly because effect takes 10 to 20 minutes. Oral (PO) dose: start with 200 mg bid if converting from IV; otherwise, start 100 mg PO bid and increase 100 mg/dose q 2 days, maximum 2400 mg/day.[1-4]

Side effects: Fatigue, dizziness, orthostatic hypotension[1,3]

Hydralazine (Apresoline)

Action: Direct arteriolar smooth muscle vasodilator; may act through NO or calcium[1,3]

Contraindication: Liver metabolism; slow acetylators should not receive >200 mg/day—may induce lupus-like syndrome.[1,3]

Rx: 10 to 20 mg q 15 to 20 minutes, maximum 40 mg; repeat prn[1,3,4]

Side effects: Nausea/vomiting, headache, increased intracranial blood flow, reflex tachycardia[1,3]

Esmolol (Brevibloc)

Action: Short-acting selective β-1 antagonist; metabolized by red blood cell (RBC) esterase, urinary excretion; may lower ICP[1,3]

Contraindication: Avoid in congestive heart failure (CHF)[1]

Rx: Mix 5 g/500 mL normal saline (NS), give IV 500 µg/kg loading dose over 1 minute, follow with 4 minute infusion starting with 50 µg/kg/minute. Repeat loading dose and increment infusion rate by 50 µg/kg/minute q 5 minutes. Rarely >100 µg/kg/minute required. Doses >200 µg/kg/minute add little.[1,2,4]

Side effects: Dose-related hypotension; resolves within 30 minutes of discontinuation (D/C). Less bronchospasm than other β-blockers.[1,2]

Diltiazem (Cardizem)

Action: Slow calcium-channel antagonist; relaxes vascular smooth muscle without reflex tachycardia[1]

Contraindications: Sick sinus syndrome, wide complex tachycardia, Wolff-Parkinson-White (WPW) syndrome, second-degree or greater atrioventricular (A-V) block and concurrent β-blockers[1,3]

Rx: 20 mg IV over 2 minutes; 0.25 mg/kg. May repeat 1 × in 15 minutes if response is inadequate. Not suggested as a drip for neurosurgical patients.[1]

Side effects: Hepatitis, edema, blurred vision, flushing, injection site reaction[1,3]

Nifedipine (Procardia)

Action: Short-acting calcium-channel blocker. Decreases systemic vascular resistance; increases cardiac index, cerebral blood flow (CBF) (by 10–20%), glomerular filtration rate (GFR), and Na^+ retention[1,3]

Contraindications: Hypersensitivity, acute myocardial infarction (MI)[1,3]

Rx: PO 10 to 20 mg, faster onset with sublingual/buccal administration (puncture capsule) or if chewed. If no response after 20 to 30 minutes, give additional 10 mg.[1,3,4]

Side effects: Flushing, headache, palpitation, edema, reflex tachycardia[1,3]

Nicardipine (Cardene)

Action: The only second generation IV dihydropyridine calcium channel blocker.

Contraindications: Can often cause neurologic worsening in patients with stroke, intracerebral hemorrhage, and subarachnoid hemorrhage. Nicardipine IV drip is the relative large volume of fluid needed (up to 150 cc/hour). Has been shown to increase intracranial pressure in some limited animal and human studies.

Rx: Nicardipine drip 25 mg/250 cc in 250 cc of normal saline (NS), on a pump for a concentration of 0.1 mg/mL. Induction at a rate of 0.2 µg/kg/min, or 5 mg/hour (50 mL/hour), and may be increased in increments of 2.5 mg/hour every 5 to 15 minutes, depending upon the need to rapidly or gradually control blood pressure, to a maximum of 15 mg/hour (150 mL/hour). Once the desired level is achieved decrease rate to 3 mg/hour (30 mL/hour). Nicardipine drip is not compatible with sodium bicarbonate injection or lactated Ringer's solution.

Side effects: Dizziness, fainting, unusual weakness, lightheadedness, headache, flushing, nausea, vomiting, tiredness, swelling of the ankles/feet, frequent urination, shortness of breath, irregular heartbeat, joint/muscle pain, tingling of the hands/feet, mood changes, ringing in the ears

Angiotensin II Receptor Blockers

(Candesartan, Cilexetil, Eprosartan, Irbesartan, Losartan, Mesylate, Olmesartan, Telmisartan, Valsartan)

Action: Angiotensin II receptor blockers; allows blood vessel wall relaxation and dilation, reducing blood pressure, and increases release of sodium and water into urine

Contraindications: Hypersensitivity, pregnancy.

Rx: The oral dosage depends on the specific medication used.

Side effects: Headache and dizziness. Other side effects may be diarrhea, stomach problems, muscle cramps and back and leg pain, insomnia, nasal congestion, cough, sinus problems, and upper respiratory infection. Less likely to cause a cough when compared to angiotensin-converting enzyme blockers.

Enalaprilat (Vasotec)

Action: Angiotensin converting enzyme (ACE) inhibitor; may lower ICP[1,3]

Contraindication: Pregnancy[1]

Rx: Initially, start IV 1.25 mg slow over 5 minutes, then 1.25 to 5 mg q 6 hours response seen in 15 minutes; may repeat 0.625 mg in 1 hour if response is inadequate. Maximum 5 mg q 6 hours.[1,3,4]

Side effects: Hyperkalemia ~1%; can cause renal insufficiency, angioedema, agranulocytosis[1,3]

Clonidine (Catapres)

Action: Inhibits sympathetic outflow by acting on cardiovascular control receptors in the medulla oblongata[1,3]

Contraindication: Hypersensitivity[1]

Rx: Rapid control: 0.2 mg PO, then 0.1 mg PO q 1 hour; stop at 0.8 mg total or if orthostatic. Maintenance dose: 0.1 mg PO bid or tid; increase slowly to maximum 2.4 mg/day (usual 0.2–0.8 mg/day). Patch 0.1 mg, 0.2 mg, 0.3 mg/week titrate to desired effect; maximum 0.6 mg/week.[1,3,4-]

Side effects: Tachycardia rare; mild confusion/sedation; fluid retention, dry mouth, constipation, rebound hypertension[1]

Hypotension

The appropriate evaluation of the patient's volume status and monitoring, including central venous pressure (CVP), Swan-Ganz catheterization, and arterial line, are essential to treat hemodynamic instability. IVF is always first line.[2]

Dopamine (Inotropin)

Action: Primarily a vasoconstrictor; 25% of dopamine given is rapidly converted to norepinephrine (NE). At doses >10 µg/kg/minute, α, β, and dopaminergic effect (essentially giving NE). At 2 to 10 µg/kg/minute, primarily β-1, positive inotrope. At 0.5 to 2.0 µg/kg/minute, primarily dopaminergic, vasodilating renal, mesenteric, coronary and cerebral vessels, positive inotrope.[1,3]

Contraindication: Pregnancy class C[1,3]

Rx: Mix 800 mg/250 mL NS, central line. Start with 2 to 5 µg/kg/minute and titrate for response; maximum 20 µg/kg/minute.[1-4]

Side effects: Tachycardia, peripheral vasoconstriction, arrhythmias, hyperglycemia[1,3]

Dobutamine (Dobutrex)

Action: Racemic mixture: L-isomer is α-agonist, D-isomer nonspecific; β-agonist comparable to dopamine and nitroprusside[1,3]

Contraindication: Hypertrophic cardiomyopathy[1]

Rx: Mix 500 mg/250 mL NS. Usual range 2.5 to 10.0 µg/kg/minute; rarely, doses up to 40 µg used. To prepare: Put 50 mg in 250 mL D5W to yield 200 µg/mL.[1-4]

Side effects: Tachycardia, possibly platelet function inhibition[1,3]

Norepinephrine (Levophed)

Action: β-1 and α-1 receptor agonist[1]

Contraindications: Hypertrophic obstructive cardiomyopathy, tetralogy of Fallot (right ventricular [RV] outflow tract obstruction)[1,3]

Rx: Mix 4 mg/250 mL NS. Initial rate 0.5 to 1.0 µg/minute. Average 4 to 16 µg/minute; maximum 30 to 47 µg/minute[1,3]

Side effects: Vasoconstriction (splanchnic and renal), arrhythmias[1]

Phenylephrine (Neosynephrine)

Action: Pure α vasoconstrictor; causes reflex increase in parasympathetic tone with resultant slowing of pulse. Useful in hypotension associated with tachycardia.[1-3]

Contraindication: Spinal cord injuries

Rx: Mix 40 mg/500 mL NS to yield 80 μg/mL; rate of 8 mL/hour = 10 μg/minute. Pressor range: Initial 100 to 180 μg/minute; maintenance 40 to 60 μg/minute[1-3]

Side effects: Cardiac output and renal blood flow may decrease.[1]

Inamrinone (Inocor)

Action: Inotrope-vasodilator; inhibits phosphodiesterase III; resembles dobutamine hemodynamically with less tachyphylaxis[1,3]

Contraindication: Thrombocytopenia[1,3]

Rx: 0.75 mg/kg IV slow bolus over 2 to 3 minutes, then 5 to 30 μg/kg/minute infusion. May rebolus 0.75 mg/kg IV slow 30 minutes after starting therapy.[1,3,4]

Side effects: Vasodilation hypotension, 2% thrombocytopenia, and hepatotoxicity[1,3]

Epinephrine (Adrenaline)

Action: Nonspecific adrenergic agonist has β-2 activity unlike NE and twice as potent ionotrope.[1,3]

Contraindications: Hypertrophic obstructive cardiomyopathy, tetralogy of Fallot (RV outflow tract obstruction)[1,3]

Rx: 0.5 to 1.0 mg of 1:10,000 solution IVP; may repeat q 5 minutes (may bolus per endotracheal tube). Drip: Start at 1 μg/minute; titrate up to 8 μg/minute (to prepare: put 1 mg in 100 mL NS)[1,3,4]

Side effects: Vasoconstriction (splanchnic and renal), arrhythmias[1]

Isoproterenol (Isuprel)

Action: Nonselective β-receptor agonist, potent inotrope (β1), and peripheral vasodilator (β2); second-line agent after dopamine for bradycardia unresponsive to atropine[1,3]

Contraindications: Digitalis bradycardia, angina[1]

Rx: Mix 1 mg/500 ml NS = 2 μg/mL; start at 2 μg/minute, titrate up to 10 μg/minute[1,4]

Side effects: Tachycardia, vasodilation, increased myocardial oxygen demand[1,3]

◆ Electrolytes/Intravenous Fluids

Electrolytes function within a narrow therapeutic range to promote health and ameliorate disease. Increasing amounts of electrolytes are needed at times of stress but still less than would cause further harm.

Sodium and Intravenous Fluids

Phosphorus

Hyper: Phos-Lo (calcium acetate) 2 tablets NG/PO tid with meals[1,3]

Action: Combines with dietary phosphate to form insoluble calcium phosphate[1]

Contraindications: Hypersensitivity to components, hypercalcemia, renal calculi[1]

Side effects: Hypercalcemia[1]

Hypo: Potassium phosphate 1 to 2 g qid divided NG/IV tid[1,4]

Action: Elevates serum phosphorus and serum potassium levels[1]

Contraindications: Hyperphosphatemia, hyperkalemia, hypocalcemia, hypomagnesemia, renal failure[1]

Side effects: Diarrhea, nausea, stomach pain[1]

Calcium

Hyper: Treat aggressively with 0.9 NS infusion to correct volume deficit. Follow with loop diuretic (i.e., furosemide 20–40 mg IV/PO q 2–4 hours). May use zoledronate 4 mg IV over 15 minutes qid if unresponsive to loop diuretic.[1,4]

Hyper: Calcium gluconate 2.25 to 14 mEq slow IVP or 500 to 2000 mg PO bid/tid. Calcium chloride 500 to 1000 mg slow IVP q 1 to 3 days.[1,4]

Action: Elevation of serum calcium[1,3]

Contraindications: Hypersensitivity, hypercalcemia[1,3]

Side effects: Extravasation necrosis, hypotension[1,3]

Magnesium

Hypo: Magnesium sulfate 1 g of 20% solution IM q 6 hours × 4 doses or 2 g IVP over 1 hour (note: monitor for hypertension); 1 g will raise serum magnesium 0.4 mEq/dL.[1,4]

Action: Elevation of serum magnesium[1]

Contraindications: Heart block, serious renal impairment, myocardial damage, hepatitis, Addison's disease[1]

Side effects: Hypotension, asystole, CNS depression, diarrhea, decreased neuromuscular transmission[1]

Potassium

Hyper: Treat with D5W, IV calcium and insulin administration if severe. Kayexalate (sodium polystyrene) 1 g/kg up to 15 to 60 g PO q 6 hours prn.[1,4]

Action: Exchanges sodium ions for potassium ions in the intestines[1]

Contraindications: Hypersensitivity, hypernatremia[1]

Side effects: Hypokalemia, hypocalcemia, hypomagnesemia, sodium retention[1]

Hypo: Potassium chloride 20 to 40 mEq PO bid or 10 to 20 mEq IVP over 1 hour (note: monitor for cardiac arrhythmias)[1,4]

Action: Elevation of serum potassium and serum chloride[1]

Contraindications: Severe renal impairment, untreated Addison's disease, hyperkalemia, severe tissue trauma[1]

Side effects: Diarrhea, nausea and vomiting, bradycardia, hyperkalemia, weakness, dyspnea[1]

◆ Blood Products

Patients in the NICU should have a CBC checked daily. Blood products should be administered as needed to keep hemoglobin at ~10.0 mg/dL. Platelets and plasma should be administered on a case-by-case basis. Generally, INR should be kept at 1.3 or below, platelet count >100,000.[2]

Packed Red Blood Cells

Each unit of packed red blood cells (PRBC) will raise hemoglobin by 0.8 mg/dL.

Fresh frozen plasma

Plasma transfusion is indicated in patients with documented coagulation factor deficiencies and active bleeding, or who are about to undergo an invasive procedure with suspected coagulation factor deficiencies. Deficiencies can be secondary to congenital or acquired diseases such as liver disease, warfarin anticoagulation, disseminated intravascular coagulation, or massive replacement with red blood cells and crystalloid/collid solutions.

One unit is approximately 250 mL and must be ABO compatible but not Rh factor compatible. The usual dose is 4 units to improve coagulation status by increasing factor levels of at least 10%. However, the amount will vary depending on the patient's size and clotting factor levels.

Platelets

Platelets are indicated in patients with disorders of hemostasis. Platelets are collected from pooled random donors for from a single donor. If given pooled platelets, the dosage is 4 to 6 units, whereas if given from a single donor a standard pack is equivalent to 4 pooled units and a large pack is equivalent to 6 pooled units. Functional platelet count should be maintained above 100,000/microliter for patients undergoing neurosurgical procedures. Abnormal platelet function can be seen with medications such as aspirin, and with kidney disease, liver disease, malignancy, sepsis, and tissue trauma. If platelet dysfunction is present, the patient will require higher levels of platelets to achieve hemostasis. The number of units required to increase the number of platelets is dependent upon weight, being anywhere from 5000/microliter per unit for 200 lb/91 kg to 22000/microliter per unit for a 50 lb/23 kg patient.

Cryoprecipitate

Contains fibrinogen, von Willebrand factor, factor VIII, factor XIII, and fibronectin. It comes in concentrates of 6 units. Each unit provides about 350 mg of fibrinogen. Usually 6 bags or 1 pooled bag is given, which raises the fibrinogen by 1560 mg or 45 mg/dl. Cryoprecipitate is also used to make fibrin glue.

◆ Antiepileptic Medications

Phenytoin (Dilantin)

Action: Modulates voltage-gated Na and Ca neuron channels and enhances Na/K adenosinetriphosphatase (ATPase) neuronal and glial activity. Reduced repetitive firing in neurons caused by slowing in the rate of recovery of channels due to enhanced inactivation of Na central nervous system (CNS) depressant, reduces seizure propagation, induces cerebellar-vestibular dysfunction; also weak antiarrythmic, inhibits insulin release.[1-3]

Contraindication: Hypersensitivity to medication; class C pregnancy[1,3]

Rx: Loading dose 15 to 20 mg/kg IV. Do not exceed 50 mg/minute IV. Usual 1 g load IV slow over 1 hour, then maintenance of 100 mg IV tid. Always check levels after 3 days. Phosphenytoin formulation can be given faster IV because it does not contain propylene glycol. Before infusion, it should be diluted in 5% dextrose in water or 0.9% NS to a concentration of 1.5 to 25.0 mg/mL (phenytoin equivalents; PE). To avoid hypotension, do not exceed 150 mg PE/minute. For seizure prophylaxis, loading dose is 16 to 18 mg/kg IV or intramuscularly (IM). Daily maintenance dose is 4 to 6 mg PE/kg/day IV or IM, divided into 2 or more doses.[1-4]

Side effects: Hypotension, hyperglycemia, arrhythmia, peripheral neuropathy, gingival hyperplasia, megaloblastic anemia (rare), hepatotoxicity (rare), Stevens-Johnson syndrome[1]

Valproic Acid (Depakene)

Action: Inhibitor of γ-aminobutyric acid (GABA) transaminase and glutamate decarboxylase[1,3]

Contraindication: Pregnancy[1]

Rx: 600 to 3000 mg/day; start at IV/PO 10 to 15 mg/kg/day. If dose >250 mg per day, it should be divided.[1,4]

Side effects: Gastrointestinal (GI) upset, pancreatitis, liver failure if <2 years of age, teratogenic, drowsiness, hyperammonia, hair loss, weight gain, tremor[1]

Carbamazepine (Tegretol)

Action: Blocks voltage-dependent Na channel in neuronal cell membrane; hepatic metabolism. Before starting, check complete blood count (cbc), platelet count, and serum Fe. Do not start or stop if white blood (cell) count (WBC) < 4, hematocrit (HCT) < 32, platelet count (Plt) < 100, reticulocyte (Retic) < 3, Fe >150.[1,3]

Contraindication: Hepatic failure or insufficiency[1]

Rx: 200 to 400 PO bid-qid[1,4]

Side effects: Aplastic anemia, ataxia, drowsiness, transient diplopia, Stevens-Johnson syndrome, syndrome of inappropriate antidiuretic hormone (SIADH), hepatitis[1]

Phenobarbital (Luminal)

Action: Opens postsynaptic Cl ion channels, decreasing Na and Ca influx[1,3]

Contraindication: Multiple drug interactions[1,3]

Rx: IV/PO/IM loading 20 mg/kg/day; slow maintenance 30 to 250 mg/day divided bid/tid; therapeutic level 15 to 30 μg/mL[1,3,4]

Side effects: Cognitive impairment, paradoxical hyperactivity[1,3]

Primidone (Mysoline)

Action: Same as phenobarbital[1,3]

Contraindication: Multiple drug interactions[1]

Rx: Start 125 mg/day × 1 week; increase slowly to avoid sedation, 250 to 1500 mg/day, divide bid[1]

Side effects: Fewer side effects, more significant in seizure control; loss of libido[1]

Ethosuximide (Zarontin)

Action: Antiseizure[1]

Contraindication: Hypersensitivity to succinimides; use with caution in pregnancy.

Rx: Oral/nasogastric (NG) only 500 to 1500 mg/day. In children, start at 250 mg/day, titrate up to 500 mg/day divided bid.[1]

Side effects: Lethargy, hiccoughs, headache, Stevens-Johnson syndrome, systemic lupus erythematosus (SLE)–like syndrome, psychotic behavior[1]

Clonazepam (Klonipin)

Action: Benzodiazepine used short term in acute setting; not for long-term use.[1,3]

Contraindication: Long-term use[1]

Rx: Start IV/nasogastric [NG] at 1.5 mg/day, divided tid, increased by 0.5 mg q 3 days. Usual dosage range 1 to 12 mg/day; maximum 20 mg/day.[1,4]

Side effects: Ataxia, drowsiness behavior changes[1]

Gabapentin (Neurontin)

Action: Unknown[1,3]

Contraindication: Hypersensitivity[1]

Rx: Start 300 mg PO/NG q HS (hold for loose stools); increase slowly over 3 days to 300 to 600 mg until therapeutic[1]

Side effects: Dizziness, ataxia, fatigue, nystagmus, viral infection[1,3]

Lamotrigine (Lamictal)

Action: Inhibits release of glutamate and voltage-sensitive Na channels[1,3]

Contraindication: Hypersensitivity to pregnancy class C[1]

Rx: Start 50 mg PO qid × 2 weeks, then bid × 2 weeks[1,4]

Side effects: Headache, fatigue, nausea/vomiting, pancreatitis, peripheral neuropathy[1]

Levetiracetam (Keppra)

Action: Unknown[1,3]

Contraindication: Hypersensitivity[1]

Rx: PO/NG 500 mg bid, titrate to effective maximum 3000 mg daily[1]

Side effects: Somnolence, weakness[1]

Pentobarbital (Nembutal)

Action: Short-acting barbiturate, depressing cortical activity[1,3]

Contraindications: Hypersensitivity, hepatic impairment, dyspnea, porphyria, pregnancy[1,3]

Rx: For induction of coma: Loading dose of 10 mg/kg IV over 30 minutes, then 5 mg/kg q hour × 3 doses, then maintenance 1 mg/kg/hour titrating to

1–2 burst per page. For status epilepticus: IV start at 65 to 95 mg/minute, titrate up to 1400 mg total dose.[1,2,4]

Side effects: Bradycardia, hypotension, syncope, rash, exfoliative dermatitis, Stevens-Johnson syndrome[1]

◆ Corticocosteroids

Many animal models have demonstrated that corticosteroids stabilize cell membrane structures, stabilize the blood–spinal cord barrier reducing vasogenic edema, enhance blood flow in the spinal cord, inhibit endorphin release, prevent free radical accumulation, and moderate the inflammatory response. However, corticosteroids have many side effects and must be used with caution. These side effects include sepsis, pneumonia, death due to respiratory complications, and other complications.
  See **Table 19–1**.

Dexamethasone (Decadron)

Action: Decreases inflammation by suppressing immune response, inhibiting polymorphonuclear (PMN) neutrophil leukocytes migration[1–3]

Contraindications: Hypersensitivity, active untreated infections[1,3]

Rx: Brain tumor protocol for cerebral edema: 10 to 20 mg loading dose, then 4 to 10 mg q 6. Minimal 10 day taper for weaning.[2]

Table 19–1   Corticosteroids[1–4]

Name	Approximate equivalent dose (mg)	Relative anti-inflammatory potency	Relative mineralo-corticoid potency	Biologic half-life (hours)
Betamethasone	0.6–0.75	20–30	0	36–54
Cortisone	25	0.8	2	8–12
Dexamethasone	0.75	20–30	0	36–54
Fludrocortisone	–	10	125	18–36
Hydrocortisone	20	1	2	8–12
Methylprednisolone	4	5	0	18–36
Prednisolone	5	4	1	18–36
Prednisone	5	4	1	18–36
Triamcinolone	4	5	0	12–36

*These are multiple values standing for "number of times more potent."

Side effects: Cushing's syndrome, hypersensitivity reactions, immuno-suppression, insomnia, agitation, vertigo, psychosis, delirium, pseudotumor cerebri, increased appetite[1-3]

Methylprednisolone (Solu-medrol)

Action: Decreases inflammation by suppressing immune response, inhibiting PMN migration[1,3]

Contraindications: Hypersensitivity, active untreated infections[1]

Rx: Spinal shock protocol: 30 mg/kg IV over 15 minutes, followed 45 minutes later by infusion of 5.4 mg/kg/hour × 23 hours[1,2]

Side effects: Cushing's syndrome, hypersensitivity reactions, immuno-suppression, insomnia, agitation, vertigo, psychosis, delirium, pseudotumor cerebri, increased appetite[1-3]

◆ Nonsteroidal Anti-inflammatory Drugs

Nonsteroidal anti-inflammatory drugs (NSAIDs) inhibit isoforms of the enzyme cyclooxygenase (COX 1-3) blocking prostaglandin synthesis. NSAIDs alone may be given for pain that is 4 or less. They should be with held back for 4 to 10 days after mild bleeding and not given at all with severe bleeding, and they should be given with a stomach protectant and adequate hydration to help prevent side effects. NSAIDs belong to multiple drug groups with each group affecting individual patients differently. Therefore, if one group of NSAIDs does not work consider treatment with another. When pain is 4 to 8, NSAIDs can be given with other pain-altering medications.
See **Table 19–2**.

◆ Sedatives

Propofol

Action: Enhances synaptic inhibition mediated by GABA[1,3]

Contraindications: Allergy to egg or soybean. Reduce doses for elderly, hypovolemic, or those with concomitant use of narcotics.[1,3]

Rx: Sedation: IV bolus 0.1 to 1.0 mg/kg, titrate slowly to the desired effect (onset of slurred speech); infusion 20 to 75 µg/kg/minute, monitoring

Table 19–2 Nonsteroidal Anti-inflammatory Drugs[1–4]

Generic name	Dose	Frequency (hours)	Maximum daily dose	Class
Acetaminophen	*10–75 mg/kg/day	4–6	4000 mg	Para-aminophenol, COX–3 inhibitor
Aspirin	5–100 mg/kg/day	4–6	8000 mg	Salicylate
Celecoxib	200–400 mg	12–24	800 mg	COX-2 inhibitor
Choline magnesium trisalicylate	30–60 mg/kg/day	8–12	4500 mg	Salicylate
Diclofenac	25–75 mg	6–8	200 mg	Pyrroleacetic acid
Diflunisal	250–500 mg	8–12	1500 mg	Salicylate
Flubiprofen	50–100 mg	6–8	300 mg	Propionic acid
Ibuprofen	5–50 mg/kg/day	4–6	3200 mg	Propionic acid
Indomethacin	25–75 mg	8	200 mg	Indoleacetic acid
Ketoprofen	12.5–75.0 mg	6–8	300 mg	Propionic acid
Ketorolac	30–60 mg	IV, PO 6–8	150 mg	Pyrroleacetic acid
Meloxicam	7.5–15 mg	24	15 mg	Benzothiazine
Naproxen	250–500 mg	6–8	1500 mg	Propionic acid
Oxaprozin	600–1200 mg	8–12	1800 mg	Propionic acid
Piroxicam	10–20 mg	24	20 mg	Benzothiazine

COX-2, cyclooxygenase-2; COX-3, cyclooxygenase-3; IV, intravenous; PO, orally.

respiratory/cardiac function continuously. Anesthetic induction: IV 2 to 4 mg/kg (give slowly over 30 seconds in 2–3 divided doses). Anesthetic maintenance: IV bolus 25 to 50 mg, then infuse at 100 to 200 µg/kg/minute. Antiemetic: 10 mg IV.[1-3] May also be used for burst suppression but ability to provide neuronal protection is controversial.

Side effects: Hypotension from myocardial depression, decreases systemic vascular resistance (SVR). Depresses laryngeal reflexes more than barbiturates or etomidate. Pain on injection into small veins, histamine release with rapid injection, anaphylaxis.[1,3]

Midazolam (Versed)

Action: Binds to GABA receptors containing gamma subunits, half-life 1.5 to 3 hours[1,3]

Contraindications: Hypersensitivity, narrow-angle glaucoma, pregnancy[1]

Rx: Conscious sedation: Slow IVP 1 to 2 mg over 2 minutes (do not exceed 2.5 mg with initial dose), wait 2 to 3 minutes, repeat to total of 0.1 to 0.15 mg/kg. IM preop: 0.07 to 0.08 mg/kg (5 mg/70 kg) ~1 hour preop. Induction general anesthesia: Initial dose slow IVP. For unpremedicated average adult age <55 years: 0.25 mg/kg; for >55 years, American Society of Anesthesiologists (ASA) class I or II 0.2 mg/kg; for ASA class III or IV, 0.15 mg/kg. To maintain, repeat 25% initial dose.[1,3] May also be used for burst suppression but ability to provide neuronal protection is controversial.

Side effects: Decreased tidal volume/respiratory rate, hypotension, drowsiness, oversedation, nausea and vomiting[1]

Lorazepam (Ativan)

Action: A benzodiazepine with antianxiety, sedative, and anticonvulsant effects which interacts with the γ-aminobutyric acid (GABA)-benzodiazepine receptor complex.

Contraindications: Hypersensitivity to benzodiazepines or their vehicles (polythylene glycol, propylene glycol, and benzyl alcohol). It should not be used in patients with acute narrow-angle glaucoma, or in non-intubated patients with sleep apnea syndrome or severe respiratory insufficiency. The use of Ativan injection intra-arterially is contraindicated because, as with other injectable benzodiazepines, inadvertent intra-arterial injection may produce arteriospasm resulting in gangrene, which may require amputation.

Rx: Mild sedation: IV 0.5 to 2 mg (0.044 mg/kg). Conscious sedation: up to a total of 4 mg (0.05 mg/kg). Can also be used IM reaching peak concentration in 3 hours. Orally 0.5 to 1 mg 2 to 3 times per day.

Can also be used for burst suppression but ability to provide neuronal protection is controversial.

As with benzodiazepines, its action can be reversed with flumazenil (Romazicon) but resedation may occur. Flumazenil action begins less than 2 minutes after administration and peaks in 6 to 10 minutes. The initial dosage is 0.2 mg IV repeated at 1 minute intervals to a maximum of 1mg.

Side effects: Respiratory depression, fetal damage.

Pentobarbital (Nembutal)

Action: Fast acting barbiturate with 3 to 4 hour duration of action.

Contraindications: Hypersensitivity, status asthmaticus, severe cardiovascular disease, porphyria.

Rx: Load intravenous 10 mg/hour. Give as 2.5 mg/kg/hour slowly every 15 minutes for 4 doses. Hold if blood pressure drops inappropriately. Then continue at 10 mg/kg/hour for 3 additional hours. Next continue maintenance dose at 1 to 3 mg/kg/hour. Titrate for 1 to 2 burst per page. If the loading dose achieves burst suppression then continue at maintenance dose. Watch for inadequate blood pressure/cerebral perfusion pressure. If using to salvage brain function, ICP should decrease within the hour after burst suppression has occurred. Check daily complete blood count (cbc) and blood cultures to monitor for infection and sepsis. Check pentobarbital level 1 hour after completing loading dose and daily thereafter. May also be used for burst suppression but ability to provide neuronal protection is controversial.

Side effects: Hypotension, inability to rapidly diagnose infection

Haldol

Action: Blocks postsynaptic D_1 and D_2 receptors in the brain; depresses reticular activating system; depresses hypothalamic hormones[1,3]

Contraindications: Hypersensitivity, Parkinson's disease, severe cardiac or hepatic disease, bone marrow suppression, coma[1]

Rx: Sedation: IV/IM/IVPB (intravenous piggyback); may repeat bolus doses after 30 minutes until calm achieved, then administer 50% of the maximum dose every 6 hours. Agitation: mild 0.5 to 2.0 mg; moderate 2.5 to 5.0 mg; severe 10 to 20 mg.[1]

Side effects: Hypotenstion/hypertension, anxiety, extrapyramidal and dystonic reactions, pseudoparkinsonian reactions, tardive dyskinesia, neuromalignant syndrome, akathisia[1]

Thiopental (Pentothal)

Action: Short-acting barbiturate[1,3]

Contraindications: Hypersensitivity, status asthmaticus, severe cardiovascular disease, porphyria[1,3]

Rx: Adults: Initial concentration should not exceed 2.5%. Give 50 mg test dose moderately rapid IVP; if tolerated, give 100 to 200 mg IVP over 20 to 30 seconds (500 mg may be required in large patient).[1,3,4] May also be used for burst suppression but ability to provide neuronal protection is controversial.

Side effects: Dose-related respiratory depression, myocardial depression, hypotension in hypovolemic patients, irritation if extravassated, intraarterial injection—necrosis, agitation if injected slowly[1]

Etomidate

Action: Potentiates GABA and depresses reticular activating system[1,3]

Contraindication: Hypersensitivity

Rx: IV induction: 0.1 to 0.6 mg/kg. Infusion: 0.25 to 1.00 mg/minute (5 to 20 mg/kg/minute). Continuous infusion not recommended. Rectal: In children 6 months to 6 years old, 6.5 mg/kg produces reliable hypnosis in 4 minutes but maintains a rapid recovery without any untoward effects.[1] May also be used for burst suppression but ability to provide neuronal protection is controversial.

Side effects: Pain on injection into small veins, high incidence of thrombophlebitis (24% compared with thiopental 4%), myoclonus. Lowers seizure threshold, nausea and vomiting, adrenocortical suppression.[1]

Ketamine

Action: Direct effect on the cortex and limbic system, producing cataleptic-like state, dissociated from surroundings[1]

Contraindications: Increased ICP, hypertension, hypersensitivity, aneurysms, thyrotoxicosis, CHF, angina[1,3]

Rx: 1 to 2 mg/kg IV over 1 to 2 minutes or 4 mg/kg IM induces 10 to 20 minute dissociative state.[1] May also be used for burst suppression but ability to provide neuronal protection is controversial.

Side effects: Concurrent atropine minimizes hypersalivation; hallucinations, vivid dreams, hemodynamic instability[1]

◆ Anticoagulants

Most neurosurgical intensive care unit (NICU) patients are immobilized for one reason or another. Deep venous thrombosis (DVT) prophylaxis should be implemented as soon as possible. Always begin with sequential compression devices and thigh-high compression stockings. Patients who will be long-term immobilized should be considered for anticoagulation drugs. Depending on the pathology, patients with traumatic intracranial hemorrhage (ICH) with no sequelae 72 hours posthemorrhage may be started on anticoagulation drugs.[2]

Heparin

Action: Prevents the conversion of fibrinogen to fibrin[1,3]

Contraindications: Hypersensitivity, severe thrombocytopenia, uncontrolled bleeding[1]

Rx: 5000 units subcutaneous (SQ) tid[1,3,4]

Side effects: Bleeding, vasospasm, thrombocytopenia, bruising[1,3]

Lovenox

Action: Prevents the conversion of fibrinogen to fibrin[1,3]

Contraindications: Hypersensitivity to pork products, uncontrolled bleeding[1]

Rx: Prevention: 40 SQ qid. Treatment, DVT or PE: 1 mg/kg bid[1,3,4]

Side effects: Bleeding, fever, bruising[1,3]

◆ Pain Medications

The most commonly prescribed medications for severe pain are opioids, which stimulate mu, kappa, delta and nociceptin/orphanin FG (N/OFQ) receptor. The first and most widely used opioids are the group that stimulates the mu receptor; these include morphine, demerol, dilaudid, and fentanyl. Clinically, the effect of opioids is to raise the pain threshold, increasing the minimal intensity needed to feel pain. At the anatomic level, opioids act by inhibiting nociceptive transmission to the spinal cord, activating descending inhibitory pathways, and altering higher center activity of pain perception. Just as NSAIDs belong to different groups with considerable variability in efficacy, opioid groups vary in ability to treat pain, even in the same individual.

Lidocaine Patch (Lidoderm 5%)

Action: Topical analgesic[1]

Contraindications: Hypersensitivity, broken skin barrier; but still can place adjacent to incision[1]

Rx: Place 1 to 3 patches 12 hours per day (12 hours on, 12 hours off); when using on fresh surgical incision, apply both sides but not over.[1]

Side effects: Local edema, erythema, urticaria, anaphylaxis[1,3]

Acetaminophen (Tylenol)

Action: Suspected to be cyclooxygenase-3 (COX-3) inhibitor at very high doses[1,3]

Contraindications: Hypersensitivity, chronic alcohol abuse, impaired liver function[1,3]

Rx: Adults: 650 to 1000 mg PO/PR (far point of accommodation) q 4 to 6 hours, not to exceed 4000 mg/day; children: 10 to 15 mg/kg PO/PR q 4 to 6 hours[1,3,4]

Side effects: Hepatic toxicity[1,3]

Equianalgesic Doses for Severe Pain

See **Table 19–3**.

Ketorolac (Toradol)

Action: Inhibits prostaglandin synthesis; only parenteral nonsteroidal anti-inflammatory drug (NSAID) approved for use in pain control in the United States[1,3]

Contraindication: Hypersensitivity to NSAIDs, active peptic ulcer disease, recent GI perforation, renal impairment, bleeding. Do not use prophylactically before major surgery.[1,3]

Rx: 10 mg PO q 4 to 6 hours; IM/IV 30 to 60 mg q 6 to 8 hours, use only continuously for 72 hours. Acute pain after surgery when bleeding is controlled: 120 mg in 500 cc normal saline to run at 10 cc/hour until completed over 50 hours. Must have initial loading dose of 30 to 60 mg IV. Stomach protectants must be given.[1,3]

Side effects: Bleeding time prolonged by platelet function inhibition, gastric mucosal irritation, and erosion, even though given in IV or IM form. Side effects are worse in the elderly and with prolonged use.[1,3]

Nalbuphine (Nubain)

Action: Kappa agonist, mu antagonist[1,3]

Contraindications: Hypersensitivity, head injury, impaired pulmonary or liver function, pregnancy, elderly patients[1]

Rx: IV 0.15 to 2.5 mg/kg q 3 to 6 hours

Side effects: Respiratory depression, severe bradycardia, severe hypotension, sedation, headache, dysphoria[1,3]

Butorphanol (Stadol)

Action: Kappa agonist, mu agonist and antagonist[1,3]

Contraindications: Hypersensitivity; substance abuse; impaired liver, renal, and pulmonary function. Use caution in head-injured patients and CNS depression.[1,3]

Rx: IV 2 mg, IM 0.5 to 4.0 mg q 3 to 4 hours, 0.25 to 32.0 mg/day maximum; intranasal (IN) 1 mg spray q 3 to 6 hours[1]

Side effects: Respiratory depression, substance abuse, severe hypotension, severe bradycardia, sedation, nausea/vomiting[1,3]

Tramadol (Ultram)

Action: Affects mu opioid receptors[1,3]

Contraindications: Hypersensitivity, ethanol intoxication, substance abuse history. Use caution with head-injured patients, those with CNS infections or lesions, and patients with elevated ICP.[1–3]

Rx: 50 to 100 mg PO q 4 to 6 hours prn[1]

Side effects: Hypoventilation, constipation, bradycardia. Large dose given rapidly may cause chest wall rigidity, dysconjugate gaze, headaches.[1,3]

Codeine

Action: Weak opioid[1]

Contraindications: Hypersensitivity, respiratory depression, paralytic ileus. Use caution in patients with elevated ICP, seizure disorder, or head injury.[1]

Rx: Adults: 30 to 60 mg IM/PO q 3 hours; children: 0.5 to 1 mg/kg/dose q 4 to 6 hours[1]

Side effects: Respiratory depression, CNS depression, hypotension, bradycardia, syncope, cardiac arrest, elevated ICP, seizures, paralytic ileus, dependency, shock, anaphylactoid reactions. More common side effects include dizziness, nausea and vomiting, sedation, and constipation.[1]

Hydrocodone

Action: Moderate opioid[1,3]

Contraindications: Hypersensitivity, respiratory depression, paralytic ileus, CNS depression, head injury, elevated ICP, seizure disorder[1,3]

Rx: Available in 5.0, 7.5, and 10.0 mg doses with acetaminophen dose, 1 or 2 tablets PO q 4 to 6 hours; not to exceed 60 mg hydrocodone in 24 hours, not to exceed 4000 mg acetaminophen per 24 hours[1,3]

Side effects: CNS depression, respiratory depression, dependency, paralytic ileus, increased ICP, hypotension, nausea and vomiting, sedation[1,3]

Fentanyl

Action: Binds to mu opiate receptor in the CNS, inhibits pain pathway. Opiate potency 100 × morphine. In small doses, lasts 20 to 30 minutes. Supplied in concentration 50 µg/mL. Increases CBF.[1,3]

Contraindications: Hypersensitivity, increased ICP, respiratory depression, pregnancy[1,3]

Rx: 25 to 100 µg (0.5–2.0 mL) IVP, repeat prn. Also available as transdermal patch, which is changed every 72 hours, delivering 25, 50, 75, or 100 µg/hour.[1]

Side effects: Hypoventilation, constipation, bradycardia. Large dose given rapidly may cause chest wall rigidity, dysconjugate gaze.[1]

Morphine

Action: Binds to mu opiate receptor in the CNS; inhibits pain pathway, increases CBF[1,3]

Contraindications: Hypersensitivity, increased ICP, respiratory depression[1,3]

Rx: Drip: mix 100 mg/100 mL NS, start 2 mg q hour, titrate to effect maximum 10 mg q hour. IVP: start 2 mg q 1 to 2 hours, increase prn.[1–4]

Table 19–3   Equianalgesic Dose for Severe Pain[1–4]

Drug	Receptor agonist or antagonist	Route	Dosage	Dosage frequency (hours)	Half-life (hours)
Morphine	Mu	IV	0.1 mg/kg	3–4	2.1–2.6
		IM	0.2 mg/kg	3–4	
		PO	0.3 mg/kg	3–4	
Ketamine	Mu	IV	5 µg/kg/minute	3–4	
Hydromorphone	Mu	IV, IM	0.015 mg/kg	3–6	2.6–3.2
			0.5–1.0 mg/hour		
		PO	0.06 mg/kg	3–6	
Fentanyl	Mu	IV	25–50 µg/hour		3.7
		TC	25–100 µg/hour, 600–7200 µg	72 hour patch	3.7
Oxycodone	Mu	PO	0.2 mg/kg	3–4	
Hydrocodone	Mu	PO	0.2 mg/kg	3–4	
Meperidine	Mu	IV	0.75 mg/kg	2–3	3
		IM	75 mg		3
		PO	300–400 µg		3
Levorphanol	Mu	IM	0.02 mg/kg	4–6	3
		PO	0.04 mg/kg	6–8	11
Buprenorphine	Mu	IV	0.4 mg/kg	6–8	11
		SL	2–24 mg	6–8	5
Codeine	Mu	IV	1 mg/kg	6–8	5
		IM	1 mg/kg	6–8	3
		PO	1 mg/kg	3–4	3

Drug	Mechanism	Route	Dose		
Tramadol	Mu	PO	50–100 mg	6	
Nalbuphine	Kappa agonist, mu antagonist	IV	0.15–2.50 mg/kg	3–6	5
Butorphanol	Kappa agonist, mu agonist and antagonist	IV, IM	2 mg 0.5–4.0 mg 0.25–32.0 mg/day maximum	3–4	3
		IN	1 mg spray, 1–4 mg/day	3–6	
		IV			
Thyrotropin-releasing hormone					
Naloxone	Binds mu receptor without stimulation; also binds kappa and delta	IV	0.4 mg every 2–3 minutes		1
Pentazocine	Kappa; mu agonist and antagonist	PO	50 mg	4–6	4
Propoxyphene hydrochloride	Mu	PO	65 mg	4–6	9

IM, intramuscularly; IN, intranasal; IV, intravenous; PO, orally; SL, sublingual; TC, transcutaneous.

Side effects: Respiratory depression, miosis, hypotension, bradycardia, apnea, pulmonary edema, dysconjugate gaze[1,3]

◆ Antiemetics

Nausea and vomiting are frequent problems for patients in the NICU due to stimulation of the chemoreceptor trigger zone (CRTZ). Phenothiazine derivatives, such as Phenergan, should be avoided in general, due to a lowering of the seizure threshold.[2]

Ondansetron (Zofran)

Action: Selective 5-hydroxytryptamine (5HT)–receptor antagonist; blocks serotonin on vagus nerve terminals and in the CRTZ[1,3]

Contraindication: Hypersensitivity to ondansetron[1]

Rx: 4 to 8 mg IV q 6 to 8 hours prn nausea/vomiting[1,2]

Side effects: Malaise, fatigue, headache[1]

Granisetron (Kytril)

Action: Selective 5-HT-receptor antagonist. Blocks serotonin both peripherally and centrally at CRTZ.[1,3]

Contraindication: Hypersensitivity to granisetron[1]

Rx: 1 mg PO q 12 hours or 2 mg PO q 24 hours[1]

Side effects: Headache, constipation, dizziness, insomnia, anxiety[1,3]

Trimethobenzamide (Tigan)

Action: Inhibits CRTZ[1,3]

Contraindications: Hypersensitivity to trimethobenzamide or benzocaine. Injection contraindicated in children.[1,3]

Rx: 250 to 300 mg PO tid/qid, 200 mg IM/PR tid/qid[1]

Side effects: Hypotension, depression, coma, disorientation, jaundice, muscle cramps, blurred vision[1,3]

◆ Reversal Agents

Flumazenil

Action: Competitively inhibits benzodiazepine at receptor sites[1,3]

Contraindications: Pregnancy, patients chronically treated with benzodiazepines where antagonism may provoke a withdrawal syndrome and/or seizures. May provoke a panic attack.[1]

Rx: 0.2 mg IV q minute × 1 to 5 doses; maximum dose 1 mg, 3 mg/hour[1]

Side effects: Seizures—high risk in patients on benzodiazapines for long-term sedation, hypoventilation, arrhythmias, and resedation[1,3]

Naloxone

Action: Oxymorphone derivative, competitively binds to opioid receptors, half-life (t½) ~4 to 60 minutes[1,3]

Contraindication: Hypersensitivity; may cause acute withdrawal from opioids in individuals who are physically dependent.

Rx: Load: 1 to 4 μg/kg, infuse at rate of 5 to 15 μg/kg/hour. Titrate IV in small doses 20 to 40 μg.[1,4]

Side effects: Severe unmasked pain can lead to sympathetic and cardiovascular stimulation: hypertension, dysrhythmias, pulmonary edema, and cardiac arrest.[1,3]

Naltrexone

Action: Oxymorphone derivative, competitively binds to opioid receptors, t½ > 10 hours[1]

Contraindication: See naloxone.

Rx: Oral: 100 mg or greater[1,3]

Side effects: See naloxone

Case Management

The patient must be fully resuscitated with 0.9% normal saline. Initially attempts should be made to increase his cerebral perfusion pressure with fluids, and if not successful, with vasopressive medications. A chemistry panel, complete blood count, and coagulation profile should be obtained. After resuscitation, if the patient's GCS remains 8 or less and the coagulation profile is in the normal range with or without the use of blood products, an ICP monitor and drain should be inserted. There is no indication for steroids in the treatment of isolated severe head injury. Sedation could be administered to help control respiratory rate if necessary. Pain medication must be administered when appropriate. An anti-epileptic medication could be started if the patient is at a higher risk of seizures and if a seizure event would likely worsen brain injury.

References

1. Lacy CF, Armstrong LL, Goldman MP, Lance LL. Drug Information Handbook. 11th ed. Hudson, OH: Lexi-Comp; 2003
2. Greenberg MS. Handbook of Neurosurgery. 5th ed. New York: Thieme; 2001
3. Murray L, ed. Physician's Desk Reference. 59th ed. Montvale, NJ: Thompson PDR; 2005
4. Green SM, ed. Tarascon Pocket Pharmacopoeia. Lompoc, CA: Tarascon Publishing; 2005

20
Nutrition

Dan Miulli

Case Study

A 60-year-old male (154 lb [70 kg], 5 ft 5 in [166 cm]) was in a motor vehicle accident and suffered a traumatic subarachnoid hemorrhage. His Glasgow Coma Scale (GCS) score is 7. The patient was in the neurosurgical intensive care unit (NICU) for 2 days, intubated, with a heart rate of 90.

See page 286 for Case Management.

◆ Need for Nutrition

At the moment of neurologic injury, only half of the damage that is going to happen occurs. After admission to the medical system, when the remainder of the harm can occur, is when the biggest impact in care can be made. *Guidelines for the Management of Severe Head Injury*[1] provides information for the optimal care of patients with severe head injuries, from appropriate oxygenation, blood pressure, and intracranial pressure (ICP) to nutrition. Much of the information given in this chapter is drawn from this source.

Adequate nutrition is critical to maintaining internal systems, meeting the metabolic demands of increased activity in illness, and helping in the repair and healing of wounds. Considering all the secondary insults occurring in the patient while in the NICU, nutrition may play an even larger role than once imagined, especially if it is considered not as an adjunct but as a necessary therapy.[2–4]

Nutritional management is a high priority in the NICU setting. Injury to the central nervous system (CNS) can stem from trauma, metabolic disorders, stroke, ischemia, neoplasm, and neuromuscular dysfunction, all of which in the acute stage can significantly increase metabolic needs. Yet nutritional support has not been considered a primary treatment modality; subsequently, the incidence of malnutrition in NICU patients may be as high as 50%.[5] Thus, in all admissions to the NICU, nutrition must be addressed in the management of CNS-injured patients.

Contrary to what was once thought, after neurologic injury, there is a profound systemic hypermetabolic reaction that results in the rapid depletion of whole-body energy stores. If not attended to, catabolic injury cascade results in the degradation of the integrity of gastrointestinal (GI) mucosa, loss of muscle mass, reductions in systemic protein stores and synthesis, and compromise of both humoral and cellular immune competence. Nutrition can help the patient with neurologic injury by improving ventilator function, speeding wound healing, and fighting secondary infections.

◆ Undernutrition

The results of not adequately feeding patients are the following:

- ◆ Loss of gastrointestinal mucosa integrity
- ◆ Reduction in muscle mass
- ◆ Reductions in systemic protein stores and synthesis
- ◆ Compromise of both humoral and cellular immune competence
- ◆ Decrease in the absolute number of circulating T cells
- ◆ Promotion of cutaneous anergy
- ◆ Depression of the production of new antibodies in response to a novel antigen

Undernutrition is dangerous; as outlined in the preceding list, it has been shown to decrease the absolute number of circulating T cells, promote cutaneous anergy, and depress the production of new antibodies in response to a novel antigen. The depression of the immune response caused by undernutrition can significantly increase the probability and virulence of infectious complications in surgical patients.

Energy and fat stores allow the body to function for a long time without devastating effects. The earliest studies from Studley[6] show that a 30% preoperative weight loss led to a 10-fold increased morbidity and mortality following gastric surgery. By extrapolation, using fuzzy logic, there is the assumption that a 15% weight loss in the bedfast patient is of little consequence, bearing in mind a 30% weight loss is potentially very deleterious. Nutritional problems are usually only discussed after visual signs of weight loss, which is the reason nutrition during the first several days to as long as 2 weeks following the injury has not been studied. Three randomized class I studies have evaluated the relationship between caloric intake and patient outcomes.[7–10] Rapp et al[9] showed that the consequence of severe undernutrition for patients for a 2 week period after injury was an increased mortality rate when compared with those individuals who had full caloric replacement by 7 days. In Young et al's study,[10] there was no difference in those patients who were fed parenterally at 3 days when compared with those fed enterally at 9 days.

The preceding chapter discusses weight and weight loss. It is necessary to know how to determine weight in order to determine if there is weight loss. The ideal body weights for people with a medium frame are the following:

- *Men:* 106 lb (48 kg) for a height of 5 ft (150 cm); add 6 lb (2.73 kg) for each additional inch (2.5 cm)
- *Women:* 100 lb (45.5 kg) for a height of 5 ft (150 cm); add 5 lb (2.27 kg) for each additional inch (2.5 cm)
- *For both:* Subtract 10 lb (4.55 kg) for small frame; add 10 lb (4.55 kg) for large frame.

When protein calorie malnutrition occurs, there is a depletion of skeletal and visceral muscle in a 30:1 ratio. The measured level of the serum protein albumin can approximate visceral muscle stores. Mortality risk increases by ~37% for each gram deficit of serum albumin. Decreased albumin is also responsible for altering colonic resorption of water and salt, manifested by edema and ascites, causes gastric stasis, prolonged small bowel retention, delayed wound healing, and increased wound infection. When a patient has not been fed or when a patient has been hypermetabolic because of neurologic injury, a nutritional blood test panel should be obtained that includes albumin, prealbumin, transferrin, total iron-binding capacity, and serum creatinine. To further help with nutritional assessment, there should be strict monitoring of total input and output as well as daily weights (**Table 20–1**).

Nutrition must not be thought of as preventing large stores of excess fat from being lost but as a form of therapy. At the same time, nutrition must not be haphazardly given, for it has side effects just as any drug does. The nutritional formula must be beneficial and aid in treatment of the neurologically injured patient.

Table 20–1   Nutritional Assessment[2–4]

Test for nutrition	Normal values	Meaning of low value
Serum albumin	3.5–5.5 g/dL	<3.5 g/dL: compromised protein status, fluid overload, stress
Prealbumin (transthyretin)	14.0–42 mg/dL after 60 years/o 20% lower	<14.0 mg/dL: protein depletion
Transferrin	215–415 mg/dL	<200 mg/dL: malnutrition
Total iron-binding capacity	270–400 μg/dL	<270 μg/dL: compromised protein status
Serum creatinine	0.6–1.6 mg/dL	< 0.6 mg/dL: muscle wasting due to calorie deficiency
Total input and output	Euvolemic to slightly hypervolemic	Dehydration and resultant hypotension
Daily weights		Loss of fluid or undernutrition

◆ Hypermetabolism following CNS Injury

Patients have an inflated hypermetabolic response to CNS injury. Hadley et al[7,8] demonstrated a mean resting energy expenditure 46% above the normal predicted basal metabolic rate in a study of 45 head-injured patients. Most other investigators who measured metabolic expenditure in rested comatose patients also demonstrated ~120 to 250% metabolic rate of the predicted normal basal metabolic rate. During these times, to meet the needs of the increased energy production, there is a marked increase in gluconeogenesis and hepatic protein synthesis and an increased utilization of proteins, carbohydrates, and fats. The increased utilization of fats, carbohydrates, and proteins not only makes supplying nutrition difficult, but it also accelerates the development of malnutrition in patients who are not being fed. In the CNS-injured patient, there is a change in the ratio of nutrients required, an increased demand for protein and lipid calories, and a relative decrease in carbohydrate needs. These requirements must be taken into account when designing a nutritional formula for the CNS-injured patient.

The basic requirements in neurologic injury are

- ◆ Increased metabolism
- ◆ Increased proteins
- ◆ Increased lipids
- ◆ Decreased carbohydrates

The adaptive response to CNS injury is an increase in catecholamines, cortisol, and glucagons, with a subsequent increase in metabolism and hyperglycemia.[8] Both gluconeogenesis and lipolysis continue. Even with hyperglycemia, 75 to 90% of energy is still supplied by fat oxidation. In moderation, fat oxidation is not a major problem; however, when there is decreased blood return and continued fat oxidation, there is free radical production and further neurologic damage. Although protein is required for the repair of the injured brain, the changes in catecholamines, cortisol, and glucagon lead to proteolytic metabolism. Catecholamines are released and, in turn, stimulate the release of adrenocorticotropic hormone, growth hormones, glucagons, and insulin. Catabolic hormones, such as glucagons, cortisol, and catecholamines, cause utilization of alternate energy sources when there are no further nutrients supplied. As the injury continues, stress increases and proteolysis persists, making it impossible to achieve a positive nitrogen balance in the early period after CNS injury. Even if CNS-injured patients are paralyzed or put into barbiturate comas, they still require 100 to 120% of the resting energy expenditure.[11] The increase in resting energy suggests that a major part of the elevated metabolic expenditure is due to muscle tone.[12]

The normal responses to CNS injury are

- ◆ Increased catecholamines
- ◆ Increased cortisol

Table 20–2   GI Losses following CNS Injury[2–5]

GI loss	Sodium mEq/L	Chloride mEq/L	Potassium mEq/L
Gastric	60	100	10
Bile	140	100	10
Pancreas	140	75	10
Small bowel	100	100	20
Diarrhea	60	45	30

CNS, central nervous system; GI, gastrointestinal.

♦ Increased glucagons
♦ Proteolysis
♦ Gluconeogenesis
♦ Lipolysis
♦ Increased adrenocorticotropic hormone, growth hormones, and insulin

In addition to the loss of protein stores throughout the body, injury results in other changes, such as electrolytes being lost from GI tract secretions. Just as protein stores must be replaced, electrolytic losses must be replaced in nutritional therapy (**Table 20–2**).[2]

♦ How Much Nutrition Is Needed?

The ballpark figures for determining normal caloric requirements is 30 kcal per kg per day for GCS >13 to 15, 35 kcal per kg per day for GCS = 8 to 12, and 40 to 45 kcal per kg per day for GCS = 3 to 7. Indirect calorimetry performed with the aid of a portable metabolic cart once a day for the first several days is the most accurate way to determine the patient's resting energy expenditure and nutrition requirements. This method is unnecessary, however, because the general energy requirements can also be determined using the Harris-Benedict equation (**Table 20–3**), although that formula has a systematic error rate of 5 to 15% overestimation.

Clifton et al[13] simplified the adjustment factors, correcting the Harris-Benedict overestimation. They showed that the required percentage of resting energy expenditure of total calories calculated from part I of the Harris-Benedict formula can be estimated accurately using GCS, heart rate (HR), and days since injury. The percentage of required energy expenditure as determined using the Clifton equation is

$$152 - [14 \times GCS] + 0.4 \times HR + 7 \times \text{the day since injury.}$$

Table 20–3 Harris-Benedict Equation for Determining General Energy Requirements[2–5,7–9]

Men

Part I: [66.47+(13.75 × weight in kilograms) + (5.0 × height in centimeters) – (6.76 × age in years)] = basal calories

Part II: Multiply basal calories by adjusted activity factor, then by injury factor = the required energy expenditure in total calories per day

Women

Part I: [655.10 + (9.65 × weight in kilograms) + (1.85 × height in centimeters) – (4.68 × age in years)] = basal calories

Part II: Multiply basal calories by adjusted activity factor, then by injury factor = the required energy expenditure in total calories per day

Source: From Page CP, Hardin TC. Nutritional Assessment and Support: A Primer. Baltimore, MD: Williams & Wilkins; 1989.
Activity factors: confined to bed: 1.2; out of bed: 1.3.
Injury factors: minor surgery: 1.1; major surgery: 1.2; infection, mild: 1.2; infection, moderate: 1.4; infection, severe: 1.8; trauma, skeletal: 1.35; head injury, with steroids (increase metabolism): 1.6; head injury, blunt: 1.35; burns, 40% 1.5; burns, 100%: 1.95.[2–4]

In the first 2 weeks after injury, energy expenditure rises regardless of neurologic course, but its extent beyond this is unknown. The hypermetabolic response is also prolonged in patients who have other major organ system trauma. This hypermetabolism can be exaggerated for up to 1 year in severe head-injured patients; however, this should not be thought of as the norm.

In the neurologically injured patient, the resting energy requirements will be supplied by muscle breakdown or other body stores of proteins, fats, and carbohydrates (**Table 20–4**).

Initially in the neurologically injured patient, often the hypermetabolic state is combined with undernutrition, compromising protein synthesis and resulting in lean muscle mass catabolism for essential amino acids. As the hypermetabolism/hypercatabolic process continues, nitrogen is lost through the urine and feces. There is essentially no nitrogen gained through normal levels of nutrition, but a great deal of nitrogen is lost, leading to a negative nitrogen balance. For each gram of nitrogen in the urine and feces, 6.25 g of protein has been catabolized. Nonfed patients with severe brain injury continue to lose 14 to 25 g of nitrogen per day. The maximum excretion occurs during the second week. The average nitrogen loss of a head injury patient is

Table 20–4 Resting Energy Requirements[2–4]

Substrate Providing Calories	Energy (kcal/g)
Muscle	1
Carbohydrate	4
Protein	4
Fat	9

0.2 g of nitrogen per kilogram per day, which will result in a 10% loss of lean mass in 7 days.[8] This is about double or triple the loss in the normal person. Unlike the Studley[6] article, which showed that a 30% preoperative weight loss led to increased morbidity and mortality following gastric surgery, there are no studies that examine nitrogen loss or nitrogen replacement with outcome; therefore, nitrogen balance may not be a major issue. Nonetheless, a study by Clifton et al[14] examined two matched groups of comatose head injury patients and determined that the level of nitrogen intake should be 20% of the core composition of a 50 kilocal/kg/day feeding protocol. For the hypermetabolic patient, 20% is the maximal protein content of most enteral feedings; it is also the maximal amino acid content of most parenteral formulations.

Any feeding has to take into consideration fluid requirements, which average 35 cc per kilogram per 24 hours, more in athletes and less in the elderly. Another way to measure normal fluid requirements (average 35 cc/kg, elderly 30 cc/kg) is

- 100 mL/kg for first 10 kg in 24 hours, then
- 50 mL/kg for next 10 kg in 24 hours, then
- 20 mL/kg for remainder weight in kg in 24 hours age < 60 years
- 15 mL/kg for remainder weight in kg in 24 hours age > 60 years

The protein content of the fluid should be 1.0, 1.5, or 2.0 kcal/mL to meet partial nutritional needs and to continue a fluid euvolemic state. There are many physiological circumstances that require increased fluids from the normal amount. Fever increases fluid requirements by 12.5% for each 1°C above normal, sweating 10 to 25%, and hyperventilation 10 to 60%.[15]

Fluid types must also be used judiciously. The deleterious effects of hypotonic intravenous (IV) solutions on brain injury have been known since 1919[16]; therefore, immediately after neurologic problems have been detected, IV hypotonic fluid such as lactated Ringer's (Na = 130 mEq/L; 273 mOsm/L), dextrose 5% in water (D5W), and 0.45% sodium chloride (0.45NS) should be avoided. Decreasing IV fluids 1 mEq/L decreases osmotic pressure 38.6 mm Hg[16] and can lead to brain edema. It is also known, though, that hypertonic saline solutions lower ICP.[17,18]

There have been multiple class I investigations of the amount of feeding, the route of feeding, the use of steroids, and nitrogen balance, but none of these studies have looked at patient outcome or complications. Even the evidence of what to feed the CNS-injured patient remains unclear. The formulas must be specifically tailored; even the ingredients once thought to be the foundation of nutritional therapies need to be reexamined. High osmolar total parenteral nutrition (TPN) increases brain edema after cryogenic injury in animals[19] because of changes in serum osmolarity. The increased edema does not occur with lower osmolarity TPN. Besides hyperosmolar nutrition causing worse outcome after CNS injury, hyperglycemia is well recognized as worsening outcome after CNS injury and must be avoided.[20–23] It has even been suggested that hypoglycemia may be neurocytoprotective.[24–26] Hyperglycemia is common in trauma patients, even without supplementation, and is exacerbated by the administration of any TPN, hyper- or iso-osmolar.[10] Therefore, TPN should not be given during the first 48 hours after CNS injury, and serum glucose concentrations must be closely monitored and treated vigorously and kept below 110 mg/dL.

Nutritional treatments should not deliver less than the minimal daily requirement; As nutritional science matures, nutritional requirements in specific diseased states will be developed.

◆ The Gut Benefits from Nutrition

Early nutritional support increases CD4 cells, the CD4:CD8 ratio, and the T-lymphocyte responsiveness to concanavalin A (ConA), which assists immune function in patients sustaining CNS injury.[27] For nutrition delivery to the body to optimally occur in a physiological manner, the GI tract cells must be functioning. A functioning GI tract is necessary to protect against infection and sepsis from its own bacteria, particularly after CNS injury or surgical stress. If the gut is maintained, there will be no bacterial overgrowth, no proliferation of specific pathogens within the bowel, and no penetration of the pathogens into the bowel wall. Furthermore, with nutrition, the GI tract will remain the principal organ in the regulation of interorgan amino acid exchange, with glutamine being the most important amino acid available to the GI cells. After CNS injury, the GI tract cells' uptake of glutamine increases despite decreased oral intake and decreased delivery of glutamine to the intestinal mucosa. Glutamine is the most abundant amino acid in the blood, possibly because it is a precursor for purines and pyrimidines. When there is no added nutrition available, glutamine must come from another source; it originates from the muscle catabolism.

In summary, the primary benefits of maintaining GI mucosa with glutamine nutrition are the following:

- ◆ Protects against infection and sepsis from GI bacteria
- ◆ Prevents the proliferation of specific pathogens within the bowel
- ◆ Prevents penetration of the pathogens into the bowel wall
- ◆ Maintains the gut as the principal organ in the regulation of interorgan amino acid exchange
- ◆ Necessary for protein production
- ◆ Necessary for nitrogen transport and ammonia excretion
- ◆ Prevents muscle degradation
- ◆ Decreases hypermetabolism

In undernutrition, muscle undergoes proteolysis and releases essential glutamine into the circulation, supplying the basic requirements for GI enterocytes and for renal aminogenesis. However, the GI cells quickly use the glutamine from the muscle, thereby decreasing the circulating glutamine level available to other cells of the body for protein production, nitrogen transport, and ammonia excretion. In functioning cells throughout the body, glutamine is catabolized by mitochondrial glutaminase to glutamate and ammonia; once released into the circulation and across the blood–brain barrier, it can destroy brain cells. However, not all glutamine by-products are neurotoxic; alanine, for example, is used by the liver for gluconeogenesis, and ammonia is converted to urea. Circulating glutamine is necessary for the gut to prevent infection; is necessary to cells for protein synthesis; is important for nitrogen and carbon transport, as well as ammonia excretion; is the major substrate for gluconeogenisis and renal angiogenesis; and is a fuel source for rapidly replicating cells. However, too much glutamine can be a problem. Although the by-products of glutamine metabolism can cause neurologic problems, there is no evidence that an exogenous supply to the gut increases neurologic injury when the kidneys and liver are functioning. Therefore, the net overall requirement is for glutamine to be provided during CNS injury as soon as possible at appropriate levels to maintain homeostasis.

◆ How to Feed CNS-Injured Patients

Patients can be fed using the stomach (gastric), the small intestines (enteral), and the veins (IV) (parenteral). Each method has advantages and disadvantages. Multiple issues affect each type of feeding. Enteral feeding in the neurologically impaired patient is often complicated by medications such as phenobarbital, morphine, and other narcotics that delay gastric emptying. Ott et al[28] found that for a mean of 15 days, more than 50% of head-injured patients did not tolerate enteral feedings because of delayed gastric emptying. However, gastric feeding does not have to be the method of choice when utilizing the GI tract. There has been one class I report and one class II report indicating better tolerance of enteral feeding with a jejunal rather than gastric administration. Enteral feeding does have advantages over IV (parenteral) feeding. It is more cost effective, safer, has fewer complications, and is more physiologic than parenteral nutrition.

Indications for enteral nutrition are

- ◆ Malnourished patients expected to be unable to eat > 5 to 7 days
- ◆ Nourished patients not able to eat for 7 to 9 days
- ◆ Patients who are unable to consume adequate amounts of kilocalories to prevent macronutrient and micronutrient deficiencies

Contraindications to enteral nutrition are

- ◆ Severe acute pancreatitis
- ◆ High output proximal fistula

- Inability to gain access
- Patients expected to eat within 5 to 7 days
- Intractable vomiting and diarrhea
- Aggressive therapy not indicated

Using the gastrointestinal tract has physiologic superiority, stimulating gut hormones, gastric acid buffering, and buffering supplements into the blood. The advantages of enteral feeding are decreased hyperglycemia, decreased infection and sepsis, and decreased cost. Enteral feeding maintains the gut mucosa integrity, prevents infection, promotes protein synthesis, transports toxins, and decreases hypermetabolism. The only advantage of parenteral nutrition can be seen when enteral feeding cannot be tolerated; immediately preoperatively, with the need for intentional bowel rest, and with bowel dysfunction, the IV route must be used for a short time. IV nutrition can also supplement enteral nutrition when not enough calories and proteins are being provided. Parenteral nutrition aggravates brain edema in laboratory animals and may cause elevated liver or pancreatic enzymes. Lebkowski[29] showed that neither parenteral nor enteral nutrition in severely head-injured patients made any difference in outcome. However, the same study also demonstrated that no nutrition made any difference in outcome.

The neurologically injured patient often is treated in the flat bed position, especially if spinal injuries have occurred or vasospasms are present. Most of the time the head of the bed is tilted at 30 to 45 degrees or titrated to the best ICP. When the head of the bed is flat, the patient is at risk of aspiration. If aspirations are suspected, tube feedings should be held until the tube can be placed into the small intestine. Intubation does provide a degree of protection, especially if a subglottic suction endotracheal tube is used. However, a recent study demonstrated ulcers in an animal model; therefore, its use cannot be recommended.[30] When there is a concern about possible aspiration, gastric reflux, or a tracheal-esophageal fistula, food coloring can be added for 24 hours to feedings for investigation. In the past, blue food coloring and methylene blue have been added to enteral feedings to detect aspiration. Increased absorption and systemic levels of drugs such as methylene blue can occur when there is increased intestinal permeability. The blue dye then interferes with normal adenosine triphosphate (ATP) production and ultimately inhibits mitochondrial respiration, leading to shock, metabolic acidosis, and cell death.[31] Therefore, its use cannot be recommended.

Severely head-injured patients who remain comatose have swallowing difficulties and may be fed either parenterally or enterally. Prolonged use of a naso- or orogastric tube should be avoided because of the risk of mucosa ulceration and sinus disease. If the patient is expected to have feeding difficulties for 1 month or more, a percutaneous endoscopic gastrostomy (PEG) tube should be placed.

Eventually, established feedings should approximate the normal bolus manner of feeding instead of continuous feedings,[32,33] although initially, continuous feedings are better tolerated in the critically injured patient.[34] If given the choice of gastric or duodenal feeding versus jejunostomy, the more proximal area should be used because a patient receives fewer calories via the more distal jejunostomy tube. This was exemplified by Opeskin and Lee[35] in the case of a healthy 16-year-old severely head-injured patient being fed by jejunostomy tube who died because of malnutrition. She had hyperperistalsis that caused the jejunostomy tube to migrate even more distally, resulting in less nutrition being absorbed.

The gut may provide the most efficient and safe route of fluid administration and should be used as the first choice when there are no contraindications. For example, when diabetes insipidus is suspected, an enteric feeding tube can be used to provide the patient water when IV water would never be considered.

Once again, no class I studies have looked at patient outcome, but there are multiple class II to IV studies that provide evidence of outcome. Borzotta et al[36] demonstrated that neither enteral nor TPN was effective in changing outcome. In the past, when compared with enteral nutrition, TPN was thought of as a superior means of nutrition because of the misconception that the bowel was atonic. However, Hadley et al[7] demonstrated that aggressive enteral feeding could be accomplished early and effectively despite bowel atony. Grahm et al[37] added support to using enteral routes when they demonstrated that enterally fed patients had statistically significant lower rates of hospital-acquired infection and sepsis, and shorter stays in the ICU, than patients receiving the same caloric and nitrogen supplements by TPN. The researchers passed a malleable nasojejunal feeding tube directly into the proximal jejunum with the aid of bedside fluoroscopy. They used the nasojejunal feeding tube in spite of a history of blunt abdominal trauma, the use of barbiturates, narcotics, and other agents, and compared the results with TPN. The minor differences that tended to favor enteral nutrition were less hyperglycemia, less of a difference in osmolarity loads causing edema, and lower cost. Enteral nutrition preserved gut mucosa, stimulated complex circulatory hormonal mechanisms that are intrinsic to the human digestive system, and preserved the secretion of the immunoglobulin A (IgA) immune system. Thus the use of enteral nutrition tends toward improved efficacy. Furthermore, enteral feedings are best accomplished if the tube is placed in the jejunum, decreasing chances of aspiration and improving GI tract motility.

Postpyloric enteral feeding requires the following:

- Bowel sounds must be present.
- Bowel movements or flatus is not necessary.
- Nasoduodenal feeding tube must be placed.
- Certain feeding tubes must be confirmed by abdominal x-ray.
- Head of bed must be maintained at a tilt of 30 degrees or greater.
- Check gastric residuals by oral gastric tube; do not aspirate through a small or pliable duodenal tube.

♦ Bolus flush the feeding tube with at least 30 cc water every 4 hours to prevent clogging.

Small intestinal feedings can reduce the risk of aspiration. In addition to a decrease in infection rates with early enteral feedings, the occurrence of bacterial translocation, or the passage of bacteria across the intestinal wall, is also decreased.

As outlined above, when starting tube feedings, determine first that there are bowel sounds, confirm the placement of certain tubes by abdominal x-ray, place the head of the bed at 30 degrees or more, then determine the total amount of calories or the goal calories and the amount of liquid in milliliters to be given per hour for 24 hours. Begin tube feedings at 10 to 50 cc per hour, full strength. Check for gastric residuals after the first 2 hours, then after every 4 hours for 3 cycles. If the amount of feeding formula residual is greater than 50% of the feedings delivered during the cycle, hold the feedings for 1 hour and recheck every hour until there is less than 50% of the feedings delivered during the last cycle. It is often difficult as well as inaccurate to measure residuals with pliable feeding tubes. If feedings are tolerated, increase the amount 20 to 40 cc every 8 hours until the goal is reached. Make sure that the feeding tube is flushed with 30 cc of water every 4 hours to prevent clogging.

When tube feedings have reached the goal amount and are well tolerated, bolus feeding may begin. Give feedings during normal waking hours every 4 hours. Start with double the hourly rate of the continuous tube feedings. Flush with at least 30 cc water after every bolus, then clamp the feeding tube. Next, follow the same guidelines for checking residuals with continuous feedings. Check for gastric residuals after the first 2 hours, then after every 4 hour cycle. The cycles of bolus feedings may be increased to every 6 hours if fluid requirements dictate. If the amount of residual feeding formula in the gut is greater than 50% of the feedings delivered during the cycle, hold the feedings for 1 hour and recheck every hour until there is less than 50% of the feedings delivered during the last cycle; resume when appropriate.

Discontinue enteral feedings only when oral intake is appropriate. If possible, wean the tube feedings to oral intake; this is often easier with bolus-type delivery. However, some patients do not tolerate oral intake if a nasal feeding tube is in place.

Occasionally, diarrhea occurs with tube feedings. Likely causes are elixir medications containing sorbitol, magnesium-containing antacids, oral antibiotics, phosphorus supplements, cimetidine, metopramide, lactulose, pseudomembranous colitis, and gastrointestinal disorders. When diarrhea starts, measure stool *Costridium difficile* titers, especially if the stool is very malodorous. Then increase fiber by considering the addition of pectin or psyllium; however, psyllium will clog the feeding tube. When treating diarrhea, do not initially give antidiarrheal agents before the cause is known; otherwise, it will slow down the elimination of the offending agent and prolong the diarrhea. Do not stop the tube feedings for any length of time, and do not change formulas.[4]

◆ What Should CNS-Injured Patients Be Fed?

Nutrition is a form of therapy. It must be safe, it must prevent secondary injury, and it should improve outcome. Nutrition decreases the risk of infection, maintains the gut mucosa integrity, promotes protein synthesis, transports toxins, prevents muscle degradation, and decreases hypermetabolism. To decrease complications, nutrition should be made slightly acidic because gastric alkalinization significantly increases the risk of nosocomial ammonia in long-term ventilated patients.[38] The brain requires ~20% of the body's resting energy expenditure, and although dependent on glucose, it will utilize ketones under conditions of significant deprivation. Ritter et al[39] randomized 20 severely head-injured patients to receive Osmolyte HN (Ross Laboratories, Columbus, OH) or carbohydrate-free tube feeds. The experimental tube feed contained 2060 kcal/L, 129 g/L of protein, and 175 g/L of fat. In these patients, blood glucose and blood lactate were lower, arterial ketones were higher, and daily nitrogen loss was lower. Unfortunately, the investigators did not measure outcome.

To be well rounded, in addition to proteins, enteral nutrition must contain fat and possibly some carbohydrates. Each should be added in moderation. Carbohydrates should not be overly used because hyperglycemia leads to a worse outcome in CNS injury. Large amounts of administered carbohydrates/glucose have several negative effects. First, they will raise the carbon dioxide production because of their relatively high respiratory quotient of 1. The respiratory quotient of protein oxidation is 0.8; fat oxidation, 0.7. The higher respiratory quotient of carbohydrates will result in increased ventilation needs and decreased ability to be weaned. High serum glucose levels will also stimulate lipogenesis and result in hepatic steatosis. Additionally, high glucose increases the resting energy expenditure due to the thermic effect of the large doses of administered carbohydrates.

The use of tight glucose control 80 to 110 mg/dL improves mortality and morbidity. This can be accomplished with a Humulin regular sliding scale IV dosage or much more accurately with an insulin continuous infusion. Continuous infusion of insulin has been shown to provide more steady states, approximating physiological conditions.[40–44]

Fats

In addition to carbohydrates, fats must be included in feedings. Although Roth et al[45] described how a fat emulsion containing 20% intralipid caused life-threatening hemophagocytosis, hypertriglyceridemia, and creaming plasma after a 3 day period of parenteral nutrition in a 21-year-old, fats are important. They provide 8 kcal per gram of fat and normally make up 10% or less of the consumed calories in the modern diet. Diets should contain medium-chain fatty acids because they are well tolerated and do not increase deleterious plasma lipoproteins. Essential fatty acids are required, with each type having advantages and disadvantages. Diets rich in omega-6 polyunsaturated fatty acids, such as those obtained from corn, safflower, and sunflower oils, diminish the immune response to infection, trauma, or tumor growth, as documented by Alexander and Peck.[46] Arachidonic acid, a by-product of fats, breaks down and stimulates oxygen-free radicals and further damage. In contrast, diets abundant in omega-3 polyunsaturated fatty acids, such as those found in coldwater fish oils, stimulate the immune response to infection and trauma and activate the rejection of foreign bodies.

Proteins

Proteins are very important in nutrition and must supply the enormous need for specific amino acids. Saito et al[47] demonstrated that arginine is important in neurologic injury. When arginine comprised 2% of the total nonprotein calories in burn-injured animals, it increased survival, improved delayed hypersensitivity, and reduced susceptibility to infection. Arginine is thymotrophic and improves cellular immunity by increasing thymic lymphocytes sensitivity. It also improves wound healing and decreases nitrogen release.[8] Amino acids are vital for neurologic healing; for example, inosine has been shown to stimulate axonal growth.[48] However, not all amino acids benefit head-injured patients. Theoretically, glutamine and glutamate from the diet can cross a disrupted blood–brain barrier and exacerbate glutamate neurotoxicity immediately after primary injury or during secondary injury, and can lead to the loss of cells in the ischemic penumbra. This has not been proven in human subjects, however. In general, after injury, protein catabolism leads to increased nitrogen levels and an increased production of ammonia. However, the levels of nitrogen that lead to increased ammonia and neuronal damage are not known. It is recommended that nitrogen to nonprotein calories in the human diet range from 1:75 to 1:185. Enteral feedings should contain at least 15% of calories as smaller protein by the seventh day after injury. The optimal amount of protein per kilogram of body weight in the neurologically injured patient is unknown. Normal nutrition suggests 1.5 g/kg, studies suggest 2.5 g/kg,[49] but it may be as high as 4.5 g/kg. Proteins, electrolytes, and dextrose add osmolarity. Most feedings should have an osmolarity around 300 so that it does not add to edema at lower osmolarities or leak across the damaged blood–brain barrier as higher osmolarity would.

In addition to the main building blocks of carbohydrates, fats, and protein, there should be 1 to 2 calories per milliliter to decrease the fluid load. The nutritional formula should be high in zinc, as this is associated with improved neurologic recovery rate and improved protein levels in patients with severe closed head injury.[50] The formula should also be low in iron and high in desferrioxamine. Desferrioxamine prevents the damage associated with free radical generation and reperfusion injury. It inactivates the iron-dependent enzyme ribonucleotide reductase that has been shown to decrease infarct size and improve functional recovery.[51] A creatine-enriched formula was shown to help prevent secondary neurologic energy in an animal model.[52] Additionally, the nutritional formula must contain vitamins and other elements. Glucose loads should be low because of problems with hyperglycemia; large doses of glucose will suppress lipolysis and prevent mobilization of stored linoleic acid. It may also be prudent to add human growth hormone.[53] This has no effect on nitrogen imbalance in highly stressed immobilized patients after severe head injury, but it significantly enhances serum protein concentrations.

◆ Disease-Specific Formulas

Immune-enhancing formulas with glutamine, arginine, omega-3 fatty acids, and nucleotides have been used recently in critically ill patients. Glutamine and arginine have been shown to decrease infection rates and promote wound healing in the critically ill,[54] but they are contraindicated in patients with hepatic and renal failure. Arginine supplementation has immune-enhancing benefits, including increased rate of protein repletion, improved collagen synthesis and wound healing, and enhanced T cell function.

The goal of pulmonary formulas is to reduce carbon dioxide production. These formulas are low in carbohydrates and have a high (50%) fat content. Care must be taken to avoid overfeeding. Total calorie intake has more of an impact on respiratory function than specialized pulmonary formulas.

Hepatic formulas are low in protein to minimize ammonia production. These formulas contain large amounts of the branched chain amino acids valine, leucine, and isoleucine, and low amounts of aromatic amino acids. They assist in treating encephalopathy, especially from ammonia.

Special diabetic formulas are high fiber, low carbohydrate, and high fat to provide nutrition support to patients with hyperglycemia; they may be considered in all neurologically injured patients. However, because of delayed gastric emptying in a head trauma patient, close monitoring of tube feeding tolerance is recommended.

Absorption may be enhanced with the use of elemental formulas if intestinal atrophy or loss of absorptive surface has occurred.

The characteristics of an optimal nutritional formula in the treatment of an acute neurologic injury are

- ◆ One to 2 calories per milliliter, depending on the need for euvolemia or hypervolemia
- ◆ Slightly acidic
- ◆ Small intestine placement
- ◆ Osmolarity 300
- ◆ High protein containing arginine, inosine, and glutamine
- ◆ Fatty acids with medium chain and omega-3 and polyunsaturated fatty acids
- ◆ Very low or absent carbohydrates

- Fiber (25–35 g/day)
- High magnesium initially
- High zinc
- Desferrioxamine
- Creatine
- Low potassium initially
- Low calcium (800–1500 mg/day initially)
- Low iron

◆ Total Parenteral Nutrition

The advantage of parenteral nutrition can be seen when enteral feeding cannot be tolerated immediately preoperatively, with the need for intentional bowel rest and with proven severe bowel dysfunction. IV nutrition can also supplement enteral nutrition when not enough calories and proteins are being provided.

TPN is drug therapy delivered to the IV system without the benefit of the GI buffering system. It must contain the appropriate medications to provide optimal nutrition. Electrolytes, protein, fats, and vitamins are required for health and are provided in most nutritional supplements, but they must be added to IV TPN. The amount that the physician prescribes is dependent upon sex, age, organ losses, and diseased states. The normal requirements thus vary by the same criteria, but general guidelines are given in **Table 20–5**.

Often electrolytes are prescribed in different units, and the conversion must be known. IV fluids are given in milliequivalents, and dietary supplements are given in milligrams (**Table 20–6**).

The requirements in the average healthy individual are not the same in the debilitated individual. When providing TPN, the amount of electrolytes must be adjusted for 1000 kcal of TPN (**Table 20–7**).

Typical central IV TPN must be adjusted for diseased state, determining the beneficial compounds added. The fluid requirements must also be obtained according to the disease state and whether euvolemia or hypervolemia is beneficial. Peripheral administration requires adjustment to prevent peripheral vein injury. As such, the amount of amino acids in peripheral IV feedings should be 35 g, dextrose 70 g, sodium chloride 15 mEq, and heparin 200 units (**Table 20–8**).

Prior to beginning TPN, make sure that the central venous access line has one port labeled for only TPN. Central line TPN usually contains 70% dextrose, 10% amino acids, and 20% fat emulsion. If peripheral access is chosen, the amount of dextrose is decreased to 20%, amino acids to 8.5%, and fats to 10%. As with the administration of all IV medication, the TPN must be delivered at a constant rate. The TPN delivery system must be maintained

Table 20–5 General Guidelines to Normal Nutritional Requirements [2–5,15]

Nutrient	Recommended daily allowance	Nutrient	Recommended daily allowance
Sodium	60–150 mEq 1.0–1.7 mEq/kg	Zinc	15 mg 2.5–5.0 mg IV
Potassium	70–150 mEq 0.9–1.3 mEq/kg	Copper	2–3 mg 0.5–1.5 mg IV
Chloride	60–150 mEq 1.0–1.7 mEq/kg	Chromium	55–70 µg 10–15 mg oral
Magnesium	0.35–0.45 mEq/kg	Manganese	2–5 mg 0.15–0.8 mg IV
Calcium	800–1500 mg 0.2–0.3 mEq/kg	Selenium	55–70 µg 125 µg IV
Phosphorus	7–30 mmol/1000 kcal 3–4 g	Iron	10–15 mg
Vitamin A	3300 IU	Fatty acids	0.1 g/kg
Vitamin D	200–400 IU	Protein	0.8–4 g/kg
Vitamin E	10 IU	Glucose	100 g/m^2
Vitamin C	100 mg	Fiber	25–35 g
Vitamin K	64–80 µg	Cystine	13 mg/kg
Folacin	400 µg	Isoleucine	23 mg/kg
Niacin	40 mg	Leucine	40 mg/kg
Riboflavin	3.6 mg	Lysine	30 mg/kg
Thiamine	3 mg	Methionine	13 mg/kg
Vitamin B$_6$	4 mg	Phenylalanine	39 mg/kg
Vitamin B$_{12}$	3–5 µg	Tyrosine	39 mg/kg
Pantothenic acid	15 mg	Threonine	15 mg/kg
Biotin	60 µg	Tryptophan	6 mg/kg
		Valine	20 mg/kg

IU, international unit; IV, intravenous.

sterile. Document the patient's height, weight, age, sex, heart rate, and GCS; the days since injury; the total caloric goal; and the fluid desired. There are specific TPN formulas commercially available. Start TPN at 50 cc per hour, and increase every 8 hours until the goal can be reached in 24 hours. When discontinuing the TPN, taper the infusion rate by 50% every 30 minutes for 1 hour to prevent hypoglycemia.

TPN is a direct assault on the liver and pancreas and bypasses the stomach, providing electrolytes directly to the bloodstream. TPN causes fatty liver, cholestasis, GI atrophy, and gastric hyperacidity. Therefore, multiple tests should be monitored when delivering TPN (**Table 20–9**).

Table 20–6   Electrolyte Requirements in Different Units [2–5,15]

Electrolyte	MEq	mmol	mg
Sodium NaCl (1 g)	1	1	23
	43	43	1000
	17 Na	17 Na	393 Na
Potassium	1	1	39
	26	26	1000
Calcium	1	0.5	20
	50	25	1000
Magnesium	1	0.5	12
	82	41	1000
Phosphorus	2	1	31
Chloride	1	1	35
	29	29	1000

Table 20–7   Recommended Electrolyte Requirements in Total Parenteral Nutrition* [2–5,15]

Electrolyte	mEq
Sodium	5–10
Potassium	20–40
Phosphorus	10–15
Magnesium	8
Calcium	5

*For each 1000 kcal of TPN, add recommended milliequivalents of electrolyte.
TPN, total parenteral nutrition.

◆ Changing Metabolic Conditions

Formulas must have the ability to change under different metabolic conditions. For example, magnesium is important early in injury treatment, preventing vasospasms and the spread of glutamate neurotoxicity. However, it is not beneficial after 7 to 10 days, when recovery is expected and when cell transmission is needed.

Table 20–8   Typical Central Total Parenteral (IV) Nutrition Formula (not recommended for peripheral administration)[2–5,14,15]

Ingredients	Average amount (per liter)
Carbohydrate dextrose	250 g
Lipids 20%	250 mL
Amino acids	60 g
Sodium given as:	
Sodium chloride	60 mEq
Sodium acetate	60 mEq
Sodium phosphate	60 mEq
Potassium given as:	
Potassium chloride	60 mEq
Potassium acetate	60 mEq
Potassium phosphate	60 mEq
Magnesium sulphate	16–24 mEq/day
Calcium gluconate	10–15 mEq/day
Multivitamins	10 mL
Vitamin C	1000 mg
Vitamin K	10 mg/week
Trace elements	4 mL
Insulin	At least 15 units/day
Zinc, extra	10 mg
Heparin	1000 units

Table 20–9   Test for Patients Receiving Total Parenteral Nutrition[2–5,14,15]

Serum electrolytes, glucose, BUN, creatinine, calcium, magnesium, phosphorus	Daily
Albumin, prealbumin, transferrin, total iron-binding capacity, hepatic enzymes, bilirubin, triglycerides, prothrombin time, WBC	Weekly

BUN, blood urea nitrogen; WBC, white blood (cell) count.

◆ Additional Concerns for Nutrition

Nutritional therapy must be customized for clinical conditions (**Table 20–10**).

At times, the neurologically injured patient may not have been fed for 1 to 3 days, is inactive, and may often receive narcotics, all of which individually can result in decreased gut motility. Therefore, initial admitting orders for the NICU should include a stool softener such as docusate sodium or the combination capsule casanthranol/docusate sodium. Appropriate bowel

Table 20–10   Different Nutritional Requirements in Clinical Conditions

Syndrome of inappropriate antidiuretic hormone	Decreased fluids
Cerebral salt wasting	Increased salt
Diabetes insipidus	Decreased salt and increased fluids
Ventilators	Increased phosphorus
Initial head injury	Increased magnesium
Vasospasms	Increased magnesium

movement prevents abdominal distention, pain, anxiety, nausea, and vomiting. Therefore, treat constipation appropriately. Always consider abdominal injury in the multitrauma patient; if not present and if stool softeners do not result in regularly scheduled bowel movements, then bisacodyl suppositories and enemas should be given every other day unless a bowel movement has occurred.

There is no benefit to giving metoclopramide in patients with severe neurologic injury to stimulate gastric motility. It does not prophylactically improve gastric tolerance;[55] furthermore, it can cause CNS effects such as neuroleptic malignant syndrome, parkinsonian symptoms, dystonic reactions, and restlessness.

Case Management

A soft nasal feeding tube should be placed into the proximal small intestine because the patient is expected to have a decreased mental status for an extended time but will be able to orally feed in <30 days. An enteral nutritional formula with continuous feedings should be used days 1 through 7 after neurologic injury. The formula should have water content 110% of normal or 35 mL/kg/day. The general caloric requirements for 70 kg/GCS = 7 is 40 kcal/kg, yielding 2800 kcal/day. The Harris-Benedict equation predicted required calories would be 6.47 + (13.75 × 70 kg) + (5.0 × 66 cm) – (6.76 × 60) = 1547.37 calories. The 1547.37 calories would be multiplied by the activity bedridden factor (1.2) and the trauma factor (1.35), yielding a total 2506.74 calories. Adjusted instead by the Clifton equation, the percentage of resting energy requirement is 152 – (14 × GCS of 7) + (0.4 × the heart rate of 90) + (7 × the second day since injury), giving a predicted increased metabolism of 104% of normal, yielding 1609 kcal. The nutritional therapy should have an osmolarity of 300 mOsm, and pH 7.5 to 7.8. The patient should have frequent finger stick glucose monitoring and a continuous insulin drip to keep blood glucose less than 110 mg/dL.

◆ Summary

Neurologic injury initiates a cascade of local and systemic metabolic responses. Patients become hypermetabolic, hypercatabolic, and hyperglycemic and develop decreased immune competence and altered GI function. New methods of enteral feeding, such as percutaneous placements of tubes or fluoroscopic placements of proximal jejunostomy tubes, allow early feeding and adequate nutrition. Evidence indicates that early small bowel feeding of patients with acute head injury results in decreased incidence of infection and shorter NICU stays. Optimal nutritional support for improving neurologic recovery continues to be established. It is more likely that this will be a dynamic state, changing from person to person, and over time, depending on the clinical circumstances. There are many advantages to early feeding. Early feeding should not be based on preventing a loss of weight, but should be based using the nutrition as a form of therapy. However, nutrition should not have detrimental effects; it must not cause secondary injury. Nutritional formulas cannot contain hyperosmotic/hyperglycemic solutions, omega-6 polyunsaturated fatty acids, iron, and glutamate, as well as an abundance of amino acids that will be converted into ammonia. Nutritional formulas should adhere to the motto, Do no harm. Because there is no sound evidence that early feeding before 7 days improves outcome, feedings should be given as soon as the benefits are not outweighed by the risks.

References

1. Guidelines for the Management of Severe Head Injury. New York: Brain Trauma Foundation; 2000
2. Page CP, Hardin TC. Nutritional Assessment and Support: A Primer. Baltimore, MD: Williams & Wilkins; 1989
3. Morgan SL, Weinsier RL. Fundamentals of Clinical Nutrition. 2nd ed. St. Louis, MO: Mosby; 1998
4. Heimburger DC, Weisner BL. Handbook of Clinical Nutrition. 3rd ed. St. Louis, MO: Mosby; 1997
5. Christman JW, McCain RW. A sensible approach to the nutritional support of mechanically ventilated critically ill patients. Intensive Care Med 1993;19:129–136
6. Studley HO. Percentage of weight loss: a basic indicator of surgical risk in patients with chronic peptic ulcer. JAMA 1936;106:458–460
7. Hadley MN, Grahm TW, Harrington T, et al. Nutritional support and neurotrauma: a critical review of early nutrition in forty-five acute head injury patients. Neurosurgery 1986;19:367–373
8. Hadley MN. Hypermetabolism following head trauma: nutritional considerations. In: Barrow D, ed. Complications and sequelae of head injury. New York: Thieme and American Association of Neurological Surgeons; 1992:280
9. Rapp RP, Young B, Twyman D, et al. The favorable effect of early parenteral feeding on survival in head-injured patients. J Neurosurg 1983;58:906–912
10. Young B, Ott L, Haack D, et al. Effect of total parenteral nutrition upon intracranial pressure in severe head injury. J Neurosurg 1987;67:76–80

11. Magnuson B, Hatton J, Zweg TN, Young B. Pentobarbital coma in neurosurgical patients: nutritional considerations. Nutr Clin Pract 1994;9:146–150
12. Clifton GL, Robertson CS, Choi SC. Assessment of nutritional requirements of head injury patients. J Neurosurg 1986;64:895–901
13. Clifton GL, Robertson CS, Hodge S, et al. The metabolic response to severe head injury. J Neurosurg 1984;60:687–696
14. Clifton GL, Robertson CS, Contant DF. Enteral hyperalimentation in head injury. J Neurosurg 1985;62:186–193
15. Matarese LE, Gottschlich MM. Contemporary Nutrition Support Practice: A Clinical Guide. Philadelphia: WB Saunders; 1998
16. Weed LH, McKibbin PS. Experimental alteration of (brain) bulk. Am J Physiol 1919; 48:531–555
17. Prough DS, Whitley JM, Taylor CL, et al. Regional cerebral blood flow following resuscitation from hemorrhagic shock with hypertonic saline: influence of a subdural mass. Anesthesiology 1991;75:319–327
18. Schmoker JD, Zhuang J, Shackford SR. Hypertonic fluid resuscitation improves cerebral oxygen delivery and reduces intracranial pressure after hemorrhagic shock. J Trauma 1991;31:1607–1613
19. Waters DC, Hoff JT, Black KL. Effect of parenteral nutrition on cold-induced vasogenic edema in cats. J Neurosurg 1986;64:460–465
20. Chopp M, Welch KM, Tidwell CD, Helpern JA. Global cerebral ischemia and intracellular pH during hyperglycemia and hypoglycemia in cats. Stroke 1988;19: 1383–1387
21. Kalimo H, Rehncrona S, Soderfeldt B, et al. Brain lactic acidosis and ischemic cell damage, II: Histopathology. J Cereb Blood Flow Metab 1981;1:313–327
22. Fahn S, Rowland L, Davis J. Cerebral Hypoxia and Its Consequences. New York: Raven Press; 1979:195–213
23. Pulsinelli WA, Waldman S, Rawlinson D, Plum F. Moderate hyperglycemia augments ischemic brain damage: a neuropathologic study in rat. Neurology 1982;32:1239–1246
24. Marie C, Bralet AM, Gueldry S, Bralet J. Fasting prior to transient cerebral ischemia reduces delayed neuronal necrosis. Metab Brain Dis 1990;5:65–75
25. Siemkowicz E, Hansen AJ. Clinical restitution following cerebral ischemia in hypo-, normo- and hyperglycemic rats. Acta Neurol Scand 1978;58:1–8
26. Strong AJ, Miller SA, West IC. Protection of respiration of a crude mitochondrial preparation in cerebral ischaemia by control of blood glucose. J Neurol Neurosurg Psychiatry 1985;48:450–454
27. Sacks GS, Brown RO, Teague D, Dickerson RN, Tolley EA, Kudsk KA. Early nutrition support modifies immune function in patients sustaining severe head injury. JPEN J Parenter Enteral Nutr 1995;19:387–392
28. Ott L, Young B, Phillips R, et al. Altered gastric emptying in the head-injured patient relationship to feeding intolerance. J Neurol 1991;74:738–742
29. Lebkowski WJ. Does hyperalimentation improve outcome in patients with severe head injury? Rocz Akad Med Bialymst 1994;39:117–120
30. Berra L, Panigada M, De Marchi L, et al. New approaches for the prevention of airway infection in ventilated patients: lessons learned from laboratory animal studies at the National Institutes of Health. Minerva Anesthesiol 2003;69:342–347
31. Maloney J, Metheny N. Controversy in using blue dye in enteral feeding as a method of detecting pulmonary aspiration. Crit Care Nurse 2002;22:84–85
32. Pender SM, Courtney MG, Rajan E, McAdam B, Fielding JF. Percutaneous endoscopic gastrostomy results of an Irish single unit series. Ir J Med Sci 1993;162: 452–455
33. Kiel MK. Enteral tube feeding in a patient with traumatic brain injury. Arch Phys Med Rehabil 1994;75:116–117
34. Rhoney DH, Parker D, Formea CM, Yap C, Coplin WM. Tolerability of bolus versus continuous gastric feeding in brain-injured patients. Neurol Res 2002;24:613–620
35. Opeskin K, Lee KA. Failure of a feeding jejunostomy. Med Sci Law 1993;33: 263–266
36. Borzotta AP, Pennings J, Papasadero B, et al. Enteral versus parenteral nutrition after severe closed head injury. J Trauma 1994;37:459–468

37. Grahm TW, Zadrozny DB, Harrington T. Benefits of early jejunal hyperalimentation in the head-injured patient. Neurosurgery 1989;25:729–735
38. Tryba M, Cook DJ. Gastric alkalinization, pneumonia, and systemic infections: the controversy. Scand J Gastroenterol Suppl 1995;210:53–59
39. Ritter AM, Robertson CS, Goodman JC, et al. Evaluation of a carbohydrate-free diet for patients with severe head injury. J Neurotrauma 1996;13:473–485
40. Finney SJ, Zekveld C, Elia A, Evans TW. Glucose control and mortality in critically ill patients. JAMA 2003;290(15):2041–2047
41. Mesotten D, Van den Berghe G. Clinical potential of insulin therapy in critically ill patients. Drugs 2003;63(7):625–636
42. Van den Berghe G, Wouters PJ, Bouillon R, et al. Outcome benefit of intensive insulin therapy in the critically ill: insulin dose versus glycemic control. Crit Care Med 2003;31(2):359–366
43. Preiser JC, Devos P, Van den Berghe G. Tight control of glycaemia in critically ill patients. Curr Opin Clin Nutr Metab Care 2002;5(5):533–537
44. Van den Berghe G, Wouters P, Weekers F, et al. Intensive insulin therapy in the critically ill patients. N Engl J Med 2001;345(19):1359–1367
45. Roth B, Grande PO, Nilsson-Ehle P, Eliasson I. Possible role of short-term parenteral nutrition with fat emulsions for development of haemophagocytosis with multiple organ failure in a patient with traumatic brain injury. Intensive Care Med 1993;19:111–114
46. Alexander JW, Peck MD. Future prospects for adjunctive therapy: pharmacologic and nutritional approaches to immune system modulation. Crit Care Med 1990;18:S159–S164
47. Saito H, Trocki O, Wang S, et al. Metabolic and immune effects of dietary arginine supplementation after burn. Arch Surg 1987;122:784–789
48. Chen P, Goldberg DE, Kolb B, Lanser M, Benowitz LI. Inosine induces axonal rewiring and improves behavioral outcome after stroke. Proc Natl Acad Sci U S A 2002;99:9031–9036
49. Wilson RF, Dente C, Tyburski JG. The nutritional management of patients with head injuries. Neurol Res 2001;23:121–128
50. Young B, Ott L, Kasarkis E, et al. Zinc supplementation is associated with improved neurologic recovery rate and visceral protein levels of patients with severe closed head injury. J Neurotrauma 1996;13:25–34
51. Hershko C. Control of disease by selective iron depletion: a novel therapeutic strategy utilizing iron chelators. Baillieres Clin Haematol 1994;7:965–1000
52. Scheff SW, Dhillon HS. Creatine-enriched diet alters levels of lactate and free fatty acids after experimental brain injury. Neurochem Res 2004;29:469–470
53. Behrman SW, Kudsk KA, Brown RO, Vehe KL, Wojtysiak SL. The effect of growth hormone on nutritional markers in enterally fed immobilized trauma patients. JPEN J Parenter Enteral Nutr 1995;19:41–46
54. Bower RH, Cerra FB, Bershadsky B, et al. Early enteral administration of a formula (Impact) supplemented with arginine, nucleotides, and fish oil in intensive care unit patients: result of a multicenter, prospective, randomized, clinical trial. Crit Care Med 1995;23:436–449
55. Marino LV, Kiratu EM, French S, Nathoo N. To determine the effect of metoclopramide on gastric emptying in severe head injuries: a prospective, randomized, controlled clinical trial. Br J Neurosurg 2003;17:24–28

21
Fluid Management
Dan Miulli

Case Study

A 60-year-old female presents with a loss of consciousness, right-sided weakness, and a Glasgow Coma Scale (GCS) score of 9. Her husband found her in the morning on the kitchen floor. She was wearing her nightclothes, and her husband does not know when or if she made it into the bedroom to sleep. She has a past medical history of mild chronic obstructive pulmonary disease (COPD) and hypertension. She was and still is intubated because of mild respiratory difficulties. In the field, dextrose 5% in water (D5W) intravenous fluids (IVFs) were started because of presumed dehydration.

See page 309 for Case Management.

◆ Need for Intravenous Fluids

The body is composed of 50 to 70% water and requires euvolemia to survive optimally and to overcome illness. The understanding of sodium and water balance is key to managing the patient in the neurosurgical intensive care unit (NICU). Although water content is different in individuals, in general, men have a higher percentage of body fluid, and in either sex, the amount decreases with age. Fifty-five to 75% of the body's total fluid is intracellular, and 25 to 45% is extracellular. The extracellular fluid is located in intravascular plasma (25%) and interstitial spaces (75%). Therefore, in a 70 kg man, of the 48 L of total body fluid, $\frac{8}{12}$ is intracellular (32 L), $\frac{3}{12}$ is interstitial (12 L), and $\frac{1}{12}$ is intravascular (4 L).

Fluid balance is extremely complicated, governed by antidiuretic hormone (ADH) (also known as arginine vasopressin [AVP]), aldosterone, and the natriuretic peptides: brain (BNP), atrial (ANP), and C-type (CNP). The main control of fluid balance is the tonicity made mostly by sodium, with the minor constituents chloride and bicarbonate ions of the extracellular fluid adding to the remainder. Potassium, magnesium, and phosphate constitute intracellular ions and tonicity. The hormones mentioned react to as little as a 1 to 2% change in vascular tonicity.

◆ Hormone Control of Fluids

ADH/AVP is made in the magnocellular part of the supraoptic nuclei of the hypothalamus and conveyed to the posterior pituitary, where it is secreted. It binds to the distal renal collecting tubules to stimulate water reabsorption and to make concentrated urine in response to opioids, barbiturates, and carbamazepine, as well as high osmolality, hypovolemia, stress, hypoglycemia, and pain. ADH/AVP is a potent vasoconstrictor. In addition to affecting renal tubule cells, it affects brain cells. ADH/AVP V receptors appear to control fluid entry into the brain cell by activation of aquaporin-2, allowing fluid into the cell, which, if increased excessively, increases brain edema and infarction.[1]

Aldosterone is released in response to baroreceptors sensing hemorrhage, decreased intravascular volume, or decreased blood pressure. The baroreceptors stimulate rennin angiotensin, leading to aldosterone release and causing sodium resorption followed by water retention.

Natriuretic peptides not only cause renal sodium loss and fluid loss, but they also reduce water and sodium in areas of brain edema by directly reducing brain cell water and brain capillary permeability.[2,3] ANP increases cerebral blood flow and causes significant cerebral vasodilation. It is also produced in the hypothalamus and is found in the median eminence, midbrain, choroid plexus, and spinal cord.[4] BNP fibers are found along the carotid, middle cerebral, posterior communicating, and anterior cerebral arteries (**Table 21–1**).[5]

Normally, a person is able to drink and will become thirsty when the osmoreceptors in the anterior hypothalamus become stimulated ~295 mOsm/kg. However, when the patient is comatose from stroke, trauma, tumor, infection, or other devastating neurologic disease, the physician must prescribe appropriate fluids. The average dose of IVF can be approximated several ways using a general or graduated, weight-based formula (**Table 21–2**). There are several physiological circumstances that require increased fluids above the normal amount (**Table 21–3**).[4]

Table 21–1 Hormone Control of Fluids[5,63–66]

Hormone	Fluid action	Vessel action
ADH/AVP	Water reabsorption increased	Vasoconstriction
Aldosterone	Sodium reabsorption increased	Vasoconstriction
Natriuretic peptide ANP, BNP, CNP	Renal sodium loss Renal and brain water loss	Vasodilation

ADH, antidiuretic hormone; ANP, atrial natriuretic peptide; AVP, arginine vasopressin; BNP, brain natriuretic peptide; CNP, C-type natriuretic peptide.

Table 21–2   Daily and Hourly Fluid Requirements: Graduated, Weight-Based Formulas[4,63–66]

Daily Fluid Requirements*
100 mL/kg for the first 10 kg in 24 hours, then
50 mL/kg for the next 10 kg in 24 hours, then
20 mL/kg for remainder weight in kg in 24 hours age <60 years
15 mL/kg for remainder weight in kg in 24 hours age >60 years
* For 70 kg male, age 55: (1000 + 500 + 1000)/24 = 104 cc/hour
Hourly Fluid Requirements*
4 cc/hour for the first 10 kg
2 cc/hour for the next 10 kg
1 cc/hour for remainder weight in kg
* For 70 kg male, age 55: 110 cc/hour
Daily Fluid Requirements, Average*
Average 35 cc/kg, elderly 30 cc/kg
* For 70 kg male, age 55: 2450/24 = 102 cc/hour

If these conditions are not taken into consideration, a patient will become hypovolemic. Volume status can be approximated using the following clinical criteria:

- Heart rate: >110 beats/minute
- Systolic blood pressure (SBP): <90
- Dry mucosal surface
- Crackling heard in lungs
- Evidence of skin edema or turgor
- Central venous pressure (CVP): <6 to 8 mm Hg
- Urine specific gravity: <1.010 or >1.030
- Urine color: clear or amber
- Urine output: <0.5 cc/kg/hour
- Daily weight change: increase or decrease of 1 kg
- Input and output, 8 hours: <500 cc (24 hours: <1500 cc)

Table 21–3   Increased Fluid Requirements, by Percent*[4,63–66]

Fever: 12.5% for each 1°C above normal
Sweating: 10 to 25%
Hyperventilation: 10 to 60%

* A 70 kg male, age 55, requiring 110 cc/hour who has an elevated temperature 1°C and is sweating may require 135 to 151 cc/hour.

Each value by itself may not be diagnostic, but when weighted, it can lead to a clearer idea of fluid balance.

◆ Osmolality, Osmolarity, and Tonicity

Just knowing the fluid balance of the patient or even the cell will not allow proper maintenance. The amount of solutes concentrated in fluid is also vital. Osmolality is a measure of the number of osmotically active particles measured in osmoles or milliosmoles per kilogram of solvent (mmol/kg or mOsm/L). A highly concentrated osmotic solution will have a high osmolality. That is, it will have more osmotically active particles per unit of solvent than a solution with a low osmolality.

Osmolarity is the total quantity (concentration) of dissolved substances in a solution both penetrating and not penetrating the semipermeable membrane.

Tonicity reflects only the concentration of nonpenetrating solutes in the extracellular space compared with the nonpenetrating solute concentration inside the cell.

The intracellular space is a large reservoir, accounting for $8/12$, or 32 L, of fluid, and can easily control the solutes in the extracellular volume of $3/12$, or 12 L. An iso-osmotic cell has an osmolarity of 300 mOsm; that is, it contains 300 mOsm of penetrating and nonpenetrating solutes. When the extracellular fluid also contains 300 mOsm of penetrating and nonpenetrating solutes, the extracellular solution is isotonic, and the cell will not change fluid volume. When the extracellular solution contains 250 mOsm (equivalent to lactated Ringer's solution) of penetrating and nonpenetrating solutes, the extracellular fluid is hypotonic, and the cell will swell as the fluid rushes into the large cellular reservoir in an attempt to make the extracellular space isotonic. If the extracellular solution contains 921 mOsm concentration (equivalent to 3% saline) of penetrating and nonpenetrating solutes, the extracellular solution is hypertonic, and the cell will shrink; fluid will rush out in an attempt to make the extracellular space isotonic.

In reality, the cell contains different amounts of penetrating and nonpenetrating solutes compared with the interstitial and intravascular fluid. A cell may have 300 mOsm of nonpenetrating solutes and 20 mOsm of penetrating solute such as urea, causing it to be hyperosmotic (320 mOsm). If the extracellular fluid has 300 mOsm of nonpenetrating solutes, the extracellular solution is isotonic, and the cell will not change fluid volume. The tonicity is always the relationship of the nonpenetrating solutes across the cellular membrane. Even though the cell's osmolarity is 320 mOsm (300 mOsm nonpenetrating and 20 mOsm penetrating solutes), the extracellular solution is isotonic because it has the same concentration of nonpenetrating solutes as the cell. There are multiple osmotically active components, or osmoles, of solute concentrated in body fluid, expressed as mOsm/L. The intracellular penetrating solute concentration, such as urea and ethanol,

Table 21–4   Normal Concentrations of Components in Intra- and Extracellular Fluid[4,63–66]

Component	Intracellular fluid (mOsm/L)	Extracellular fluid (mOsm/L)
Sodium	5–15	135–145
Potassium	140–150	3.5–5.0

does not affect fluid movement because the penetrating solutes will equilibrate across the semipermeable membrane.[6]

The nonpenetrating particles or solutes making up the tonicity of the intravascular fluid are inorganic ions of sodium, chloride, bicarbonate, and potassium, as well as organic osmolytes of amino acids, sorbitol, and methylamines, among others. These osmoles do not easily cross the cell membrane, are restricted to the extracellular or intracellular compartments by the semipermeable cellular membrane, and therefore drive the fluid shifts or the tonicity of the fluid. Compounds such as ethanol, urea, and other solutes easily cross the intravascular boundary and therefore do not significantly add to the tonicity of the fluid, although they do add to the osmolarity.

Sodium is the major component of intravascular fluid whose regulation is closely tied to the volume of the same intravascular fluid. It is the main determinate of tonicity or effective osmolality, which determines where fluid will move. The normal plasma osmolality is 280 to 290 mOsm/L (although some sources suggest as low as 275 to as high as 295 mOsm/L) and is closely controlled by thirst osmoreceptors in the anterolateral hypothalamus. Intracellular components consist of potassium and other tightly regulated anions, leading to an osmolality of 300 mOsm/L, driving fluid into the cell. Tonicity affects fluid movement. The normal concentrations of intra- and extracellular components in osmoles are given in **Table 21–4**.

From the average extracellular concentrations, the daily requirements of those same constituents can be deduced (**Table 21–5**).

Table 21–5   Average Daily Requirements of Extracellular Components (for 70 kg [154 lb] man)[4,63–66]

Component	mEq/L	mEq/kg	Change in mEq
Sodium	60–150	1.0–2.0	80–120
Potassium	55–80	0.5–1.3	50–100
Chloride	60–150	1.0–1.7	80–120
Calcium		0.2–0.3	6–10
Magnesium			20
Phosphorus			30
Glucose			100–200

◆ The Blood–Brain Barrier and Intravenous Fluids

The blood–brain barrier has an effective pore size of 8 angstroms (Å) and is impermeable to sodium, ions, water-soluble compounds, and protein, but is permeable to lipophilic substances and gases. The majority of substances are actively transported across the brain capillary endothelial cell to the brain interstitial space. The cerebrospinal fluid (CSF) flows along a gradient to the ventricle and is absorbed through the arachnoid villi, where a pressure differential allows it to pass into the venous sinus. Likewise, the larger reservoir, the cellular fluid, is actively transported into the brain interstitial space and follows the same pathway. Ninety-one percent of the circulating fluid is in the intracellular and interstitial spaces; this is the area where fluid and solute need to be regulated.

The optimal treatment would be to actively remove solutes out of the cell into the brain interstitial space, through the ventricles, and into the blood. This would be accomplished with high-tonicity, low-osmolality fluid flowing from the brain capillary endothelial cell into the interstitium, increasing the tonicity of the interstitial fluid with nonpermeable sodium. Low molecular weight solutes would then leave the damaged swollen brain cell, followed by water. The damaged cell contains increased osmoles of H^+ and K^+. Therefore, if ion exchange mechanisms are functioning, lower interstitial solutes of H^+, K^+, and others would simultaneously draw the cellular toxins out of the cell into the CSF, followed by water, then drained out of the ventricle into the venous system; simulating CSF ventricular dialysis.

Inhibiting CSF formation or decreasing intravascular volume does not decrease intracellular and interstitial edema. Decreasing edema is accomplished by removing CSF.

During times of trauma and disease, the cell may be swollen in an initial response to dilute the solute toxins. There is additional swelling when fluid increases in the brain interstitial space in an attempt to dilute those increased solutes that entered through the broken blood–brain barrier. If the interstitial fluid does not drain out of the ventricle, the brain will swell, compressing blood vessels and leading to further ischemia.

The brain initially attempts dialysis by opening the blood–brain barrier, allowing water and solutes to enter the brain interstitium attempting to have a hypo-osmolar, hypertonic solution, so that solutes may leave the cell, followed by the increased cellular water.

The blood–brain barrier, which is formed by the cerebral capillary endothelial cells, contains channels regulated by aquaporins through which water flows somewhat passively down an osmotic gradient. The cerebral capillary endothelial cells are different in function and regulation from those of the brain arteriole or venule. The other brain fluid barrier, albeit much smaller in area, is between the blood and CSF and consists of the choroid plexus epithelium. Tight gap junctions, low pinocytic activity, and specific energy-dependent membrane transporters regulate the passage of substances into and through the capillary endothelial cells to the brain interstitial fluid. Substances can freely diffuse into the capillary endothelial cells if they are gases, lipid soluble, and have a molecular weight less than 400 to 600 daltons (Da). However, most substances, such as choline, glucose, glutamate, and lactate, are associated with either a carrier-mediated transport system or solutes such as cationized albumin, insulin, insulin-like growth factor (IGF), and transferrin. Others are associated with a receptor-mediated transport system. Both systems transport substances through the capillary endothelial cell into the brain interstitial space.

The intact blood–brain barrier only mildly restricts the passive diffusion of water from a cellular hypotonic solution to an interstitial hypertonic space through aquaporin-regulated channels. In the adult, the blood–brain barrier regulates most common IVF types. However, the brain damaged by trauma, ischemia, tumors, and increased pressure does not have an intact blood–brain barrier, nor is the barrier intact with changes in normal brain homeostasis that occur with edema, hyperventilation, mannitol infusion, hyperthermia, hypotension, hypertension, or tumor necrosis factor secretion. During these times of stress, when the blood–brain barrier is open, vasogenic edema has begun, and the brain is at further risk of damage if the incorrect therapeutic fluids are used. The damaged brain does not benefit from dehydration hypovolemia but from a euvolemic to slightly hypertonic state.[7,8] In addition to vasogenic edema from an opened blood–brain barrier, the more common cellular cytotoxic edema forms in an effort to combat further injury, diluting the cellular toxins accumulated because of decreased blood and plasma flow (e.g., hydrogen ions and potassium). Therefore, dehydration hypovolemia becomes deleterious for combating cytotoxic edema. Euvolemia must be maintained to flush the toxins from the cell. The cell must maintain an osmotic gradient in the brain interstitial space, which allows the transport of solutes and water out of the cell.

Since 1919, the deleterious effects of hypotonic solution have been known.[9] Decreasing the IVF 1 mEq/L will decrease the osmotic pressure 38.6 mm Hg; likewise, decreasing the IVF 5 mEq/L (10 mOsm/kg) will decrease the osmotic pressure 193 mm Hg. This change in fluid drive is minimal under normal homeostasis but will aggravate the swelling and increase the intracranial pressure (ICP) in an opened blood–brain barrier, a condition that occurs with tumors, ischemia, and trauma. The best fluid approximates or is slightly above normal sodium concentration and normal tonicity without having an additional glucose load. The calculated mOsm/L of individual fluids is shown in **Table 21–6**; however, it should be noted that the actual measured osmolality is ~20 mOsm/kg water less.[10] Administering hypertonic saline decreases intracellular volume from 32.0 to 30.6 L, increases interstitial volume from 12.0 to 13.2 L, and increases intravascular volume from 4.0 to 4.4 L. Normal saline has no significant change on intracellular volume, increases interstitial volume from 12.00 to 14.25 L, and increases intravascular volume from 4.00 to 4.75 L. D5W increases intracellular volume from 32 to 34 L, increases interstitial volume from 12.00 to 12.75 L, and increases intravascular volume from 4.00 to 4.25 L.[11] Therefore, normal saline should be used for resuscitation and any time there is brain damage or the potential for brain damage. D5W, half-normal saline, and lactated Ringer's solution should be avoided. Hypertonic saline must be considered during times of increasing cerebral edema (**Table 21–6**).

Table 21–6 Concentration of Sodium, Osmolarity, Osmolality, and Glucose of Available Intravenous Fluids[10,11]

Intravenous fluid	Sodium (mEq/L, or mmol/L)	Osmolarity calculated tonicity (mOsm/L)	Measured osmolality	Glucose (g/L)
Normal body fluids	142	280–290	280–290	
0.9 normal saline NaCl	154	308	282	
0.45 half-normal saline NaCl	77	154		
D5W	0	252	259	50
D5W, 0.45% NaCl	77	406		50
D5W, 0.9% NaCl	154	560		50
Lactated Ringer's solution	130	273	250	
Normosol	40	363		50
Plasmanate® plasma protein fraction (human), 5% usp	145	300		
3% NaCl	513	1030	921	
Albumin 5%	130–160	330		
Albumin 25%	130–160	330		
Hetastarch 6%	145	310	307	

D5W, dextrose 5% water.

Prescribing additives to IVFs must be done with care. Hyperglycemia at the time of primary or secondary injury aggravates ischemic insults and worsens neurologic outcome by increasing lactic acidosis. The condition is not from previously unknown or untreated hyperglycemia; rather, it is usually from reaction to trauma, stress, glucocorticoid administration, sepsis, or other causes.

Hyperglycemia causes a dose-dependent increase in the severity of ischemic and severe head injury. In one study, glucose >150 mg/dL had worse outcome than glucose < 150 mg/dL.[12] Hyperglycemia-induced lactic acidosis increases neurologic damage, increases infarct size, and causes secondary injury, a condition that appears to be a major cause of decreased outcome in patients with severe head injury.[13,14]

Therefore, under conditions of suspected brain injury, as seen with ischemia, tumors, and trauma, do not give IV solutions that would worsen edema, such as those containing dextrose, low tonicity, and low sodium.[15] Start fluid maintenance with IV normal saline to keep the patient euvolemic to slightly hypervolemic.

◆ Hypovolemia

Hypotension must be avoided at all costs, because a single episode of hypotension doubles the morbidity and mortality associated with severe head injury. Hypovolemia decreases cardiac output and nervous tissue perfusion. It may be seen with a blood urea nitrogen/creatinine (BUN/Cr) ratio greater than 15/20:1 or any other number of clinical conditions. Also, it does not improve outcome after brain injury.

The body attempts to correct hypovolemia by upregulation of norepinephrine, ADH, rennin-angiotensin II, and aldosterone, each increasing sodium reabsorption and water retention. Sodium absorption is increased in the renal proximal tubule cells by rennin-angiotensin II, and reabsorption of sodium occurs at the distal tubule and collecting duct by the stimulation of aldosterone. Norepinephrine decreases glomerular filtration rate–enhancing sodium reabsorption at the proximal tubule. However, these hormones also affect brain cell water absorption in a similar fashion, further increasing water retention in the brain interstitium and cell. Therefore, not only trauma patients but also patients with cerebral ischemia, vasospasms, and spinal cord injuries require fluid resuscitation. Euvolemia to slight hypervolemia improves outcomes in head trauma. Each effect of hypotension further worsens the effects of trauma. Daily maintenance fluids should be administered to compensate for the normal loss, for example, in a 70 kg man of 1200 to 1500 mL/day and to maintain a urine output of 0.5 to 1.0 cc/kg/hour. If there are questions concerning volume status that cannot be determined using clinical and laboratory data presented in this chapter, then a Swan-Ganz catheter should be inserted to attempt to obtain normal[16,17] or optimal values in the management of head injury (**Table 21–7**).[18]

Patients with spinal cord injury have decreased sympathetic tone, leading to vasodilation, bradycardia, hypotension, and decreased perfusion. These patients must have adequate fluid resuscitation with euvolemia and vasopressors to restore sympathetic tone. They should not be overhydrated, which would cause hyponatremia, pulmonary edema, and worsening of spinal cord edema.

Table 21–7   Invasive Hemodynamic Monitoring[18]

	Normal values (mm Hg)	Optimal values (mm Hg)
CVP	0–8	6–8
PAD	6–16	12–16
PCWP	6–14	10–14

CVP, central venous pressure; PAD, pulmonary artery diastolic pressure; PCWP, pulmonary capillary wedge pressure.

◆ Intravenous Fluids in Extremes of Pathological Conditions

When intensive care management of the neurologically injured patient begins to fail with standard fluids and treatment, additional or different IVFs may be required. When ICP or edema remains elevated, despite initial measures, mannitol or hypertonic saline may be needed.

Hypertonic solutions have been shown to lower ICP[19-21] and improve cerebral perfusion pressure (CPP),[22-25] whereas isotonic fluids do not improve ICP, as can be deduced from changes in intracellular, interstitial, and intravascular volumes, as noted above.[26] In a study by Vasser et al,[27] hypertonic saline reduced ICP in severe head injured (SHI) patients. Furthermore, 7.5% sodium chloride (NaCl) improved survival when compared with standard treatment in patients with a GCS of 3 to 8. Wade et al[28] performed a meta-analysis of SHI patients who receive hypertonic saline and demonstrated that they are twice as likely to survive as those who receive standard therapy. Hypertonic saline is more beneficial than mannitol in refractory intracranial hypertension[29,30] by creating a driving force that pulls water out of the brain cells and interstitium. Hypertonic saline has an increased concentration of sodium and chloride. In an attempt to decrease hyperchloremic metabolic acidosis, the hypertonic solution may be made with a balanced mixture of sodium chloride and sodium acetate.

There is considerable debate regarding resuscitation with colloids. However, if a 1 to 2 L fluid bolus of normal saline does not stabilize the patient or 20 cc/kg in children per advanced trauma life support (ATLS) guidelines, then colloid should be given. Crystalloids such as normal saline remain intravascular for a maximum of 2 hours, and their effect on pulmonary wedge pressure and cardiac index is small. Colloids contain high molecular weight solutes that do not readily cross the capillary wall, remain intravascular for longer periods of time, and require smaller infused volumes. Some investigators have demonstrated that colloids exacerbate pulmonary edema, decrease cardiac output, and compromise the immune system. Others believe that colloids reduce secondary brain injury. Of the colloids, blood may be the best alternative for fluid resuscitation, attempting to maintain a hemoglobin and hematocrit of 10 and 33%, respectively.[31-36] This allows maximum oxygen-carrying capacity and best viscosity.[37-40] Hemodilution to a hemoglobin and hematocrit of 10 and 33%, respectively, has been studied in the management of cerebral vasospasms, in an attempt to improve viscosity and oxygen-carrying capacity as well as cerebral blood flow.[41,42] Hematocrit lower than 30% decreases oxygen-carrying capacity beyond the improvements made because of increased viscosity. Even in ischemic stroke patients, a hematocrit of 30% optimizes infarct volume, being worse for values ≥35% and <26%.[43,44] Anemia, where the hematocrit is less than 25 to 30%, increases cerebral vasodilation, ICP, and edema.[45]

Several substances in addition to blood have been used to increase volume, such as albumin, Plasmanate (Bayer Pharmaceuticals, Yakutin, Japan), Normosol (Abbott Laboratories, Abbott Park, IL), and hetastarch. Each volume expander has risks; however, the best expander remains blood. Plasminate appears to be better than lactated Ringer's solution and causes fewer lung problems when compared with other fluids.[46,47] Normosol may have better red blood cell (RBC) protection than Plasminate.[48] Hetastarch, although it expands volume well, does have the side effect of bleeding, significantly elevating partial thromboplastin time. It therefore should not be used when hemorrhage has occurred or may occur.[49] Albumin 5, 20, or 25% may[50,51] or may not improve outcome when used in the trauma patient and may in fact increase pulmonary extravascular fluid.[52] Although 5% albumin is oncotically and osmotically equivalent to plasma, its use remains controversial. The Saline Versus Albumin Fluid Evaluation (SAFE) study[53] concluded that, in patients in the NICU, use of 4% albumin or normal saline for fluid resuscitation results in similar outcomes at 28 days. The authors looked at 6997 randomized patients. For the entire study population, there were no significant differences in deaths and number of days spent in the NICU, hospital, on ventilator, or in renal replacement therapy. However, the subgroup analysis of patients with trauma and brain injury trended toward an increased relative risk of death. There was insufficient power to make significant claims. The actual number of patients (59 of 241) receiving albumin with trauma and head injury compared with those receiving saline (38 of 251) was small (p = .009). In the analysis of death in all patients with trauma, 81 of 596 were in the albumin group, and 59 of 590 deaths were in the saline group (p = .06); however, once again, the power was too low to support significant claims. Patients with head injury constituted only 7% of the study population. The investigators concluded that there needs to be further study of trauma and head injury patients.

Mannitol has been in the neuroscience armamentarium for some time. Mannitol improves viscosity and therefore circulation. It does, however, open the blood–brain barrier and, with multiple doses, will cross into the interstitial space and increase its osmotic pull of fluids into the tissue, causing hypotonicity, contrary to the intended desire of therapy. It works on the microvasculature in several minutes, vasoconstricting, decreasing viscosity, increasing cerebral blood flow,[54–59] and acting as a free radical scavenger. Mannitol works best at high ICP, low CPP at vasodilation when autoregulation is preserved. Its plasma expansion is equal to 7.5% NaCl. The systemic capillary is permeable to water, which moves into the intravascular space to dilute mannitol, while an intact brain is not freely permeable to water to the same extent as the systemic capillary or the damaged blood–brain barrier. As an osmotic diuretic, mannitol draws in systemic water, causing hemodilution and improving shear rate and RBC deformity. The osmotic effect is delayed 15 to 30 minutes, and persists 90 minutes to 6 hours. Mannitol has a small osmotic effect in the brain, only changing the brain water content 2 to 6%. It becomes less effective after multiple doses, such as >3 or 4 doses in 24 hours. If given at higher rates, mannitol moves across the defective blood–brain barrier into tissue, exacerbating edema.[60,61] Mannitol can be used when there is suspected increased ICP, such as in the emergency room.

When given, there must be adequate fluids to support blood pressure because hypotension doubles morbidity and mortality rates associated with severe head injury. On occasion, mannitol can demonstrate an increase in ICP and a transient short-term decrease in sodium, magnesium, phosphorus, and potassium. Mannitol increases intravascular osmolality; therefore, when there is reasonable concern about osmolality, a measured recording of osmolality must be made, not a calculated recording.

Guidelines for the Management of Severe Head Injury[62] states that

> [m]annitol is effective therapy for the control of increased ICP. Intermittent bolus is probably better than continuous infusion therapy. Dose ranges are 0.25–1 gram/kg.

OPTION: Where mannitol is being used prior to ICP monitoring, where it is not titrated, you should have evidence of raised ICP present (e.g., signs of transtentorial herniation or progressive neurologic deterioration). Serum osmolarity should be kept <320 mOsm, because when greater the incidence of renal failure is increased. Euvolemia should be maintained and a Foley catheter inserted.

Diuretics

Mannitol may be the most appropriate agent for diuresis in the short term. Another agent is furosemide, which acts by inhibiting distal tubule reabsorption of sodium and water. It can also reduce ICP and CSF production. The dose varies with the degree of diuresis required, from as little as 5 mg IV every 4 to 6 hours to as high as 80 to 160 mg every 6 hours.

Acetazolamide is a carbonic anhydrase inhibitor reducing CSF production from the choroid plexus while vasodilating. It can be used during conditions of excess CSF production, which by itself causes an increased ICP. It should not be used during times of intracellular and interstitial edema. The usual dose is 125 to 250 mg tid/qid to a maximum of 2 g/day. Side effects include metabolic acidosis that should be checked with chemistry panel or arterial blood gases (ABG). Other side effects include paresthesias, altered taste, renal calculi, and nausea.

◆ Calculation of Fluid Balance

Fluid balance determination may be a difficult task in the NICU because of medications and concomitant injuries. It is important to determine fluid input and output exactly. The patient must be weighed daily using the same scale and the same clutter of material, such as sheets, blankets, pillows, sequential compression devices, and monitors. Although bothersome to the nursing staff, the most exact measurement would be to weigh without these items.

There is no concrete means to determine fluid balance. Swan-Ganz measurement may be confounded by cardiac and pulmonary changes. However, on a daily basis, the fluid balance can be determined from clinical exam and laboratory tests. The clinical exam for volume status must be part of the daily examination of the NICU patient.[64-66]

Although **Table 21–8** simplifies the calculation of fluid balance, the true determination is not simple.

Specific States of Fluid and Electrolyte Imbalance

Specific states of fluid and electrolyte imbalance can be calculated using the following equation:

$$\text{Osmolality (mOsm/L)} = 2 \times (\text{Na mEq/L} + \text{K mEq/L}) + (\text{BUN}/2.8) + (\text{glucose}/18).$$

There are three states of hyponatremia (Na < 135 mmol/L), the most common being hypotonic hyponatremia and the least common being isotonic and hypertonic (**Table 21-9**).

Isotonic hyponatremia (serum mOsm 280–290) is caused by hyperlipidemia and hyperproteinemia that increase plasma volume and dilute sodium. The expected amount of sodium reduction is equal to the current protein concentration minus 8 g/dL multiplied by 0.25. A very large protein concentration is needed to change sodium concentration significantly. Treatment consists of correcting the underlying disorder.

Hypertonic hyponatremia (serum mOsm > 290) is more commonly seen with diseases of hypertonicity, such as hyperglycemia, or after hypertonic administration of glucose, mannitol, or glycine, causing dilution of sodium. The expected amount of sodium reduction is equal to 1.45 mmol/L for each 100 mg/dL increase in blood glucose above 200 mg/dL. Treatment consists of correcting the underlying disorder.

Hypotonic hyponatremia (serum mOsm < 280) is the most common type seen in the NICU patient and itself consists of three subtypes: isovolemic, hypovolemic, and hypervolemic.

Isovolemic hypotonic hyponatremia occurs after consumption of large amounts of water in patients with mild renal impairment, potassium loss from diuretics, or gastrointestinal (GI) loss, as well as in those with tuberculosis, bronchogenic tumors, cirrhosis, aspergillosis, stress, severe pain, acute intermittent porphyria, and those receiving positive pressure ventilation. It is also associated with the use of carbamazepine, phenothiazines, antidepressants, chloropropramide, oxytocin, thiazide diuretics, sulfonylureas, and opiates, and with syndrome of inappropriate antidiuretic hormone (SIADH). (Information regarding the diagnosis, symptoms, and treatment of SIADH is given below.) Increasing intrathoracic pressure causes aortic baroreceptors to sense hypotension and respond with water retention. Most causes are treated with fluid restriction of 800 to 1500 mL/day. Lower sodium levels can be treated with sodium tablets (2 g) 3 or 4 times per day or 3% NaCl IV solution. The use of each depends on the clinical condition.

Table 21–8 Calculation of Fluid Balance[63–66]

Component (absolute value or daily change)	Positive overload (value or lose [L] pts)	Negative dry (value or gain [G] pts)
Hgb (12–16)	< 10 or L1.5 or >	> 15 or G1.5 or >
HCT (37–54)	< 30 or L4 or >	> 50 or G4 or >
Na (134–145)	< 134 or L5 or >	> 145 or G5 or >
BUN (7–18) **or (only give 1 or 2 pts)**	< 10 or L4 OR	> 18 or G4 or >
BUN (7–18)	< 5 or L7 (2 pts)	
Creatinine (0.7–1.3)	< 0.7 or L0.3 or >	> 1.3 or G0.3 or >
Serum osmolarity (280–300)	< 280 or L15 or >	> 300 or G15 or >
Heart rate		> 110 or G30 or >
SBP		< 90 or L35 or >
Orthostatics		Positive
Mucosa		Mucosa dry
Lungs	Crackles	
Skin	Edema	Turgor (2 pts)
CVP (0–8 mm Hg) (* ∇ = 6–8)	> 9 or G5 or >	< 4 or L5 or >
Urine specific gravity (1.010–1.030)	< 1.010 or L0.020 or>	> 1.030 or G0.020 or >
Urine color	Clear	Amber
Urine output		< 0.5 cc/kg/hr (2 pts)
Weight change daily	Gain > 2.2 lb	Lose > 2.2 lb
I&Os 8 hours	+500	−500
I&Os 24 hours **or (only give 1 or 2 pts)**	+1000 **or** +1500 or > (2 pts)	−1000 **or** −1500 or > (2 pts)

Note: Of a total of +17 points for positive overload, overload occurs at greater than 5 points. Of a total of −22 points for negative dry, dry occurs at less than −5 points. To determine fluid status, add positive values in column 2 and negative values in column 3.

* Average values.[16,17]
∇ Optimal value for the treatment of head injury.[18]
BUN, blood urea nitrogen; CVP, central venous pressure; HCT, hematocrit; Hgb, hemoglobin; I&Os, inputs and outputs; Na, sodium; SBP, systolic blood pressure.
2. Assuming no significant effects of vasoconstrictors or severe cardiopulmonary changes, the values of pulmonary artery diastolic pressure (PAD) below may be used to adjust fluids. Numbers preceded by + or − indicate change from previous reading.
If PAD > 17 or > +5, decrease fluids 25%. If PAD < 10 or < −5, increase fluids 50%.
If PAD > 20 or > +8, decrease fluids 50%. If PAD < 8 or < −8, increase fluids 100%.
If PAD > 23 or > +10, give diuretic, and decrease fluid 75%.
If PAD < 6 or < −10, increase fluids 100%, and give fluid bolus 300% over 1 hour; if no response, give 100% bolus colloid.

(*Continued*)

Table 21–8   Calculation of Fluid Balance (*Continued*)

Current hemodynamic parameters		
Cardiac output 4–7 PCWP 6–14* 10–14 ▽	Cardiac index 2.8–4.2 PAD 6–16* 12–16 ▽	MAP SVR 770–1500

*Average values.[16,17]
▽, optimal value for the treatment of head injury.[18]
MAP, mean arterial pressure; PAD, pulmonary artery diastolic pressure; PCWP, pulmonary capillary wedge pressure; SVR, systemic vascular resistance.

Hypervolemic hypotonic hyponatremia is the subtype of edema seen in congestive heart failure, cirrhosis, and transurethral prostatic resection (TURP). Most causes are treated with fluid restriction of 800 to 1500 mL/day and can be augmented with loop diuretic because of the higher afterload. Lower sodium levels can be treated with sodium tablets 2 g 3 or 4 times per day or 3% NaCl IV solution. The use of each depends on the clinical condition.

Hypovolemic hypotonic hyponatremia occurs when loss of fluids rich in sodium, such as bile, sweat, and fluids found in the pancreas, small

Table 21–9   States of Hyponatremia

State (Na < 135 mEq/L or mmol/L)	Subtypes	Clinical condition	Treatment
Isotonic (serum mOsm 280–290)		Hyperproteinemia, hyperlipidemia	Correct underlying disorder
Hypertonic (serum mOsm > 290)		Glucose, mannitol load	Correct underlying disorder
Hypotonic (mOsm < 280)	Isovolemic	Water intoxication	Fluid restriction
		K+ loss, diuretics, carbamazepine	Fluid restriction
		TB, cirrhosis	Fluid restriction
		SIADH	Fluid restriction
	Hypervolemic	CHF, liver disease	Fluid restriction, loop diuretic, 3% NaCl, NaCl tablets
		TURP	Multiple
	Hypovolemic	CSW	Increase volume, 3% NaCl, NaCl tablets
		D5W, 0.45% NaCl	Increase volume with 0.9% NaCl

CHF, congestive heart failure; CSW, cerebral salt wasting; D5W, dextrose 5% in water; SIADH, syndrome of inappropriate antidiuretic hormone; TB, tuberculosis; TURP, transurethral prostatic resection.

intestine, and lung, are replaced with D5W or 0.45% NaCl. The most common clinical condition of this subtype seen in the NICU patient is the syndrome of cerebral salt wasting (CSW). (Information regarding the diagnosis, symptoms, and treatment of CSW is given below.) Renal loss of sodium and low volume in CSW are opposite the condition of SIADH. CSW is seen in subarachnoid hemorrhage (SAH) of any type and is possibly due to the brain releasing natriuretic factor from the hypothalamus in an attempt to increase cerebral blood flow and cause cerebral vasodilation during times of vasospasm. Natriuretic peptides not only cause renal sodium loss and fluid loss, but they also reduce water and sodium in areas of brain edema. Natriuretic peptide fibers are found along the carotid, middle cerebral, posterior communicating, and anterior cerebral arteries, areas of highest vasospasm. CSW occurs 3 to 7 days after initial SAH, concomitant with a time of vasospasm occurrence.

Diagnosis of SIADH

The diagnosis of SIADH includes the following parameters:

- Normal or elevated intravascular volume
- Serum sodium < 134 mEq/L
- Low serum osmolality (<280 mOsm/L)
- High urine osmolality, high or normal urinary sodium (>18 mEq/L)
- Normal renal, adrenal, and thyroid function

Hyponatremia in SIADH occurs due to bronchogenic tumors, meningitis, trauma, increased ICP, tumors, and craniotomy.

Symptoms of SIADH

Symptoms of SIADH include headache, confusion, lethargy, nausea/vomiting, muscle cramps, depressed deep tendon reflexes, and seizures; these can lead to coma and death.

Treatment of SIADH

Treatment of SIADH involves slowly elevating the sodium level and restricting fluids to an amount less than urine output. In the adult, fluid intake should be restricted to 800 to 1500 mL/day. If severe SIADH is present, use 3% NaCl and furosemide. (The furosemide causes excretion of dilute urine.) If there is chronic SIADH, as seen in some alcoholics, then elevate the sodium level slowly, 8 to 10 mEq/L per 24 hours, to prevent central myelinolysis of the pons or other areas. In a chronic alcoholic patient, stop 3% NaCl when the serum sodium level reaches 125 mEq/L to prevent a relative hyperosmolar condition in this specific type of patient. The rebound relative hyperosmolar state may be the pathophysiology involved in central myelinolysis. Other treatments include phenytoin or demeclocycline 150 to 300 mg PO every 6 hours to inhibit ADH.

Diagnosis of CSW

The diagnosis of CSW includes the following parameters:

- Serum sodium < 134 mEq/L
- Low serum osmolality (<280 mOsm/L)
- Urine osmolality normal or elevated
- High urinary sodium (>18 mEq/L)
- Low CVP, pulmonary capillary wedge pressure (PCWP), and pulmonary artery diastolic pressure (PAD)
- Low vascular volume
- Dehydration

Symptoms of CSW

The symptoms of CSW include headache, confusion, lethargy, nausea/vomiting, muscle cramps, depressed deep tendon reflexes, and seizures; these can lead to coma and death.

Treatment of CSW

In treating CSW, volume replacement should include 3% NaCl IVF at 10 to 50 cc/hour and, if appropriate, salt tablets 2 to 3 g tid/qid. Fludrocortisone acetate increases sodium absorption but usually is not needed.

CSW usually ends within 2 to 3 weeks, at which time salt replacement should be discontinued.

◆ Hypernatremia

Hypernatremia occurs when serum sodium is >150 to 155 mEq/L. However, symptoms do not present until later, when serum sodium is >160 mEq/L and serum osmolality is >330 mOsm/L. At this point, the patient may exhibit confusion, lethargy, and seizure. Serum sodium >180 mEq/L can be associated with increased rates of mortality, but the mortality may be the result of a life-ending process, not necessarily of the hypernatremia.

To determine the amount of fluid needed to correct the hypernatremia, the total body water (TBW) deficit should be calculated. Normal TBW averages 60% but ranges from 50 to 70%, more in younger men and less in older women.

Fluid deficit in liters = (Na current – Na normal 140 mEq/L/140 mEq/L)
× (TBW: normal 60% of body weight [kg])

If current sodium in, for example, a 70 kg man is 170 mEq/L, the free water deficit would be

$$(170 - 140)/140 \times (0.6 \times 70)$$
$$30/140 \times 42 = 8.99 \text{ L}$$

The deficit of free water must be replaced slowly, usually one half over 24 hours and the remainder over 1 or 2 days.

As with hyponatremia, there are three states: isovolemic, hypervolemic, and hypovolemic. Isovolemic hypernatremia is seen with sweating, use of isotonic fluids to replace hypotonic losses, and diabetes insipidus with sufficient fluid replacement. In diabetes insipidus, there is an 85% loss of ADH capacity. It is seen as a familial condition; occurs idiopathically, post-trauma, and with craniopharyngioma, lymphoma, neurosarcoidosis, meningitis, autoimmune diseases, and aneurysm; is linked to the administration of mannitol, phenytoin, furosemide, hydrochorothiazide, and ethanol; is seen in brain death or impending brain death; and is associated with Wegener's granulomatosis and lymphocytic hypophysitis.

Hypervolemic hypernatremia results from the use of hypertonic solutions and mineralocorticoid excess. Hypervolemic hypernatremia is seen in hypotonic fluid loss such as in burn patients and with diarrhea, vomiting, and nasogastric suctioning. It is also seen in adrenal insufficiency, chronic renal failure, and after diabetes insipidus has started without correction. The osmotic diuresis from mannitol use or with hyperglycemia results in urine that is iso-osmotic or hyperosmotic, not hypo-osmotic as in diabetes insipidus.

When administering mannitol, the amount of osmolarity added to the serum from mannitol can be determined from the difference of the calculated serum osmolarity [mOsm/L = $2 \times$ (Na mEq/L + K mEq/L) + (BUN/2.8) + (glucose/18)] compared with the measured serum osmolality.

Diagnosis of Hypernatremia

The diagnosis of hypernatremia includes the following parameters:

- High urine output (>250 mL/hour more than input fluids)
- Large water loss in urine relative to sodium loss, with resultant high normal or above normal serum sodium
- Low urine specific gravity (<1.005)
- Low urine osmolarity (50–150 mOsm/L)
- High serum osmolality (>290–295 mOsm/L)

After craniopharyngioma or pituitary surgery, there can be different types of diabetes insipidus. For example, there can be a transient phase, which occurs 12 to 36 hours postop; a prolonged phase, in which sodium remains abnormal for months or permanently; and a triphasic phase, in which injury to the pituitary reduces ADH for 4 to 5 days. This is then followed by cell death, liberating ADH for 4 to 5 days, during which time the diabetes inspidus resolves. The final phase is defined by the absence of ADH, either short-term or prolonged.

Symptoms of Hypernatremia

Symptoms of hypernatremia include confusion, loss of consciousness, tonic-clonic seizures, and rhabdomyolysis. There is no evidence that it causes intracranial hemorrhage.

Treatment of Hypernatremia

Treatment of hypernatremia includes

- Desmopressin (DDAVP) IV 1 to 5 μg (works for 8–20 hours) or
- Arginine vasopressin intramuscularly (IM), SQ 12.5 μg (works for 4–8 hours) or
- Desmopressin (DDAVP) intranasally 1 to 5 μg (works for 12–20 hours)

Check laboratory tests and urine specific gravity every 6 hours.

Replace urine output greater than input with 0.45 normal saline, or use GI system through a feeding tube to replace with free water. Do not give free water IV if it can be avoided. The rapid correction can cause cerebral edema and permanent neurologic damage. One half of the water deficit as calculated above should be corrected in 24 hours and the remainder over 1 to 2 days; the rate of correction should not exceed 10 to 12 mmol/L/24 hours in an attempt to prevent further cerebral edema.

◆ Other Electrolyte Imbalances

Magnesium

This cation occurs both as protein bound and as a free divalent ion. Magnesium is lost with acidosis, diuresis, extracellular fluid expansion, diarrhea, alcoholism, and phosphate depletion. Low magnesium (<1.5 mg/dL) is associated with seizures, confusion, and cardiac disturbances.[63] Treatment consists of 25% magnesium sulfate 2 to 4 g every 4 hours. Magnesium may block the N-methyl-D-aspartate (NMDA) receptor, decreasing the neuroexcitotoxic reaction that occurs with brain injury; may help decrease seizures; and may help decrease cerebral vasospasm.

Calcium

Free ionized calcium is controlled by the parathyroid hormone (PTH) and vitamin D. PTH stimulates the release of calcium from the bones, reabsorption from the kidneys, and absorption from the GI tract. Hypocalcemia (<8.5 mEq/L) may be seen with phenytoin use, albumin, alkalosis, low magnesium, sepsis, pancreatitis, vitamin D deficiency, hypoparathyroidism, and rhabdomyolysis. Low serum albumin will decrease total calcium but will not affect ionized calcium. Therefore, ionized calcium should be measured, not calculated. Low calcium is associated with neuronal irritability such as seizures, confusion, paresthesias, hypotension, arrhythmias, sinus tachycardia segment prolongation, apnea, stridor, and no response to norepinephrine or dopamine. If calcium is suspected to be low, then the magnesium level should be checked and, if low, corrected. Ionized calcium levels must be checked, and low levels should be treated with 100 to 200 mg in 50 to 100 mL D5W bolus, followed by 1 to 2 mg/kg/hour infusion for 6 to 12 hours.

Potassium

Potassium is an intracellular cation whose release by the kidney is controlled by aldosterone. Only 0.4% of total body potassium is present in the plasma; therefore, intracellular stores can effectively replenish extracellular pools. During times of brain damage, cellular acidosis causes potassium to leave the cell for the intravascular space. Other causes include diabetic ketoacidosis, angiotensin converting enzyme inhibitors, β-blockers, digoxin, heparin, nonsteroidal anti-inflammatory drugs (NSAIDs), trimethoprim-sulfamethoxazole, rhabdomyolysis, and rewarming after hypothermia. Hyperkalemia ($K^+ > 5.5$ mmol/L) produces paralysis, muscle weakness, dysesthesia, and cardiac disturbances due to neuroexcitability of cellular membranes. Treatment of hyperkalemia consists of 10 mL calcium gluconate 10% solution containing 93 mg of elemental calcium. Calcium antagonizes the cardiac muscle toxicity for 20 to 60 minutes. Sodium bicarbonate, as well as insulin and glucose infusion, causes enhanced activity of Na^+–K^+ adenosinetriphosphatase, moving K^+ into the cell. This helps stabilize the neurologic and neuromuscular toxicity. However, sodium bicarbonate may bind calcium, making its action ineffective. Cation exchange resins such as polystyrene sulfonate (Kayexalate) removes 1 mEq K^+ from the body for each gram given. The usual dose is 20 to 50 g dissolved in 100 to 200 mL 20% sorbitol given every 3 hours, up to 5 doses per day. However, should there be any suggestion of renal failure, hemodialysis should be instituted as soon as possible.

Case Management

This patient should have the IVF switched to normal saline at 35 cc/kg/day, plus a 10% increase for presumed hyperventilation. She should have a computed tomography scan and laboratory tests to include a chemistry panel and ABG.

References

1. Vakili A, Kataoka H, Plesnila N. Role of arginine vasopressin V_1 and V_2 receptors for brain damage after transient focal ischemia. J Cereb Blood Flow Metab 2005; 25:1012–1019

2. Rosenberg GA, Scremin O, Estrada C, et al. Arginine vasopressin V_1-antagonist and atrial natriuretic peptide reduce hemmorhagic brain edema in rats. Stroke 1992;23:1767–1773

3. Naruse S, Takei R, Horikawa Y, et al. Effects of atrial natriuretic peptide on brain edema: the change of water, sodium, and potassium contents in the brain. Acta Neurochir Suppi (Wien) 1990;51:118–121

4. Andrews BT. Fluid and electrolyte disorder in the neurosurgical intensive care. Neurosurg Clin N Am 1994;5:707–723

5. Edvinsson L, Krause DN. Neuropeptides. In: Edvinsson L, Krause DN, eds. Cerebral Blood Flow and Metabolism. 2nd ed. Philadelphia: Lippincott Williams & Wilkins; 2002:273

6. w3.ouhsc.edu/human_physiology/Cell%20Fiz%20Discussion%20questions.htm; accessed July 2005

7. Rosner MJ, Becker DP. Origin and evolution of plateau waves: experimental observations and theoretical model. J Neurosurg 1984;60:312–324

8. Rosner MJ, Daughton S. Cerebral perfusion pressure management in head injury [abstract]. AANS, Nashville, TN, Spring 1990

9. Weed LH, McKibben PS. Experimental alteration of brain bulk. Am J Physiol 1919;48:531–555

10. Gravenstein D, Gravenstein N. Intraoperative and immediate postoperative neuroanesthesia. In: Layon AJ, Gabrielli A, Friedman WA, eds. Textbook of Neurointensive Care. Philadelphia: WB Saunders; 2004

11. Chernow B. The Pharmacologic Approach to the Critically Ill Patient. 3rd ed. Baltimore, MD: Williams & Wilkins; 1994:272–290

12. Lam AM, Winn HR, Cullen BF, Sundling N. Hyperglycemia and neurological outcome in patients with head injury. J Neurosurg 1991;75:545–551

13. Wass C, Lanier W. Glucose modulation of ischemic brain injury: review and clinical recommendations. Mayo Clin Proc 1996;71:801–812

14. Cherian L, Manny M, Vauner U, et al. Hyperglycemia increases neurological damage and behavioral deficits from post-traumatic secondary ischemic insults. J Neurotrauma 1998;15:307–321

15. Zornow MH, Prough DS. Fluid management in patients with traumatic brain injury. New Horiz 1995;3(3):488–498

16. Darovic GO. Hemodynamic Monitoring Invasive and Noninvasive Clinical Application. 3rd ed. Philadelphia: WB Saunders; 2002

17. Lefor AT. Critical Care on Call. 2002. New York: Lange Medical Books; 2002:354

18. Narayan RK, Wilberger JE, Polishock JT. Neurotrauma. New York: McGraw-Hill; 1996:87–89, 315–317

19. Prough DS, Whitley JM, Taylor CL, Deal DD, DeWitt DS. Regional cerebral blood flow following resuscitation from hemorrhagic shock with hypertonic saline: influence of a subdural mass. Anesthesiology 1991;75:319–327

20. Schmoker JD, Zhuang J, Shackford SR. Hypertonic fluid resuscitation improves cerebral oxygen delivery and reduces intracranial pressure after hemorrhagic shock. J Trauma 1991;31:1607–1613

21. Bayir H, Clark RS, Kochanek PM. Promising strategies to minimize secondary brain injury after head trauma. Crit Care Med 2003;31:S112–S117

22. Simma B, Burger R, Falk M, Sacher P, Fanconi S. A prospective, randomized, and controlled study of fluid management in children with severe head injury: lactated Ringer's solution versus hypertonic saline. Crit Care Med 1998;26:1265–1270

23. Khanna S, Davis D, Peterson B, et al. Use of hypertonic saline in the treatment of severe refractory posttraumatic intracranial hypertension in pediatric traumatic brain injury. Crit Care Med 2000;28:1144–1151

24. Munar F, Ferrer AM, de Nadal M, et al. Cerebral hemodynamic effects of 7.2% hypertonic saline in patients with head injury and raised intracranial pressure. J Neurotrauma 2000;17:41–51

25. Horn P, Munch E, Vajkoczy P, et al. Hypertonic saline solution for control of elevated intracranial pressure in patients with exhausted response to mannitol and barbiturates. Neurol Res 1999;21:758–764

26. Fisher B, Thomas D, Peterson B. Hypertonic saline lowers raised intracranial pressure in children after head trauma. J Neurosurg Anesthesiol 1992;4:4–10

27. Vassar MJ, Perry CA, Holcroft JW. Prehospital resuscitation of hypotensive trauma patients with 7.5% NaCl versus 7.5% NaCl with added dextran: a controlled trial. J Trauma 1993;34:622–632, discussion 632–633

28. Wade CE, Grady JJ, Kramer GC, Younes RN, Gehlsen K, Holcroft JW. Individual patient cohort analysis of the efficacy of hypertonic saline/dextran in patients with traumatic brain injury and hypotension. J Trauma 1997;42:S61–S65

29. Vialet R, Albanese J, Thomachot L, et al. Isovolume hypertonic solutes (sodium chloride or mannitol) in the treatment of refractory posttraumatic intracranial hypertension: 2 mL/kg 7.5% saline is more effective than 2 mL/kg 20% mannitol. Crit Care Med 2003;31:1683–1687

30. Mirski AM, Denchev ID, Schnitzer SM, Hanley FD. Comparison between hypertonic saline and mannitol in the reduction of elevated intracranial pressure in a rodent model of acute cerebral injury. J Neurosurg Anesthesiol 2000;12:334–344

31. Allcock JM, Drake CG. Ruptured intracranial aneurysm: the role of arterial spasm. J Neurosurg 1965;22:21–29

32. von Kummer R, Scharf J, Back T, Reich H, Machens HG, Wildemann B. Autoregulatory capacity and the effect of isovolemic hemodilution on local cerebral blood flow. Stroke 1988;19:594–597

33. Mead CO. A study of cerebral blood flow in experimental head injury: the beneficial effects of hemodilution. Proc Inst Med Chic 1970;28:173–179

34. Jurkiewicz J, Mempel E, Szumska J, Czernicki Z. Use of haemodilution in the treatment of cranio-cerebral injuries. [in French] Neurochirurgie 1979;25:122–123

35. Cole DJ, Drummond JC, Osborne TN, Matsumura J. Hypertension and hemodilution during cerebral ischemia reduce brain injury and edema. Am J Physiol 1990;259:H211–H217

36. Shin'oka T, Shum-Tim D, Jonas RA, et al. Higher hematocrit improves cerebral outcome after deep hypothermic circulatory arrest. J Thorac Cardiovasc Surg 1996;112(6):1610–1620, discussion 1620–1621

37. Hassler W, Chioffi F. CO_2 reactivity of cerebral vasospasm after aneurismal subarachnoid haemorrhage. Acta Neurochir (Wien) 1989;98:167–175

38. Hint H. The pharmacology of dextran and the physiological background for the clinical use of Rheomacrodex and Macrodex. Acta Anaesthesiol Belg 1968; 2:119–138

39. Ekelund A, Reinstrup P, Ryding E, et al. Effects of iso- and hypervolemic hemodilution on regional cerebral blood flow and oxygen delivery for patients with vasospasm after aneurysmal subarachnoid hemorrhage. Acta Neurochir (Wien) 2002;144:703–712, discussion 712–713

40. Duebener LF, Sakamoto T, Hatsuoka S, et al. Effects of hematocrit on cerebral microcirculation and tissue oxygenation during deep hypothermic bypass. Circulation 2001;104:1260–1264

41. Korosue K, Heros RC. Mechanism of cerebral blood flow augmentation by hemodilution in rabbits. Stroke 1992;23:1487–1493

42. Ohtaki M, Trammer BI. Role of hypervolemic hemodilution in focal cerebral ischemia of rats. Surg Neurol 1993;40:196–206

43. Lee SH, Heros RC, Mullan JC, Korosue K. Optimal degree of hemodilution for brain protection in a canine model of focal cerebral ischemia. J Neurosurg 1994;80:469–475

44. Shimoda M, Oda S, Trugane R, Sato O. Intracranial complications of hypervolemic therapy in patients with a delayed ischemic deficit attributed to vasospasm. J Neurosurg 1993;78:423–429

45. Gravenstein D, Gravenstein N. Intraoperative and immediate postoperative neuroanesthesia. In: Layon AJ, Gabrielli A, Friedman WA, eds. Textbook of Neurointensive Care. Philadelphia: WB Saunders; 2004:696–700

46. Laks H, O'Connor NE, Anderson W, Pilon RN. Crystalloid versus colloid hemodilution in man. Surg Gynecol Obstet 1976;142:506–512

47. Shires GT III, Peitzman AB, Albert SA, et al. Response of extravascular lung water to intraoperative fluids. Ann Surg 1983;197:515–519

48. Brown WJ, Kim BS, Weeks DB, Parkin CE. Physiologic saline solution, Normosol R pH 7.4, and Plasmanate as reconstituents of packed human erythrocytes. Anesthesiology 1978;49:99–101

49. Trumble ER, Muizelaar JP, Myseros JS, Choi SC, Warren BB. Coagulopathy with the use of hetastarch in the treatment of vasospasm. J Neurosurg 1995;82:44–47

50. Belayev L, Alonso OF, Huh PW, Zhao W, Busto R, Ginsberg MD. Posttreatment with high-dose albumin reduces histopathological damage and improves neurological deficit following fluid percussion brain injury in rats. J Neurotrauma 1999;16: 445–453

51. Chorny I, Bsorai R, Artru AA, et al. Albumin or hetastarch improves neurological outcome and decreases volume of brain tissue necrosis but not brain edema following closed-head trauma in rats. J Neurosurg Anesthesiol 1999;11:273–281

52. Bunn F, Lefebvre C, Li Wan Po A, Li L, Roberts I, Schierhout G. Human albumin solution for resuscitation and volume expansion in critically ill patients: the Albumin Reviewers. Cochrane Database Syst Rev 2000;2:CD001208

53. The SAFE Study Investigators. A comparison of albumin and saline for fluid resuscitation in the intensive care unit. N Engl J Med 2004;350:2247–2256

54. Andrews RJ, Muto RP. Retraction brain ischemia: mannitol plus nimodipine preserves both cerebral blood flow and evoked potentials during normoventilation and hyperventilation. Neurol Res 1992;14:19–25

55. Andrews RJ, Bringas JR, Muto RP. Effects of mannitol on cerebral blood flow, blood pressure, blood viscosity, hematocrit, sodium, and potassium. Surg Neurol 1993; 39:218–222

56. Johnston IH, Harper AM. The effect of mannitol on cerebral blood flow: an experimental study. J Neurosurg 1973;38:461–471

57. Mendelow AD, Teasdale GM, Russel T, Flood J, Murray GD. Effect of mannitol on cerebral blood flow and cerebral perfusion pressure in human head injury. J Neurosurg 1985;63:43–48

58. Meyer FB, Anderson RE, Sundt TM, Yaksh TL. Treatment of experimental focal cerebral ischemia with mannitol. J Neurosurg 1987;66:109–115

59. Shirane R, Weinstein PR. Effect of mannitol on local cerebral blood flow after temporary complete cerebral ischemia in rats. J Neurosurg 1992;76:486–492

60. Kaufmann AM, Cardoso ER. Aggravation of vasogenic cerebral edema by multiple-dose mannitol. J Neurosurg 1992;77:584–589

61. Wise B, Perkins R, Stevenson E, et al. Penetration of 14C-labelled mannitol from serum into cerebrospinal fluid and brain. Exp Neurol 1964;10:264–270

62. Guidelines for the Management of Severe Head Injury. New York: Brain Trauma Foundation; 2000

63. Ropper A, Gress D, Diringer M, et al. Fluid and metabolic derangements. In: Neurological and Neurosurgical Intensive Care. 4th ed. Philadelphia: Lippincott Williams & Wilkins; 2004:105–112

64. Layon AJ, Gabrielli A, Friedman WA. Textbook of Neurointensive Care. Philadelphia: WB Saunders; 2004

65. Suarez JI. Critical Care Neurology and Neurosurgery. Totowa, NJ: Humana Press; 2004

66. Wijdicks EF. The Clinical Practice of Critical Care Neurology. 2nd ed. Oxford: Oxford University Press; 2003

22

Ventilator Management

Dan Miulli and Javed Siddiqi

Case Study

A 43-year-old male presents after a motor vehicle accident with obvious contusions to his chest, abdomen, and head. At the scene, he easily makes quick shallow breaths, does not follow commands nor open his eyes to pain, makes incomprehensible sounds, and has flexor/decorticate posturing. His pupils are equal and briskly reactive. There is no obvious asymmetry of chest movement or chest deformity, and the abdomen is slightly distended but not hard. Should the patient be intubated?

See page 326 for Case Management.

◆ Requirements for Intubation

The patient has a Glasgow Coma Scale (GCS) score of 6: 3 for decorticate/flexor posturing, 2 for incomprehensible sounds, and 1 for not opening his eyes. The definition of severe head injury is a GCS of 8 or less and according to *Guidelines for the Management of Severe Traumatic Brain Injury*,[1] initial management and resuscitation should include intubation.

Intubation may help prevent significant secondary brain injury from hypoxia, which is oxygen (O_2) saturation <90%, partial pressure of oxygen in arterial blood (PaO_2) <60 mm Hg, apnea, or cyanosis. Stocchetti et al[2] demonstrated that hypoxic patients without hypotension had 3 times the mortality rate and 20 times the severe morbidity rate of nonhypoxic patients. Furthermore, prehospital intubation of severe trauma victims significantly reduced mortality.[3] Systematic withholding of endotracheal (ET) intubation in patients with severe head injury is not recommended. Careful and rigorous neurologic examination, including assessment of brainstem reflexes, might help to identify patients with a very high probability of death despite mechanical ventilation.[4]

Considerable national variation in the care of severely head-injured patients still persists, even though *Guidelines for the Management of Severe Traumatic Brain Injury*[1] were first published in 1995. Those that actively follow these management strategies have an associated decreased mortality rate for patients with severe head injury, with no significant difference in functional status at discharge among survivors.[5]

In addition to data supporting intubation for severe head injury, the literature supports intubation for stroke as well. However, intubation in the face of stroke still remains somewhat controversial. Magi et al[6] concluded that the likelihood of deterioration is high in acute stroke patients who present to hospital intubated and ventilated is high. However, the observed survival rate is sufficient to justify this treatment, even in cases not requiring other invasive procedures, such as neurosurgery and angiography. The severity of the ischemic event often leads to mechanical ventilation and, in two thirds of those individuals, death in the hospital; the remainder are severely disabled. In a study of a multiethnic urban population, survival was unlikely if patients were deeply comatose or deteriorated clinically after intubation. However, the authors concluded that mechanical ventilation for stroke was relatively cost effective for extending life but not for preserving quality of life.[7]

◆ Reasons for Intubation

The brain and spinal cord require O_2 and blood flow. Ischemia must be prevented at all costs. Depending on the severity and onset, in the absence of O_2, glucose and glycogen are depleted in 4 minutes. In addition to the general lack of energy substrates, there is a demand for additional energy from the injured brain, as demonstrated by an increased metabolism in the layer surrounding the penumbra and increased brain temperature. When the brain tissue partial pressure of oxygen (PO_2) is <20 mm Hg, anaerobic respiration becomes the predominant energy exchange system. This leads to glucose store–dependent lactic acidosis, decreased pH, vasodilation, mitochondrial damage, and cell death. *Guidelines for the Management of Severe Traumatic Brain Injury*[1] addresses blood pressure and oxygenation as follows:

> Hypotension ([systolic blood pressure, SBP] < 90 mm Hg) or hypoxia (apnea or cyanosis in the field, PAO_2 < 60 mm Hg, saturation < 90%) must be scrupulously avoided, if possible, or corrected immediately.

◆ Methods Used in Intubation

Prior to intubation, the patient is preoxygenated with 100% O_2 to maintain the arterial O_2 (O_2 saturation) at the highest level. Maintain cervical spine precautions by continued use of a cervical collar. Use a jaw thrust technique to keep the patient's airway open for oxygenation. Do not use a head tilt technique in a patient with any suspected spinal injuries. After suctioning the upper airway, maintain spinal immobilization and begin rapid sequence intubation with an in-line orotracheal tube, a blind nasotracheal tube, an esophageal-tracheal Combitube (Kendall-Sheridan Corp. Argyle, NY), or a laryngeal mask airway. The equipment must be available, and tube cuffs must be checked prior to delivering the paralytics. If tracheal intubation cannot be performed because of facial fractures, then intubation after cricothyrotomy or tracheotomy must be considered.

Rapid Sequence Intubation

The steps in rapid sequence intubation are as follows:

1. Preoxygenate with 100% O_2 by mask.
2. Premedicate with lidocaine 1.5 to 2.0 mg/kg intravenous (IV) over 30 to 60 seconds to help prevent a spike in increased intracranial pressure (ICP).
3. Administer a nondepolarizing paralytic, such as rocuronium, at the 10% intubating dose of 0.06 to 0.10 mg/kg to lessen fasiculations from the next drug given.
4. Administer the depolarizing agent succinylcholine at 1.5 mg/kg IV push, which acts in 30 seconds to 1 minute.
5. Attempt tracheal intubation with cricoid pressure if needed.
6. If you are unable to intubate within 20 to 30 seconds, stop and ventilate with a bag mask for 30 to 60 seconds before once again attempting oro-tracheal intubation.
7. After the tube is visualized passing through the vocal cords, confirm placement by listening to breath sounds over the lateral chest, watching the chest rise and fall, not just the abdomen, seeing a mist in the tracheal tube with expiration, and using a CO_2 detector after 5 or 6 breaths or an esophageal detector device.
8. Treat intubation-induced bradycardia with atropine 0.5 mg IV push in adults or 0.1 mg minimum in children (0.01 mg/kg).

Premedication/induction/sedation in head injury patients may prevent the increased ICP that can occur from pain or suctioning. Use drugs depending on the time requirement for intubation and the need to assess the patient via another neurologic exam after intubation (**Table 22–1**).

Paralytic prophylaxis prior to succinylcholine or a paralytic in place of succinylcholine is summarized in **Table 22–2**. Remember that, after intubation, the patient will need to have a neurologic exam. Sometimes the patient may need to be examined for brain death, for example, when the intubation was a reaction to a code. It is best to decide the neurologic status prior to intubation. However, the GCS should be determined after (not in place of) resuscitation (**Table 22–2**).

The side effects of commonly administered drugs include the following:

♦ *Succinylcholine:* depolarizing effect may increase ICP; give with prophylaxis. May cause dysrhythmia and hyperkalemia; may cause cardiac arrest in healthy children and adolescents.

Table 22–1 Drugs Used in Rapid Sequence Intubation[8–10]

Drug	Dosage IV push	Onset	Duration
Atropine	0.01 mg/kg IV children (minimum 0.1 mg)	30–60 seconds	35 minutes
Etomidate	0.2–0.6 mg/kg	1 minute	3–5 minutes
Fentanyl	2–3 µg/kg IV > 2–3 minutes	1 minute	30–60 minutes
Ketamine	2 mg/kg	30–60 seconds	15 minutes
Lidocaine	1.5–2.0 mg/kg IV	30–60 seconds	5–10 minutes
Midazolam	0.02–0.04 mg/kg	2 minutes	1–2 hours
Thiopental	3–5 mg/kg	20–40 seconds	5–10 minutes

IV, intravenous.

Table 22–2 Paralytic Agents[8–10]

Drug	Paralytic (mg/kg)	Prophylaxis (mg/kg)	Onset	Duration (minutes)
Atracurium	0.4	0.04	3–5 minutes	20–35
Pancuronium	0.1	0.01	3–5 minutes	45–60
Rapacuronium	1.5	—	60–90 seconds	15
Rocuronium	0.6–1.2	0.06	2 minutes	30–90
Succinylcholine	1–2	—	30–60 seconds	4–6
Vecuronium	0.15–0.25	0.01	2–5 minutes	25–40

◆ Pancuronium: vagolytic; can increase cardiac output, ICP, and pulse rate; reversible with neostigmine and other anticholinesterases.[8]

Ochs et al[9] evaluated the ability of paramedic rapid sequence intubation to facilitate intubation of patients with severe head injuries in an urban out-of-hospital system. They examined adults with severe head injuries who were more than 10 minutes away from the hospital when injured. The patients were premedicated with midazolam, paralyzed with succinylcholine, and given rocuronium after tube placement was confirmed. The Combitube was used as a salvage airway device. Outcome measures included intubation success rates, preintubation and postintubation O_2 saturation values, arrival arterial blood gas values, and total out-of-hospital times for patients intubated en route versus on scene. Of the 114 enrolled patients, 84% underwent successful ET intubation, and 15% required Combitube intubation, with only 1 (0.9%) airway failure. There were no complications, and blood gases were superb with paramedic-performed rapid sequence intubation of patients with severe head injuries.

Emergent Cricothyroidectomy

Emergent cricothyroidectomy should only be performed by individuals familiar with the anatomy after unsuccessful or unavailable ET intubation in an upper airway obstruction. The procedure requires a knife blade and handle, antiseptic solution, and a tracheostomy tube, a pediatric ET tube, or a 14-gauge catheter-over-needle.

The steps in an emergent cricothyroidectomy are as follows:

1. Palpate the cricothyroid membrane between the thyroid and cricoid cartilages; it is the soft space between the "Adam's apple" and the first hard ring toward the chest.
2. Make a vertical incision in the skin, then incise the cricothyroid membrane horizontally.
3. Insert the knife handle into the opening and rotate 90 degrees.
4. Pass the tracheostomy tube or pediatric ET tube through the opening and inflate the cuff of the tube.
5. Alternatively, if none of the above is available and the 14-gauge catheter-over-needle is available, puncture the cricothyroid membrane, removing the needle mounted with a 12 mL syringe, which will serve as a connector for ventilation.

The cricothyrotomy may be converted to a tracheostomy under controlled conditions in the operating room once the airway has been secured. Tracheostomies are not appropriate procedures for urgent situations.[10]

◆ Hyperventilation after Intubation

Once a patient in a coma from stroke or head injury is intubated, O_2 and CO_2 in the patient without known chronic obstructive pulmonary disease (COPD) should be kept in a specific range for the initial period of 24 hours. Oxygen partial pressure should be maintained at ~115 mm Hg and CO_2 at ~35 mm Hg.

Brain tissue oxygenation or the related cerebral perfusion pressure depends on cerebral blood flow. Therefore, treatment modalities that cause vasoconstriction and decrease cerebral blood flow, such as aggressive hyperventilation, should be questioned and modified in the management armamentarium.

Hyperventilation works by decreasing plasma PCO_2, which causes an increase in the ambient pH in or around the brain cerebrovasculature, leading to cerebral vasoconstriction, decreasing the cerebral blood flow, and, in some cases, decreasing ICP. Soon after closed head injury, cerebral blood flow is low. During the first day after injury, it is less than half that of normal individuals; it then increases for at least 3 days, except in those patients who have uncontrollable ICP.

Cerebral blood flow is generally less than 30 cc/100 g/minute during the first 8 hours after injury and may be less than 20 cc/100 g/minute during the first 4 hours after injury in patients with the worst trauma. The cerebral blood flow around contusions is lower than the global blood flow. The blood flow in punctate hemorrhages may be even lower. Individuals with severe head injury may actually have increased O_2 extraction for 24 to 36 hours, requiring at least baseline blood flow.

Cerebral blood flow has been measured with hyperventilation, and there are significant differences in and around contusions, including local variability secondary to hyperventilation-induced steal. Cerebral blood flow changes with hyperventilation; there is a 3 to 4% change in cerebral blood flow per millimeter change in PCO_2, as demonstrated by Obrist et al.[11]

When cerebral blood flow is decreased, the level at which irreversible ischemia or infarction takes place is not precisely known. The same study by Obrist et al[11] suggested that, in patients with severe head injuries, there is a depression of normal cerebral metabolism. Furthermore, the reduced cerebral blood flow that occurs may, in many cases, be appropriate for the metabolic needs of the brain. Cerebral blood flow is lowest in patients with subdural hematomas, diffuse injuries, and hypotension, and highest in those with epidural hematoma or normal computed tomography (CT) scans. There is a direct correlation between cerebral blood flow and GCS during the first 4 hours after injury, as demonstrated by Bouma et al.[12] Therefore, the consequences of cerebral-blood-flow–reducing hyperventilation become more apparent.

Aggressive hyperventilation to a PCO_2 of 25 or less has been the cornerstone in the management of severe head injury for more than 20 years because it can cause a rapid reduction of ICP. However, there are no studies showing an improvement in outcome in neurologic patients with severe head injury using hyperventilation empirically. Hyperventilation reduces ICP by causing cerebral vasoconstriction and a subsequent reduction in cerebral blood flow. As stated earlier, cerebral blood flow is reduced by 50% during the first day after severe head injury; therefore, hyperventilation can only exacerbate this already deadly condition. Raichle et al[13] looked at a group of healthy individuals treated with hyperventilation. When these individuals had their PCO_2 decreased by 15 to 20 mm Hg from normal, there was a 40% decrease in cerebral blood flow after 30 minutes. Four hours later, despite continued hyperventilation, the cerebral blood flow increased to 90% of baseline, even though the PCO_2 was still decreased, demonstrating that hyperventilation to reduce ICP may be only a temporary phenomenon. This suggests that hyperventilation, if necessary, should be used only in short bursts.

In the same study, when the original PCO_2 was quickly restored, the cerebral blood flow was increased to 31% above baseline. The quick restoration increases cerebral blood volume and, in turn, can increase ICP. Therefore, when elevating PCO_2 from below normal levels, gradually increase the PCO_2.

In the autoregulatory intact individual, there is a 3 to 4% change in cerebral blood flow per mm Hg change in PCO_2. This decrease in cerebral flow occurs less when cerebral blood flow is already reduced; also, the lower CO_2 vasoresponsivity is associated with a poorer outcome. Local CO_2 responsivity can differ from values by more than 50%. Cold et al[14] demonstrated that in some patients cerebral autoregulation is preserved with normocapnia and lost with hypocapnia. Others have found varying responses with hyperventilation. Crockard et al[15] found an increase in ICP associated with a decrease in PCO_2, and Obrist and Martin[16] found a decrease in ICP in only half of the patients treated with hyperventilation; however, over 90% of those patients also had a decrease in cerebral blood flow.

In a landmark class I study, Muizelaar et al[17] published the results of a prospective randomized clinical study in which 77 patients were randomized to a group treated with chronic prophylactic hyperventilation for 5 days after injury ($PCO_2 = 25 \pm 2$ mm Hg) or to a group that was kept normocapnic ($PCO_2 = 35 \pm 2$ mm Hg). Those patients who were treated with prophylactic hyperventilation had a significantly worse outcome than those in the normocapnic group at 3 and 6 months. The researchers did find that hyperventilation may be beneficial with hyperemia, and hyperventilation is needed in signs of acute herniation.

Guidelines for the Management of Severe Head Injury[1] recommends the following:

> In the absence of increased intracranial pressure, chronic prolonged hyperventilation therapy (PCO_2 of 25 mm Hg or less) should be avoided after severe traumatic brain injury.
>
> Guideline: The use of prophylactic hyperventilation (PCO_2 less than or equal to 35 mm Hg) therapy during the first 24 hours after severe traumatic head injury should be avoided because it can compromise cerebral perfusion during a time when cerebral blood flow is reduced.
>
> Option: Hyperventilation therapy may be necessary for brief periods when there is acute neurological deterioration or for longer periods if there is intracranial hypertension refractory to sedation, paralysis, cerebral spinal fluid drainage and osmotic diuretics. [Jugular venous oxygenation saturation, S_{jvO_2}], [arteriovenous oxygen content difference, $AVDO_2$] and cerebral blood flow monitoring may help to identify cerebral ischemia if hyperventilation, resulting in PCO_2 that is less than 30 mm Hg, is necessary.

Several studies have demonstrated that aggressive hyperventilation causes secondary brain injury from decreased brain tissue oxygenation.[17-20] The literature is also replete with documentation of improved survival for severe head injury utilizing modern treatment paradigms. The majority of physicians who are exposed to head trauma patients, explicitly emergency room doctors, are managing severe head injury patients in accordance with *Guidelines for the Management of Severe Head Injury*,[1] with the exception of avoiding prophylactic hyperventilation. It is hoped that more education and exposure to the evidence regarding prophylactic hyperventilation of severely head-injured patients may improve adherence to the hyperventilation guidelines.[21]

◆ Measuring Cerebral Blood Flow

Not all facilities have the ability to directly measure cerebral blood flow; therefore, they choose to indirectly measure it using $AVDO_2$ or S_{jvO_2}. $AVDO_2$ is indirectly a manifestation of metabolism and cerebral blood flow. The brain, which comprises approximately 2% of body weight, uses 20% of the cardiac output and 25% of the resting body glucose. It has a very small energy reserve; therefore, metabolism is tightly coupled to cerebral blood flow. Normally, metabolism is 1.5 μg/g/minute, or 3.4 mL/100 g/minute; this is the cerebral metabolic rate of O_2. Approximately 19 mL/dL of O_2 is delivered to the brain on the arterial side and ~12 to 13 mL/dL of O_2 on the venous side, yielding approximately 35% O_2 extraction, leaving an $AVDO_2$ of 6.5 mL/dL.

The brain uses 90% aerobic and 10% anaerobic respiration. This occurs through the citric acid cycle. Approximately half the energy is used for cell maintenance and half for brain function. Normally, there is a very small amount of lactate produced.

Arteriovenous Oxygen Content Difference

Isolated patients with severe head injuries were studied, keeping SBP, hematocrit, and temperature normal.[22] These patients were divided into two groups. One had mass lesions requiring surgery, and the other did not. Both were treated according to protocol: with PCO_2 > 30 mm Hg, patients were intubated, sedated, and paralyzed, and given mannitol if the ICP was elevated. Patients had jugular venous catheters inserted, and the $AVDO_2$ was calculated before and 30 minutes after treatment. In those patients who underwent evacuation of a mass lesion, their perfusion pressure was termed adequate to prevent ischemia; however, some individuals still demonstrated infarction by CT scan. ICP and cerebral perfusion pressure (CPP) were normal. The closer the $AVDO_2$, the less likely the chance of having an infarction. Likewise, in the nonsurgical group, those patients who developed an infarction also had adequate ICP and CPP after treatment, but had a larger $AVDO_2$, suggesting they required more oxygen for energy maintenance. There was a change in $AVDO_2$ in both groups that predicted the outcome. An elevated $AVDO_2$ signifies increased O_2 extraction, which is consistent with ischemia. It would seem that the failure of the $AVDO_2$ to improve with treatment was the one factor that was consistent with infarction. The ideal monitor, therefore, would give reliable continuous readings, would be portable, and would suggest a cause and appropriate therapy.

Jugular Venous Oxygen Saturation

The saturation of jugular venous O_2 is the reciprocal of $AVDO_2$. If O_2 extraction increases, the $AVDO_2$ will increase, but the S_{jvO_2} will decrease. This measurement assumes that cerebral metabolism and hemoglobin are constant, and the effective dissolved O_2 is negligible. There are limitations to SjO_2 measurements. It is contraindicated with C-spine injuries, coagulopathy, and tracheostomies. It measures hemispheric flow, which may not be constant from one side to the other, and even on one side will give measurements of general hypoxia but will not allow region-specific treatment. Changes in SjO_2 can occur after herniation has taken place. There are artifacts associated with catheter movement; placement has to be precise, not too proximal, and not against a vessel wall. SjO_2 < 50% is consistent with ischemia. Profound or prolonged episodes of desaturation are associated with a poor outcome. Desaturations are most common with low cerebral blood flow; SjO_2 < 50% is the equivalent of $AVDO_2$ exceeding 9 mL/dL.

◆ Determining the Level of Oxygen

The question of what level to keep the PO_2 and O_2 saturation is even more controversial than hyperventilation, leading to many debates between pulmonologists and neurosurgeons. The reason for the debate stems from the hemoglobin molecule and the measurements of brain tissue O_2. In whole blood, the hemoglobin molecule has an O_2 carrying capacity of 17 to 21 mL O_2/100 mL blood, when O_2 is bound to its four hemoglobin sites. However, that figure does not reflect the additional, albeit small, amounts of O_2 dissolved in the blood. That amount, the PaO_2, also reflects free oxygen molecules dissolved in plasma and not just those bound to hemoglobin. Likewise, O_2 saturation (SaO_2) alone does not reveal how much total O_2 is in the blood.

The O_2 saturation and the PO_2 can be most readily adjusted by increasing the fraction of inspired oxygen (FiO_2). O_2 and PO_2 are also affected by perfusion such as with cerebral blood flow. In general, without concomitant disease, the hemoglobin molecule is 100% saturated at a PO_2 of 80 mm Hg, 75% saturated at a PO_2 of 40 mm Hg, and 50% saturated at a PO_2 of 27 mm Hg. In addition to the fact that blood plasma carries extra O_2, red blood cells reach only 85% of the brain cells, the remainder being dependent upon the circulating plasma. O_2 does not always bind to the hemoglobin molecule in the same manner. There is a decreased affinity of hemoglobin for O_2 with increasing temperature, increasing PCO_2, 2,3-diphosphoglycerate (DPG), and decreasing pH. This makes it harder for the hemoglobin to bind to O_2 (requiring a higher partial pressure to achieve the same O_2 saturation), but it makes it easier for the hemoglobin to release bound O_2.

Therefore, the debate hinges on the following: arterial hemoglobin saturation of 100% is the upper limit of usefulness; increasing the FiO_2 to past the maximal saturation of hemoglobin only increases the dissolved O_2 in plasma, which represents 2 to 3% of overall O_2 transport. Use of FiO_2 levels >60% may be harmful when used for longer than 24 hours in adults.

That is only half the story, however; the other half rests on studies that actually measure brain tissue oxygenation and predict outcome. In these studies, increasing PO_2 to higher levels than necessary to saturate hemoglobin, as performed in the O_2 treated cohort, improved the partial pressure O_2 supply in brain tissue ($PBtiO_2$). During the early period after severe head injury, increased lactate levels in brain tissue were reduced by increasing FiO_2.[23] Other studies have demonstrated an improved mortality rate using hyperbaric O_2. Measurements demonstrated hyperbaric O_2 reduces mortality by 50% and improves aerobic metabolism.[24–26] The treatment PO_2 varied from keeping PO_2 = 150 mm Hg[27] to a simple approach of ventilation with

100% O_2 for at least the first 6 to 18 hours after any severe head injury when metabolic demand is greatest.[23]

◆ How Brain Tissue Oxygenation Is Measured

There are two favored technologies for measuring brain tissue oxygenation: the Licox sensor (Integra Neuro Sciences, Plainsboro, NJ), and the Codman Neurotrend (Codman and Shurtleff, Inc., Raynham, MA) cerebral tissue monitoring systems. The Licox probe (~0.5 mm in diameter) can be inserted through a standard twist drill hole into a nonlesion, where there should be a steady $PBtiO_2$, or into a lesion area with a low but dynamic $PBtiO_2$. The Neurotrend system measures four areas of brain metabolism and tracks physiological information about the progression of secondary injury at the cellular level, which may indicate the onset of ischemic injury, as observed in 80% of trauma-related deaths. These measurements have shown that by increasing FiO_2 beyond 80%, there continues to be an increase in $PBtiO_2$.[28-32] Specifically, increasing FiO_2 from 30 to 100% increased $PBtiO_2$ to a steady state of 40 mm Hg.[33] Not only does $PBtiO_2$ improve, but also the outcome improves.[34-37]

When investigating hyperventilation using one of these cerebral metabolism sensors, a PCO_2 = 27 to 32 mm Hg decreases $PBtiO_2$ in severe head injury patients.[38-40]

Increasing the PaO_2 to levels higher than needed to fully saturate hemoglobin apparently can increase PO_2, especially when it is low. This effect can continue over a period of several hours. Improved outcome is characterized by

◆ Brain tissue O_2 > 33 ± 11 mm Hg
◆ Brain tissue CO_2 < 48 ± 7 mm Hg
◆ Brain tissue pH > 7.19 ± 0.11

Poor outcome is characterized by

◆ Brain tissue O_2 < 10 to 15 mm Hg for > 30 minutes
◆ Brain tissue CO_2 > 60 mm Hg
◆ Brain tissue pH < 6.8[39-41]

◆ Pulmonary Problems

There are many patients on the neurology and neurosurgery service who come to the neurosurgical intensive care unit (NICU) without a severe head injury or cerebral vascular accident. These patients may develop abnormal

Table 22–3   Abnormal Breathing Patterns and Location[41–43]

Type	Pattern	Location
Cheyne-Stokes	Hyperventilation, short apnea, hyperventilation	Diffuse forebrain injury
Central neurogenic	Hyperventilation	Midbrain, thalamus
Apneustic	Prolonged pause at full inspiration	Pontine, brainstem
Ataxic	Random deep and shallow breaths	Medulla
Cluster	Irregular breaths and pauses	Low medulla

breathing patterns from masses, inflammation, or infections. **Table 22–3** lists some typical abnormal breathing patterns.

Cheyne-Stokes respirations occur when there is diffuse forebrain injury. At that time, the patient hyperventilates low PCO_2 and stops breathing, which normalizes PCO_2. This results in hyperventilation and apnea, with the period of hyperventilation being longer than apnea, causing the patient to become alkalotic. In rarely occurring central heurogenic hyperventilation, there can be a midbrain lesion, such as in the thalamus.[41] However, because of its unlikely presentation, the physician, when seeing continuous hyperventilation, should instead consider a cause of pulmonary edema or aspiration. With apneustic breathing, which is demonstrated by a prolonged pause at full inspiration, there may be a mid to caudal pontine lesion, brainstem stroke, or basilar artery occlusion. In ataxic breathing, there is very irregular breathing, with deep and shallow breaths randomly mixed. Ataxic breathing is a terminal stage usually pointing to a medullary lesion. A cluster pattern is characterized by clusters of breaths in irregular sequence with varying pauses, indicative of end-stage lower medullary failure or lesion. Each breathing pattern should be associated with a clinical condition verifying the level of the lesion. When there is no confirmatory exam, consider the many other causes of pulmonary dysfunction in the neurologic patient (**Table 22–4**).

Table 22–4   Types of Pulmonary Dysfunction in Neurologic Patients

Acute CHF	COPD/asthma	Neurogenic pulmonary edema
ARDS	Diaphragm rupture	Pneumonia
Airway obstruction	Diaphragm paralysis	Pneumothorax
Apnea	Fat/brain emboli	Pulmonary contusion
Aspiration	Hemothorax	Pulmonary edema
Atelectasis	Hyper-/hypoventilation	Tracheobronchial
Chest wall injury	Injury	V/Q mismatch

ARDS, acute respiratory distress syndrome; CHF, congestive heart failure; COPD, chronic obstructive pulmonary disease; V/Q, ventilation/perfusion.

Patients with severe neurologic problems, such as severe head injury, develop secondary problems (e.g., with electrolytes) 59% of the time, pneumonia 41% of the time, and coagulopathy 18% of the time. These secondary problems usually occur 2 to 4 days after the injury and affect approximately 3% of the outcomes.[42] Therefore, the neurocritical care specialist should be most cognizant of ways to prevent and treat such issues. Pneumonia can be attenuated early by ensuring airway protection, utilizing chest physiotherapy, and understanding nosocomial infections. Other nonpreventable associations with pneumonia include neutralization of gastric pH.

Pneumonia can initially be mistaken for pulmonary embolism, acute respiratory distress syndrome (ARDS), very early neurogenic pulmonary edema, or, in the nonintubated patient, even airway obstruction. Upper airway obstruction is common in the first 24 hours after stroke, especially if the patient remains in the supine position. The risks for obstruction prior to intubation are the same factors as for typical obstructive sleep apnea; body mass index and neck circumference appear to be the best predictors of its occurrence.[43]

The incidence of neurogenic pulmonary edema is unknown. It should be differentiated from pneumonia, aspiration, cardiac failure, and pulmonary contusion. Neurogenic pulmonary edema may occur in relation to epilepsy, meningitis, severe head injury, subarachnoid hemorrhage, or neoplasms. Early in its course, there may be dyspnea, chest pain, minor hemoptysis, tachypnea, tachycardia, fever, hypoxia, elevated SBP/pulmonary pressure, rales (not gallops), or murmurs. The chest x-ray may show bilateral central fluffy infiltrates. The etiology may be due to hydrostatic forces and permeability changes or to the release of catecholamines. If the pulmonary edema is due to increased ICP, then lower ICP and provide supportive care.

◆ Ventilator Management

Newer techniques of mechanical ventilation allow the neurocritical care specialist access to an increased number of mechanisms not previously available. In a very large study by Esteban et al,[44] who inquired into 412 medical/surgical units from the Americas and Europe, the patients requiring ventilation were on assist control (AC) in 47% of cases, synchronized intermittent mandatory ventilation (SIMV) in 46% of cases, or a combination of the two. The median tidal volume (Vt) was 9 mL/kg in AC, with a median pressure support of 18 cm H_2O. Positive end-expiratory pressure (PEEP) was not used in 31% of the patients.

Ventilator types are volume-cycled ventilation, pressure-cycled ventilation, and time-cycled pressure-limited ventilation. In each type, the Vt would be (1) constant with inspiratory pressure limits dependent upon applied pressure and the compliance of the lung and chest wall with incomplete exhalation; (2) limiting, when there is incomplete exhalation and the respiratory rate increases to compensate (used mostly in infants and small children); or (3) dependent, maintaining airway pressure at a preset maximum for a preset time with an added inspiratory pause, used where there is a problem with the lung and chest wall compliance (**Table 22–5**).

Ventilator modes are controlled mechanical ventilation (CMV), AC, SIMV pressure support, and high-frequency jet ventilation (HFJV). CMV is independent of patient breathing; it delivers a minute ventilation determined by a preset Vt and rate. It is frequently used in the pharmacologically paralyzed patient. If the patient is not paralyzed, he or she may not be able to synchronize with the ventilator and may therefore become quite agitated. AC mode delivers only full breaths through preset Vt when the patient initiates a breath by creating negative pressure. Consequently, this assists spontaneous ventilations, and anxious patients would hyperventilate. Therefore, the triggering sensitivity must be adjusted to prevent respiratory alkalosis. SIMV modes have preset rate and Vt; however, the patient can breathe spontaneously unassisted between ventilator breaths. In pressure support (PS), the ventilator provides a constant pressure, assisting the patient's own inspiration. By itself, PS does not provide a minimum minute ventilation, allowing the patient to work at breathing. HFJV delivers a minute ventilation at 50 to 300 breaths per minute at reduced mean airway pressure and therefore reduced ICP. It is used when there is high peak inspiratory pressure >70 to 80 cm H_2O. HFJV can cause injury (e.g., dryness, mucosal injury) due to the quick movement of air at high pressures.

In addition to the modes of ventilation, PS and PEEP can be added. PEEP maintains the opening of small airways at end expiration to improve PaO_2 so that a lower concentration of O_2 can be used. It also increases pleural, intrathoracic, and central venous pressure (CVP) while decreasing cardiac output, SBP, free water clearance, urine, and urine sodium; therefore, amounts of PEEP should be increased or decreased slowly. The increased end-expiratory pressure can cause barotrauma. Because PEEP increases pulmonary vascular resistance and CVP, its usage in patients with severe neurologic problems has been questioned. Studies have determined that

Table 22–5   Types of Ventilators[8–10,44]

Ventilator mode	Patient control	Parameters
CMV	Machine driven	Preset Vt and rate
AC	Patient driven, machine backup full breath	Preset Vt
SIMV	Patient driven	Preset Vt and rate
PS	Patient driven	Preset pressure
HFJV	Machine driven	Preset minute ventilation

AC, assist control; CMV, controlled mechanical ventilation; HFJV, high-frequency jet ventilation; PS, pressure support; SIMV, synchronized intermittent mandatory ventilation.

the adverse effects of PEEP are dependent upon intracranial compliance. Patients who require artificial ventilation can be safely ventilated using PEEP or an inverse inspiration:expiration ratio, if the blood pressure is monitored and a possible drop of the arterial blood pressure is treated.[45] As far as the amount of PEEP, in humans 10 cm H_2O of PEEP had no effect on ICP,[46] whereas 15 cm H_2O of PEEP in normal dogs produced mild effects that became worse if the ICP was elevated.[47]

Case Management

The patient with a severe head injury should be assessed for airway, breathing, and circulation. He should have rapid sequence intubation in the field using spinal precautions. Once intubated, the patient should initially be placed on 100% FiO_2 and ventilated at a rate to maintain a PCO_2 of 35 mm Hg. Any episode of hypoxia and hypotension must be avoided to maintain optimal cerebral blood flow and brain tissue oxygenation. Prophylactic hyperventilation should not be used unless there is evidence of increasing ICP despite all other acceptable measures. Mild hyperventilation can be used for brief periods of time.

References

1. Management and Prognosis of Severe Traumatic Brain Injury. New York: Brain Trauma Foundation; 2000
2. Stocchetti N, Furlan A, Volta F. Hypoxemia and arterial hypotension at the accident scene in head injury. J Trauma 1996;40:764–767
3. Hsiao A, Michelson S, Hedges J. Emergent intubation and CT scan pathology of blunt trauma patients with Glasgow Coma Scale scores 3–13. Prehosp Disaster Med 1993;8:229–236
4. Santoli F, De Jonghe B, Hayon J, et al. Mechanical ventilation in patients with acute ischemic stroke: survival and outcome at one year. Intensive Care Med 2001;27:1141–1146
5. Bulger EM, Nathens A, Rivara F, Moore M, MacKenzie E, Jurkovich G. Management of severe head injury: institutional variations in care and effect on outcome. Crit Care Med 2002;30:1870–1876
6. Magi E, Recine C, Patrussi L, Becattini G, Nannoni S, Gabini R. Prognosis of stroke patients undergoing intubation and mechanical ventilation. Minerva Med 2000;91:99–104
7. Mayer S, Copeland D, Bernardini G, et al. Cost and outcome of mechanical ventilation for life-threatening stroke. Stroke 2000;31:2346–2353
8. Cummins RO. ACLS Provider Manual. Dallas, TX: American Heart Association; 2002
9. Ochs M, Davis D, Hoyt D, Bailey D, Marshall L, Rosen P. Paramedic-performed rapid sequence intubation of patients with severe head injuries. Ann Emerg Med 2002;40:159–167
10. Lyerly HK, Gaynor JW. The Handbook of Surgical Intensive Care. 3rd ed. St. Louis, MO: Mosby Year Book; 1992
11. Obrist WD, Langfitt T, Jaggi J, Cruz J, Gennarelli T. Cerebral blood flow and metabolism in comatose patients with acute head injury. Relationship to intracranial hypertension. J Neurosurg 1984;61:241–253

12. Bouma GJ, Muizelaar J, Choi S, Newlon P, Young H. Cerebral circulation and metabolism after severe traumatic brain injury: the elusive role of ischemia. J Neurosurg 1991;75:685–693
13. Raichle M, Posner J, Plum F. Cerebral blood flow during and after hyperventilation. Arch Neurol 1970;23:394–403
14. Cold G, Christensen M, Schmidt K. Effect of two levels of induced hypocapnia on cerebral autoregulation in the acute phase of head injury coma. Acta Anaesthesiol Scand 1981;25:397–401
15. Crockard HA, Coppel DL, Morrow WF. Evaluation of hyperventilation in treatment of head injuries. BMJ 1973;4(5893):634–640
16. Obrist WD, Martin NA. Arteriovenous oxygen difference in head injury. J Neurosurg 1998;88:1122–1124
17. Muizelaar JP, Marmarou A, Ward J, et al. Adverse effects of prolonged hyperventilation in patients with severe head injury: a randomized clinical trial. J Neurosurg 1991;75:731–739
18. Dings J, Meixensberger J, Amschler J, Roosen K. Continuous monitoring of brain tissue PO_2: a new tool to minimize the risk of ischemia caused by hyperventilation therapy. Zentralbl Neurochir 1996;57:177–183
19. Kiening KL, Hartl R, Unterberg A, Schneider G, Bardt T, Lanksch W. Brain tissue pO_2-monitoring in comatose patients: implications for therapy. Neurol Res 1997;19:233–240
20. van Santbrink H, Maas A, Avezaat C. Continuous monitoring of partial pressure of brain tissue oxygen in patients with severe head injury. Neurosurgery 1996;38:21–31
21. Huizenga JE, Zink B, Maio R, Hill E. Guidelines for the management of severe head injury: are emergency physicians following them? Acad Emerg Med 2002;9:806–812
22. Le Roux PD, Newell DW, Lam AM, Grady MS, Winn HR. Cerebral arteriovenous oxygen difference: a predictor of cerebral infarction and outcome in patients with severe head injury. J Neurosurg 1997;87:1–8
23. Menzel M, Doppenberg EM, Zauner A, Soukup J, Reinert MM, Bullock R. Increased inspired oxygen concentration as a factor in improved brain tissue oxygenation and tissue lactate levels after severe human head injury. J Neurosurg 1999;91:1–10
24. Sukoff M. Effects of hyperbaric oxygenation. J Neurosurg 2001;95:544–546
25. Rockswold SB, Rockswold GL, Vargo JM, et al. Effects of hyperbaric oxygenation therapy on cerebral metabolism and intracranial pressure in severely brain injured patients. J Neurosurg 2001;94:403–411
26. Jain KK, Sukoff MA. Textbook of Hyperbaric Medicine. 3rd ed. Seattle: Hogrefe & Huber; 1999:351–371
27. Zauner A, Doppenberg EM, Woodward JJ, Choi SC, Young HF, Bullock R. Continuous monitoring of cerebral substrate delivery and clearance: initial experience in 24 patients with severe acute brain injuries. Neurosurgery 1997;41:1082–1091
28. van Santbrink H, Maas AI, Avezaat CJ. Continuous monitoring of partial pressure of brain tissue oxygen in patients with severe head injury. Neurosurgery 1996;38:21–31
29. Sarrafzadeh AS, Kiening KL, Bardt TF, Schneider GH, Unterberg AW, Lanksch WR. Cerebral oxygenation in contusioned vs. nonlesioned brain tissue: monitoring of $PtiO_2$ with Licox and Paratrend. Acta Neurochir Suppl (Wien) 1998;71:186–189
30. Schaffranietz L, Heinke W, Rudolph C, Olthoff D. Effect of normobaric hyperoxia on parameters of brain metabolism. Anaesthesiol Reanim 2000;25:68–73
31. Manley GT, Pitts LH, Morabito D, et al. Brain tissue oxygenation during hemorrhagic shock, resuscitation, and alterations in ventilation. J Trauma 1999;46:261–267
32. Zauner A, Doppenberg E, Soukup J, Menzel M, Young HF, Bullock R. Extended neuromonitoring: new therapeutic opportunities? Neurol Res 1998;20(Suppl 1): S85–S90
33. Menzel M, Doppenberg EM, Zauner A, et al. Cerebral oxygenation in patients after severe head injury: monitoring and effects of arterial hyperoxia on cerebral blood flow, metabolism and intracranial pressure. J Neurosurg Anesthesiol 1999; 11:240–251

34. Charbel FT, Hoffman WE, Misra M, Hannigan K, Ausman JI. Cerebral interstitial tissue oxygen tension, pH, HCO_3, CO_2. Surg Neurol 1997;48:414–417

35. van den Brink WA, van Santbrink H, Steyerberg EW, et al. Brain oxygen tension in severe head injury. Neurosurgery 2000;46:868–876

36. Zhi DS, Zhang S, Zhou LG. Continuous monitoring of brain tissue oxygen pressure in patients with severe head injury during moderate hypothermia. Surg Neurol 1999;52:393–396

37. Schneider GH, Sarrafzadeh AS, Kiening KL, Bardt TF, Unterberg AW, Lanksch WR. Influence of hyperventilation on brain tissue: PO_2, PCO_2, and pH in patients with intracranial hypertension. Acta Neurochir Suppl 1998;71:62–65

38. Imberti R, Bellinzona G, Langer M. Cerebral tissue PO_2 and $SjvO_2$ changes during moderate hyperventilation in patients with severe traumatic brain injury. J Neurosurg 2002;96:97–102

39. Carmona Suazo JA, Maas AI, van den Brink WA, van Santbrink H, Steyerberg EW, Avezaat CJ. CO_2 reactivity and brain oxygen pressure monitoring in severe head injury. Crit Care Med 2000;28:3268–3274

40. Kiening KL, Hartl R, Unterberg AW, Schneider GH, Bardt T, Lanksch WR. Brain tissue pO_2-monitoring in comatose patients: implications for therapy. Neurol Res 1997;19:233–240

41. Johnston SC, Singh V, Ralston HJ. Chronic dyspnea and hyperventilation in an awake patient with small subcortical infarcts. Neurology 2001;57:2131–2133

42. Piek J, Chesnut RM, Marshall LF, et al. Extracranial complications of severe head injury. J Neurosurg 1992;77:901–907

43. Turkington PM, Bamford J, Wanklyn P, Elliott MW. Prevalence and predictors of upper airway obstruction in the first 24 hours after acute stroke. Stroke 2002;33:2037–2042

44. Esteban A, Anzueto A, Alia I, et al. How is mechanical ventilation employed in the intensive care unit? An international utilization review. Am J Respir Crit Care Med 2000;161:1450–1458

45. Schwarz S, Georgiadis D, Schwab S, Aschoff A, Hacke W. Nervenarzt. Current concepts of intensive care of space-occupying middle cerebral artery infarct. Nervenarzt 2002;73:508–518

46. Cooper KR, Boswell PA, Choi SC. Safe use of PEEP in patients with severe head injury. J Neurosurg 1985;63:552–555

47. Cotev S, Paul WL, Ruiz BC, Kuck EJ, Modell JH. Positive end-expiratory pressure (PEEP) and cerebrospinal fluid pressure during normal and elevated intracranial pressure in dogs. Inten Care Med 1981;7:187–191

23

Seizure Disorders: Diagnosis and Management

Margaret R. Wacker

Case Study

A 23-year-old patient underwent a subfrontal craniotomy for cranio-pharyngioma. She developed transient diabetes insipidus. Several days later, her sodium level dropped from the 150s to 131 abruptly after a dose of 1-deamino-8-D-arginine vasopressin (DDAVP, or desmopressin) as the diabetes insipidus was resolving. At the same time, her phenytoin level was found to be subtherapeutic, though this was not immediately corrected, as she appeared to be doing well clinically and had no seizures. Later in the evening, her family noticed some staring spells and decreased responsiveness. This persisted, and later she was noted to have some seizure activity witnessed by the nurse. This continued, and the patient then developed nonconvulsive status epilepticus. A follow-up computed tomography (CT) scan was obtained, which showed increased edema in the region of the tumor consistent with hypoxic injury. Despite efforts to correct the electrolytes and control the seizure activity, she went on to brain death.

See page 334 for Case Management.

◆ Classification of Seizures

Seizures may occur in patients in the neurosurgical intensive care unit (NICU) as evidence of either a primary or secondary neurologic disease process. In addition, seizure thresholds may be lowered due to metabolic derangements or fever, as was the case in the case study. Seizures may also add to the injury to the brain, especially if they are recurrent, through the imposition of increased metabolic demand and/or hypoxia due to the suppression of respirations during the seizure episodes. Untreated or unrecognized status epilepticus can be fatal or cause permanent neurologic injury. Hence, efforts must be made to reduce the risk of seizures in the already neurologically compromised NICU patient.

Because many of the treatments for epilepsy are more effective for one or another seizure type, a brief review of types of seizures is necessary for choosing appropriate treatment. The International Classification of Epileptic Seizures (**Table 23–1**) is included here as a basis for the understanding of different types of seizures.[1] Generalized seizures, including those that have secondarily generalized, may affect respiration and thus be more dangerous to the patient, especially if they are recurrent.

♦ Treatment of Seizures

Anticonvulsant medications should be selected by optimizing the drug for the type of seizures the patient has or for which the patient is at risk. For

Table 23–1   International Classification of Epileptic Seizures[1,2]

1. Generalized seizures (bilaterally symmetrical and without local onset)
   a. Tonic, clonic, or tonic-clonic (grand mal)
   b. Absence (petit mal)
      i. Simple—loss of consciousness only
      ii. Complex—with brief tonic, clonic, or automatic movements
   c. Lennox-Gastaut syndrome
   d. Juvenile myoclonic epilepsy
   e. Infantile spasms (West's syndrome)
   f. Atonic (astatic, akinetic) seizures (sometimes with myoclonic jerks)

2. Partial, or focal, seizures (seizures beginning locally)
   a. Simple (without loss of consciousness)
      i. Motor (tonic, clonic, tonic-clonic; Jacksonian; benign childhood epilepsy; epilepsia partialis continua)
      ii. Somatosensory or special sensory (visual, auditory, olfactory, gustatory, vertiginous)
      iii. Autonomic
      iv. Psychic
   b. Complex (with impaired consciousness)
      i. Beginning as simple partial seizures and progressing to impairment of consciousness
      ii. With impairment of consciousness at outset

3. Special epileptic syndromes
   a. Myoclonus and myoclonic seizures
   b. Reflex epilepsy
   c. Acquired aphasia with convulsive disorder
   d. Febrile and other seizures of infancy and childhood
   e. Hysterical seizures

partial onset seizures, including those with secondary generalization, the preferred agents are carbamazepine and phenytoin. Alternative agents include valproate and many of the newer anticonvulsant agents. For absence seizures, first-choice agents are ethosuximide and valproate. Valproate is the first choice for atypical absence or atonic seizures. An alternative is lamotrigine for either absence or atypical absence/atonic seizures. Valproate is also the first choice for myoclonic seizures with the alternatives of lamotrigine, clonazepam, and clorazepate. For generalized tonic-clonic seizures, valproate, carbamazepine, and phenytoin are preferred agents, though newer antiepileptic drugs such as topiramate, lamotrigine, and zonisamide may also be useful. In general, one agent should be chosen and increased to the maximum tolerated dose before beginning polypharmacy for the treatment of seizures.

In the setting of the NICU, the mode of administration of agents needs to be considered, because many patients are unable to take medications orally. Agents currently available in the United States for intravenous (IV) administration include lorazepam (Ativan), diazepam (Valium), phenytoin (Dilantin), fosphenytoin (Cerebyx), phenobarbital, and valproate (Depacon). In addition, diazepam is available for rectal administration.

◆ Status Epilepticus

Status epilepticus is a special case of seizure activity without recovery of consciousness between seizures lasting for more than 30 minutes. There are ~100,000 cases per year in the United States.[2,3] In half of the cases, it is the initial manifestation of a seizure disorder. The most commonly affected groups are young children and patients over 60 years of age. Status epilepticus can be either generalized or partial. Generalized status can be convulsive (tonic-clonic, tonic-clonic-tonic, or clonic), absence, secondary generalized, myoclonic, or atonic. Generalized convulsive status is the most frequent type of status epilepticus, of which 75% of cases are secondarily generalized. There are a variety of causes for status epilepticus, including febrile seizures; cerebrovascular accidents; infection, such as meningitis; idiopathic, epilepsy, or subtherapeutic anticonvulsants; electrolyte imbalance; drug intoxication, especially cocaine; alcohol withdrawal; traumatic brain injury; anoxia; and tumors.

Treatment of status epilepticus is directed to stabilizing the patient by stopping seizure activity and addressing the underlying cause of the status epilepticus. Although status epilepticus is defined as seizures and interictal periods without return to baseline lasting for more than 30 minutes, any recurrent seizures without interval return to baseline should be treated aggressively. Historically, mortality from status epilepticus has been reported to be as high as 50%, although more recent data suggest it is on the order of 10 to 12%, to perhaps as high as 20%, of which only ~2% of deaths are directly attributable to the status epilepticus.[2,3] Morbidity and mortality may be due to central nervous system (CNS) injury caused by repetitive electrical discharges, systemic stress from the seizure (cardiac, respiratory, renal, or metabolic), or CNS damage from the insult that caused the status epilepticus.

Initial treatment should address the "ABCs" of airway, breathing, and circulation. This should include maintaining the airway with an oral airway or possibly intubation, the administration of supplemental oxygen, and cardiac and blood pressure monitoring. Once this has been accomplished, priorities must be to stop further seizure activity and to correct its cause.[1-6] An IV of normal saline should be started as soon as possible, and both a benzodiazepine, such as lorazepam or diazepam, and phenytoin loading dose should be administered. The role of valproate is not yet defined for use in status epilepticus, although it is a potential additional anticonvulsant, which may be used. In general, except in the case of cocaine-induced seizures, a benzodiazepine alone should not be used; rather, it should be used in conjunction with a longer-acting anticonvulsant.

Concurrently, efforts should be started to identify and correct the underlying cause. This workup should include blood work consisting of electrolytes, glucose, magnesium, calcium, anticonvulsant level, and arterial blood gas. If there is any consideration of CNS infection, a lumbar puncture should be performed unless it is contraindicated. If the patient is hypoglycemic or if glucose cannot immediately be measured, 25 to 50 mL of Dextrose 50 (D50) should be given. Fifty to 100 mg of thiamine should be given immediately prior to the D50 in patients in whom thiamine deficiency might be present. Likewise, naloxone (Narcan 0.4 mg IV pump [IVP]) should be given in the case of patients who might have taken narcotics. An electronencelphalography (EEG) monitor is helpful if available. Paralytic agents will stop the visible manifestation of the seizures, but they do not stop the dangerous electrical activity in the brain that can lead to permanent neurologic damage. Thus they should be avoided in patients with status epilepticus, except for the use of short-acting agents for intubation. In some cases of prolonged seizure activity, paralytic agents may be helpful in reducing the lactic acidosis and rhabdomyolysis caused by the seizure activity. In these cases, continuous EEG monitoring is necessary to determine whether electrical seizures are continuing and possibly causing further damage to the brain. In addition, narcotics and phenothiazines should be avoided in status epilepticus because they lower the seizure threshold (**Table 23–2**).

◆ Prophylaxis of Seizures

Evidence-based medicine guidelines are available for prophylaxis of seizures in the setting of both traumatic brain injury and brain tumors.[7,8] In other disease processes, no clear evidence-based guidelines currently exist.

Table 23–2   Protocol for the Management of Status Epilepticus[1–3]

1. Lorazepam (Ativan) 0.1 mg/kg IV up to 4 mg (average adult dose) at rate of <2 mg/minute

OR

Diazepam (Valium) 0.2 mg/kg (10 mg average adult dose) IV at 5 mg/minute

OR

Valproic acid 20 mg/kg diluted in water or vegetable oil administered rectally in pediatric patients with frequent seizures and no IV access

2. Phenytoin (Dilantin) or fosphenytoin (Cerebyx) load of 20 mg/kg IV at a maximal rate of 50 mg/minute. If phenytoin is used, cardiac monitoring should be performed and the rate slowed should arrhythmias occur.

3. If seizures continue, may give additional phenytoin up to a total of 30 mg/kg

OR

Phenobarbital IV up to a total load of 20 mg/kg. (Because phenobarbital may lower blood pressure and suppress respirations, these need to be monitored during its administration.)

OR

Paraldehyde 0.3–0.5 mg/kg in a 1% solution diluted 1:1 in vegetable oil administered rectally

4. If seizures continue, the patient should be intubated and general anesthesia instituted with pentobarbital to induce burst suppression. This should be started with a load of 15 mg/kg IV and continued at a rate of ~2.5 mg/kg/hour. Blood pressure should be closely monitored, and pressors may be needed to maintain an adequate blood pressure.

OR

Propofol can be used as an alternative to pentobarbital to induce burst suppression. A load of 40 mg is given and repeated to an induction dose of 2.0–2.5 mg/kg and maintenance of 0.1–0.2 mg/kg/minute. Similar to pentobarbital, blood pressure must be closely monitored, and pressors may be needed.

OR

Midazolam (Versed) 5–10 mg bolus at less than 4 mg/minute, followed by a 0.05–0.40 mg/kg/hour drip.

By this stage, continuous EEG monitoring should be used to titrate either pentobarbital or propofol to provide burst suppression. It should also be used to monitor the effect of treatment and should be instituted as early as is feasible in those patients with refractory status epilepticus who do not rapidly return to baseline function.

◆ Treatment of Trauma

Guidelines for the Management of Severe Traumatic Brain Injury, published by the Brain Trauma Foundation, recommends that prophylactic use of anti-convulsants is not recommended for the prevention of late seizures, though it may be useful in preventing early post-traumatic seizures.[9] Current practice based on these guidelines is to treat patients who have suffered severe head injury for 1 week to prevent early post-traumatic seizures. At that point, anticonvulsants are routinely discontinued unless the patient requires treatment for a documented seizure disorder.

◆ Tumors

The American Academy of Neurology published guidelines for the treatment of patients with brain tumors, which recommended against long-term prophylactic use of anticonvulsants, though it did not address the issue in the early perioperative period.[9] If patients are known to have suffered seizures as a result of their tumor, anticonvulsants are indicated for treatment of the seizure disorder.

In tumors and other disease processes, such as aneurysmal subarachnoid hemorrhage, there is variation in the practice of neurosurgeons. The author has tended to treat these patients with prophylactic anticonvulsants for a period of 1 week from surgery or bleed until surgery, analogous to the treatment of head injury patients. Long-term use of anticonvulsants is limited to those patients who have had seizures, as treatment of a seizure disorder rather than prophylaxis.

Case Management

The patient was found to have a subtherapeutic phenytoin level that should have been immediately corrected with a partial reloading of phenytoin. Although a CT scan was necessary to rule out intracranial hemorrhage after surgery, an EEG should have been performed as well. The vital signs may have demonstrated tachycardia and hypertension even in the face of nonconvulsive status epilepticus. If the seizures were not controlled with lorazepam and phenytoin, then the patient should have been intubated and the seizures treated with general anesthesia.

References

1. Adams RD, Victor M, Ropper AH. Principles of Neurology. 6th ed. New York: McGraw-Hill; 1997
2. Bassin S, Smith TL, Bleck TP. Clinical review: status epilepticus. Crit Care 2002;6:137–142
3. Greenberg MS. Handbook of Neurosurgery. Lakeland, FL: Greenberg Graphics; 1997
4. Bleck TP. Management approaches to prolonged seizures and status epilepticus. Epilepsia 1999;40(Suppl 1):S59–S63 discussion S64–66

5. Brown LA, Levin GM. Role of propofol in refractory status epilepticus. Ann Pharmacother 1998;32:1053–1059
6. Scottish Intercollegiate Guidelines Network. Diagnosis and Management of Epilepsy in Adults. Edinburgh, UK: Author; 2003
7. Bullock, R., Chestnut RM, Clifton G, et al. Guidelines for the management of severe traumatic brain injury. J Neurotrauma 2000;17:451–553
8. Glantz MJ, Cole BF, Forsyth PA, et al. Practice parameter: anticonvulsant prophylaxis in patients with newly diagnosed brain tumors. Report of the Quality Standards Subcommittee of the American Academy of Neurology. Neurology 2000 May 23;54(10):1886–1893
9. Brain Trauma Foundation. Guidelines for the Management of Severe Head Injury. New York: Author; 2000

24
Infections

Darryl M. Warner and Dan Miulli

Case Study

A 14-year-old, right-handed female is brought to the emergency room by paramedics with complaints of flulike symptoms over the past 3 or 4 days, followed by an abrupt change in mental status on the day of evaluation. The patient does not have any significant past medical or surgical history. Additionally, she does not have a history of recent travel. On initial evaluation, the patient is observed to be lethargic but arousable with deep stimulation. Her core temperature is 102.7°F. The remaining vital signs are normal. No nuchal rigidity is present. The patient's Glasgow Coma Scale (GCS) score is 8 without any focal neurologic deficits noted. Routine laboratory tests as well as blood cultures are drawn, with the only abnormality being a mildly elevated white blood cell count with many mononuclear cells. A computed tomography (CT) scan of the brain was interpreted as normal. What is the patient's diagnosis? What are the possible etiologies? What studies are needed to complete a thorough workup? What is the appropriate treatment?

See page 361 for Case Management.

Infections of the central and peripheral nervous systems are relatively infrequent occurrences; however, when present, they can cause significant morbidity and mortality. Rapid diagnosis and appropriate treatment are paramount to preventing death and limiting disability in these patients.[1–3] This chapter provides information needed for prompt and accurate diagnosis and treatment of nervous system infections in the intensive care setting. The chapter will focus on the diagnosis and treatment of community-acquired infections of the nervous system, with a section near the end for the discussion of iatrogenic or hospital-acquired infections.

Nervous system infections can be divided into two broad categories: infection of the structures surrounding the nervous system (meningitis), and infection of the parenchyma of the brain and/or spinal cord (encephalitis, abscess).

The main and subtypes of infection are listed here, along with the information necessary for the neurologic intensive care unit.

◆ Bacterial Infections of the Skull, Meninges, and Brain

Bacterial Meningitis

Inflammatory response to bacterial invasion of the pia-arachnoid surrounding the central nervous system (CNS)

Risk factors   Alcoholism, splenectomy, human immunodeficiency virus (HIV), diabetes, immunosuppression, malignancy, dialysis, and sickle cell disease[4–7]

Predisposing conditions   Otitis media, sinusitis, bacteremia, pneumonia, and bacterial peritonitis[4–7]

Most common organisms   Dependent on age; most spread by respiratory transmission (**Table 24–1**)

Clinical presentation   Headache, fever, nuchal rigidity, nausea/vomiting, neck or back pain; can have focal neurologic signs, altered level of consciousness, or seizures; onset of symptoms over hours to days[4–7]

Physical exam signs   Indicative of meningeal irritation
Brudzinski's sign: Passive flexion of the neck causes involuntary flexion of the knees and hips
Kernig's sign: Resistance to passive extension of the hip and knee

Table 24–1   Most Common Organisms in Bacterial Meningitis[1–5]

Organism and characteristics	Age
Streptococcus pneumoniae: Most common organism in all age groups (40–50% of cases); most common organism causing meningitis in patients with CSF leak	>7 years
Neisseria meningitidis: 20 to 30% of cases; associated with close living quarters	3–7 years
Haemophilus influenzae: Prior to Hib vaccination, most common organism in children <5 years of age; now <5% of cases	3 months–3 years
Group B *Streptococcus (agalactiae)*: Most frequent cause of neonatal meningitis; usually transmitted to infant during delivery; 10 to 15% of cases	<3 months
Escherichia coli: 15% of neonatal cases; 3% of all cases	<3 months
Listeria monocytogenes: 5 to 10% of cases of meningitis in neonates <1 month; fecal-oral transmission: transmitted via mother at the time of birth from genital or GI tract colonization	<1 month or >50 years + immuno-suppression

CSF, cerebrospinal fluid; GI, gastrointestinal; Hib, *Haemophilus influenzae* type B.

Differential diagnosis Includes viral meningitis, fungal meningitis, viral encephalitis, parenchymal abscess, epidural/subdural empyema, parasitic infection, neuroleptic malignant syndrome, and subarachnoid hemorrhage

Diagnosis and studies Cerebrospinal fluid (CSF) findings in bacterial meningitis: Opening pressure elevated, turbid, cloudy in appearance, red blood (cell) count (RBC) >200/mm³ with predominance of neutrophils, glucose decreased, and protein elevated (**Table 24–2**)

Imaging Has little role in the diagnosis of meningitis; is necessary to rule out hemorrhage, mass lesions, elevated intracranial pressure (ICP), or other nervous system infections

Lumbar puncture If ICP is elevated, then the risk of herniation after lumbar puncture is significantly increased; however, it may be valuable for the evaluation of clinical sequelae of infection, such as subdural empyema, hydrocephalus, and infarction.

Treatment Duration of treatment 10 to 14 days, depending on clinical response. Dexamethasone can be used to reduce meningeal inflammation and pain associated with nuchal rigidity, as well as the incidence of hearing loss in patients with *Streptococcus pneumoniae* or *Haemophilus influenzae* type B meningitis (**Table 24–3**)

Table 24–2 Cerebrospinal Fluid Analysis[1–5]

Parameter	Value
Opening pressure	4–15 mm Hg or 5.0–19.5 cm H_2O
Clarity	Cloudy: indicative of bacterial infection; WBC > 200/mm³ for turbid CSF
Color	Reddish: subarachnoid hemorrhage via traumatic tap; RBC > 6000/mm³ to appear red Yellowish: increased protein levels—usually > 150 mg/dL Xanthochromia: spin sample in centrifuge
Cell count and differential	WBC < 5/mm³; may be higher in neonates ↑ neutrophils = bacterial infection ↑ lymphocytes = viral or fungal etiology RBC measured in successive tubes to differentiate subarachnoid hemorrhage from traumatic tap with clearing of CSF and decrease in the number of RBCs
Biochemistry: glucose and protein levels	Glucose ⅔ blood glucose; CSF = normal values 45–60 mg/dL Glucose ↓ bacterial or fungal infections; normal in viral infections; protein = 15–40 mg/dL; ↑ not specific for type of meningitis
Gram's stain/culture and bacterial antigen panels	Only type[6–7]

CSF, cerebrospinal fluid; RBC, red blood (cell) count; WBC, white blood (cell) count.

Table 24–3 Treatment of Bacterial Meningitis[1-5]

Empiric antibiotic treatment based on most common organisms for a particular age group		
Treatment group	**Antibiotic**	**Dosage**
Initial treatment	Ceftriaxone or cefotaxime *and* Vancomycin	2 g IV q 12 hours 8–12 g/day divided q 6 hours 2–3 g IV q 8–12 hours (covers PCN-resistant *Streptococcus pneumoniae*)
PCN allergy	Chloramphenicol or imipenem *or* trimethoprim/sulfamethoxazole (use in place of cephalosporin)	1 g IV q 6 hours 160/800 mg bid
Chronic diseases, immunosuppression, or alcoholism	Add ampicillin	2 g IV q 4 hours
Neonates group B: *Streptococcus* is suspected	Ampicillin and gentamicin	
Focused antibiotic treatment based on culture results		
Streptococcus pneumoniae	Penicillin	4 million units IV q 4 hours
Neisseria meningitidis	Penicillin	4 million units IV q 4 hours
Haemophilus influenzae	Ampicillin + chloramphenicol + either ceftriaxone or cefotaxime	8–12 g/day divided q 6 hours
Group B *Streptococcus*	Penicillin	4 million units IV q 6 hours
Listeria monocytogenes	Ampicillin + gentamicin + ceftriaxone	2g IV q 12 hours

IV, intravenous; PCN, penicillin.

Osteomyelitis of the Skull

Most infections are due to direct extension from infected sinuses or intracranial empyema.

Most common organisms   S. aureus, S. epidermidis, and gram-negative bacilli

Clinical presentation   Focal pain, fever, scalp erythema, swelling, and tenderness

Differential diagnosis   Tumor, trauma, and epidural/subdural empyema

Diagnosis and studies   Skull x-ray will occasionally show inflammation and edema in infected area (Pott's puffy tumor). CT scan can demonstrate infectious changes of the skull as well as associated areas of infection.

Treatment   Consists of a combination of surgical debridement and antibiotic therapy. Surgery involves a craniectomy of infected skull, replacing it with mesh or acrylic cranioplasty ~6 to 12 months postoperatively if there are no signs of infection. Antibiotics are routinely given, such as vancomycin 1 g IV q 12 hours plus ceftazidime 2 g IV q 8 hours. The antibiotics are given for 6 to 12 weeks and are adjusted based on culture and sensitivities.

Subdural Empyema

Subdural empyema is usually the result of direct extension of local infection (e.g., sinus infection), spread via diploic veins in skull.[8] It can be seen in the epidural space and can be associated with osteomyelitis of the skull. It may also be postoperative or post-traumatic. There is a 50 to 60% morbidity rate, 10 to 20% mortality rate.[9]

Most common organisms   Aerobic and anaerobic *Streptococcus* species, *S. aureus*, and gram-negative bacilli

Clinical presentation   Fever, headache, nuchal rigidity, focal neurologic deficits, mental status changes, nausea/vomiting, and seizures

Differential diagnosis   Bacterial meningitis, viral meningitis, fungal meningitis, parasitic infection, viral encephalitis, parenchymal abscess, subarachnoid hemorrhage, HIV, and neuroleptic malignant syndrome

Diagnosis and studies   CT/MRI with contrast shows fluid collection with typical crescent shape as well as degree of mass effect or presence of midline shift. Lumbar puncture is not recommended due to suspected increased ICP and risk of herniation. When CSF is obtained, the findings are consistent with parameningeal infection. Usually there is an intraoperative culture swab (aerobic and anaerobic cultures).

Treatment   Emergent surgical evacuation via craniotomy; however, bur holes can be used in critically unstable patients if purulent material is liquefied. Antibiotics consist of vancomycin 1 g IV q 12 hours plus ceftazidime 2 g IV q 8 hours plus metronidazole 500 mg IV q 6 hours. The 4 to 6 week course of antibiotics is adjusted depending on culture and sensitivities.

Brain Abscess

Brain abscess is a localized suppurative infection of the brain parenchyma,[10] with a male predominance. There is a slightly higher rate in children 5 to 9 years and adults >60 years. The infection is usually due to hematogenous spread but can be a result of direct extension.

Predisposing conditions   Otitis media, sinusitis, mastoiditis, oral infections, lung abscess, pulmonary abnormalities, cyanotic heart disease, bacterial endocarditis, penetrating trauma, and HIV[11-13]

Most common organisms   Streptococci species—aerobic, anaerobic, microaerophilic; *Staphylococcus aureus* most common secondary to trauma, surgery, or endocarditis;[14] *Staphylococcus epidermidis, Pseudomonas aeruginosa, Enterococcus, Bacteroides, Actinomyces, Nocardia* associated with immunosuppression due to HIV disease;[15] *Mycoplasma* tuberculosis (TB)—most common cause of brain abscess in some developing countries; *Cryptococcus*—usually seen with meningitis; *Aspergillus*—seen in immunosuppressed patients from transplant; and *Toxoplasma gondii.*

Clinical presentation   Headache, fever, altered level of consciousness, visual changes, focal neurologic deficits—specific symptoms depending on location of lesion

Differential diagnosis   Bacterial meningitis, viral meningitis, fungal meningitis, parasitic infection, viral encephalitis, epidural/subdural empyema, intracerebral hemorrhage, subarachnoid hemorrhage, tumor, venous sinus thrombosis, and migraine headache

Diagnosis and studies   Routine laboratory tests (CBC, basic chemistry panel) are usually not helpful. However, erythrocyte sedimentation rate (ESR) is usually elevated and can be used to follow the therapeutic response to antibiotics. C-reactive protein is also very sensitive and may be added as a test. Lumbar puncture is not usually indicated unless meningitis is suspected. When CSF is obtained, the findings are similar to other parameningeal infections, such as elevated WBC, normal glucose, and elevated protein. Cultures are usually negative.

Imaging   Contrast-enhanced CT or MRI scans show characteristic rim-enhancing lesion with necrotic center surrounded by white matter edema. It can be difficult to differentiate from primary glial and metastatic tumors. MR spectroscopy can improve diagnostic accuracy.[16] The precise diagnosis of specific organisms requires pathological tissue from biopsy or resection.

Treatment   See **Tables 24–4** and **24–5**

Table 24–4   Differentiating Treatment for Brain Abscess: Medical versus Surgical[1–3,9–17]

Indications for medical treatment	Indications for surgical treatment
Multiple lesions	Solitary lesion
Lesions <3 cm	Lesions >3 cm
Deep lesions	Proximity to ventricle
Poor surgical candidate	Significant mass effect or midline shift >0.5 cm
	Altered mental status
	Progressive neurologic deficit

Table 24–5   Brain Abscess Management[1–3,9–17]

Antibiotics	Vancomycin 1 g IV q 12 hours + ceftazidime 2 g IV q 8 hours + metronidazole 500 mg IV q 6 hours if anaerobes suspected
Duration	6–12 weeks
Repeat imaging	2–4 weeks after beginning antibiotic therapy
Surgery	Consider if no change in size of the lesion or if neurologic deterioration
Surgical options	Stereotactic biopsy via craniotomy for resection

◆ Viral Infections of the Meninges and Brain

Viral Meningitis

Viruses are obligate intracellular parasites that can only replicate within a cell. They contain either deoxyribonucleic acid (DNA) or ribonucleic acid (RNA), and infection occurs via hematogenous spread as part of a systemic infection or neuronal spread via nerve cells.

Most common organism   *Enterovirus* consisting of echovirus, coxsackievirus is the most common viral CNS infections type in the United States. It is transmitted by fecal-oral spread.

Clinical presentation   Headache, fever, nausea/vomiting, nuchal rigidity, photophobia. However, patients are usually not as ill as with bacterial meningitis.

Differential diagnosis   Bacterial meningitis, fungal meningitis, viral encephalitis, parenchymal abscess, epidural/subdural empyema, severe frontal or sphenoid sinusitis, vaccination, intrathecal administration of drugs, HIV, subarachnoid hemorrhage, migraine headache, parasitic infections, sarcoidosis, and neuroleptic malignant syndrome. The diagnosis of viral meningitis is usually one of exclusion.

Diagnosis and studies   CSF findings in viral meningitis: Opening pressure usually normal; CSF usually clear/colorless; WBC elevated but usually <200/mm^3. There is initially a predominance of neutrophils with a shift toward mononuclear cells after 12 to 24 hours. The glucose is normal, and the protein is elevated. Gram's stain and routine cultures are negative; for this reason, viral meningitis is also referred to as aseptic meningitis. Viral cultures for *Enterovirus* are positive in 30 to 50% of cases; therefore, serological testing for the diagnosis of *Enterovirus* is not recommended. Polymerase chain reaction (PCR) can be used for diagnosis, but it is available only in specialized laboratories and is expensive.

Imaging   Usually unremarkable

Treatment   Currently there is no treatment for enteroviruses.

Viral Encephalitis

Most common organisms   The majority of epidemic cases of encephalitis are caused by arboviruses with spread by vector transmission (infected mosquitoes).

Arbovirus types are St. Louis encephalitis, California encephalitis, western equine encephalitis, eastern equine encephalitis, West Nile virus, and La Crosse encephalitis.

Herpes simplex virus is a latent virus found in dorsal root ganglion; it is spread via the neuronal route. The majority of cases are caused by type I virus. CNS infection involves the mesial temporal lobes bilaterally, with one side affected worse than the other. Autopsy studies show a predilection of the olfactory and limbic systems.[17]

Clinical presentation   Most common presentation is altered level of consciousness in the setting of acute febrile illness with possible focal neurologic signs.

Differential diagnosis   Bacterial meningitis, viral meningitis, fungal meningitis, parasitic infection, epidural/subdural empyema, parenchymal abscess, tumor, subdural hematoma, HIV, lupus cerebritis, adrenal leukodystrophy, Reye's syndrome, and neuroleptic malignant syndrome

Diagnosis and studies   CSF analysis similar to aseptic meningitis; viral cultures of arboviruses and herpes simplex virus are available only at specialized laboratory. Electroencephalogram (EEG) can show characteristic periodic lateralizing epileptiform discharges (PLEDs) in the case of herpes simplex encephalitis (HSE).

Imaging   Critical for diagnosis of encephalitis. Focal hyperintense lesions seen in inconsistent distribution on T2-weighted images and FLAIR (fluid attenuated inversion recovery) sequences on magnetic resonance imaging (MRI), especially in eastern equine encephalitis, asymmetric bitemporal distribution possibly with hemorrhage in HSE

Treatment   No known treatment for arbovirus infections; HSE can be treated with acyclovir 10 mg/kg IV q 8 hours for 14 to 21 days. If viral encephalitis is suspected, empiric treatment with acyclovir is indicated, as better outcomes are seen with early institution of antiviral therapy.

◆ Fungal Infections of the Meninges and Brain

Fungal Meningitis

Most common organisms   *Blastomyces*, *Coccidioides*, *Cryptococcus*, and *Histoplasma*

Most common organisms (immunocompromised)   *Aspergillus*, *Candida*, and Mucorales

Cryptococcus meningitis

Most common fungal pathogen of CNS; increased incidence of infection with increasing immunosuppression, especially when CD4 <200. Initial transmission is respiratory that subsequently disseminates into many organ systems, including CNS. Remains latent.

Clinical presentation   Two to 3 week history of headache, fever, nuchal ridgity combined with lethargy, confusion, nausea/vomiting, and rarely focal neurologic defects

Differential diagnosis   Bacterial meningitis, viral meningitis, viral encephalitis, parasitic infection, subarachnoid hemorrhage, and neuroleptic malignant syndrome

Diagnosis and studies   CSF analysis consistent with fungal etiology (e.g., elevated WBC with lymphocytic predominance, glucose decreased, and protein elevated). India ink stain; latex agglutination tests are ~95% diagnostic.

Imaging   Not usually helpful with diagnosis, but can rule out mass lesions or intracranial hemorrhage

Treatment   Amphotericin B 0.5 to 0.8 mg/kg/day IV with flucytosine 37.5 mg/kg q 8 hours. Treat for 6 weeks. After treatment is completed, need to use fluconazole as maintenance 400 mg/ day for 2 to 3 months.

Histoplasma meningitis

Mostly found in Ohio and Mississippi river valleys; widely disseminated in soil. Respiratory transmission. Disseminated disease can be seen in immunosuppressed patients due to HIV, lymphoma, or iatrogenic cause. May cause mass lesions in parenchyma (histoplasmomas).[18]

Clinical presentation   Similar to *Cryptococcus*

Differential diagnosis   Similar to *Cryptococcus*

Diagnosis and studies   CSF consistent with fungal meningitis; serology positive in 60 to 90% with CNS disease, cultures positive <30%

Treatment   Amphotericin B 0.7 to 1.0 mg/kg/day IV. Treat for 8 to 12 weeks. In patients with HIV, after treatment with amphotericin B is completed, use itraconazole 200 mg/day indefinitely. Despite aggressive treatment, there is ~20% mortality.

Coccidioides immitis meningitis

Endemic in the San Joaquin valley in central California, where it occurs in soil. There is respiratory transmission. It can present as a mass lesion in the brain parenchyma.

Predisposing factors   Pregnancy, immunosuppression, and HIV

Clinical presentation   Similar to *Cryptococcus* and *Histoplasma*

Differential diagnosis   Similar to *Cryptococcus* and *Histoplasma*

Diagnosis and studies   CSF consistent with fungal etiology. The most reliable method of diagnosis is detection of complement fixing antibody in CSF.[19] Culture is usually negative.

Treatment   Fluconazole 400 to 800 mg/day; if no clinical response, then amphotericin B 0.1 to 0.3 mg/day intrathecal via Ommaya reservoir. Treat for ~2 years after CSF is normalized. For HIV patients, treatment is lifelong. Without treatment, Coccidioides meningitis is uniformly fatal within 2 years.[20]

Blastomyces dermatitidis meningitis

Distributed along the Mississippi River; exists in moist soil. There is respiratory transmission. Most cases have evidence of systemic infection. CNS is involved in 6 to 33% of patients with disseminated disease.[21] A mass lesion forms in the brain parenchyma more frequently than other fungal infections.

Clinical presentation   Fever, cough, myalgias, arthralgias, and pleuritic chest pain

Differential diagnosis   Bacterial meningitis, viral meningitis, bacterial abscess, and parasitic infection

Diagnosis and studies   Culture from pulmonary secretions or tissue biopsy

Imaging   CT/MRI is not usually helpful unless a mass lesion is present.

Treatment   For pulmonary infection, use itraconazole 200 to 400 mg/day; if infection is severe, use amphotericin B 0.7 to 1.0 mg/kg/day. Treatment is for 6 months. CNS disease requires treatment with maximal dose amphotericin B.

Zygomycoses: Rhizopus, Mucor, and Rhizomucor

Zygomycoses invade the CNS by hematogenous spread or direct invasion. CNS mucormycosis can cause infarction, abscess formation, and mycotic aneurysms.

Predisposing factors   Diabetes and neutropenia

Clinical presentation   Headache, fever, sinus pain; rhinitis symptoms can progress to cellulitis, proptosis, and cavernous sinus thrombosis

Diagnosis and studies   Culture of surgical specimen/swab

Treatment   Surgical debridement combined with amphotericin B 1 mg/kg/day

Aspergillus

Majority of cases occur in immunosuppressed transplant patients with prolonged neutropenia. It begins as pulmonary disease and disseminates to CNS via hematogenous spread. There can be direct extension from maxillary and ethmoid sinuses. It is associated with cavernous sinus thrombosis and the formation of mycotic aneurysms.

Treatment   Surgical debridement and high-dose amphotericin B

◆ Tuberculosis of the Meninges and Brain

Tuberculosis Meningitis

Respiratory transmission; latent organisms reactivate to cause infection months to years after primary infection. There is hematogenous spread to the meninges and brain parenchyma, preferentials involving optic chiasm, pons, and cerebellum.

Predisposing conditions   Consists of immunosuppression, alcohol abuse, intravenous drug abuse (IVDA), and HIV

Clinical presentation   Slowly progressive fever, headache, and meningismus. Can also cause lethargy, mental status changes, seizures, and cranial nerve palsies.

Differential diagnosis   Bacterial meningitis, fungal meningitis, viral meningitis, parasitic infection, viral encephalitis, lupus cerebritis, and neuroleptic malignant syndrome

Diagnosis and studies   Purified protein derivative (PPD) skin testing;[22] chest x-ray may show active or chronic TB infection. CSF analysis is the most useful diagnostic test;[23] it can demonstrate WBC elevation with lymphocytic predominance. Glucose is decreased, protein is elevated. Acid-fast smear positive <23% of the time; cultures positive in 40 to 70% of cases. Serological test to detect mycobacterial antigens and PCR to detect antibodies in CSF should be performed.

Imaging   Contrast-enhanced CT/MRI can demonstrate meningeal inflammation as well as TB exudate around the basal cisterns. Magnetic resonance angiography (MRA) can detect vasculitic changes common with TB meningitis.

Treatment   If TB meningitis is suspected, start antibiotic therapy empirically consisting of isoniazid 300 mg daily, rifampin 600 mg daily, ethambutol 15 to 25 mg/kg/day, pyrazinamide 25 mg/kg/day plus pyridoxine. Treat for 1 year. Can supplement with dexamethasone in patients with extreme neurologic compromise.[24] In patients with neurologic compromise, 70 to 80% survival rate; ~50% will have neurologic morbidity, including seizures, hemiparesis, hydrocephalus, and organic brain syndrome.

Tuberculoma

Mass lesions in brain parenchyma caused by mycobacteria TB. Autopsy studies have shown ~70% to have multiple lesions.

Predisposing factors   Immunosuppression and HIV disease

Clinical presentation   Fever, headache, seizures, and focal neurologic deficits

Differential diagnosis   Bacterial abscess, fungal abscess, parasitic infection, subdural/epidural empyema, viral encephalitis, lymphoma, toxoplasmosis, tumor, intracerebral hemorrhage, and subarachnoid hemorrhage

Diagnosis and studies   PPD skin test, CSF analysis consistent with parameningeal infection; pathological tissue needed to rule out malignancy or other infectious conditions. Acid-fast bacilli (AFB) stain positive in ~60%, whereas ~60% will grow in culture

Imaging   Contrast-enhanced CT/MRI can show single or multiple homogenously enhancing lesions.

Treatment   As for TB meningitis

Spinal Tuberculosis

May accompany meningitis or exist alone. TB exudate surrounds spinal cord, causing symptoms due to cord compression and infarction due to vasculitic changes of vessels.

Clinical presentation   Symptoms can be sudden or indolent; can include weakness, paresthesias, radiculopathy. Sensory level demonstrated in about two thirds of patients.[25]

Differential diagnosis   Spinal epidural abscess, spinal cord tumor, spinal stenosis, disk herniation, spondylotic myelopathy, HIV, myelopathy, and multiple sclerosis

Diagnosis and studies   PPD skin test. CSF consistent with parameningeal infection. Blood cultures are negative; however, biopsy/culture swab is necessary for definitive diagnosis.

Imaging   MRI is modality of choice; it will show epidural or subdural exudate surrounding and compressing spinal cord.

Treatment   Surgical decompression of spinal cord; incision and drainage of abscess. Antibiotic treatment for 1 year with usual anti-TB medications

◆ Parasitic Infections

Most common organisms *Taenia solium* (cysticercosis), *Echinococcus multilocularis* (echinococcus), *Plasmodium falciparum* (malaria), and *Treponema pallidum* (syphilis)

Cysticercosis

Widespread in Central and South America; infection of brain with larval cysts of *Taenia solium* (pork tapeworm). There are two mechanisms of infection: (1) fecal-oral spread with ingestion of eggs and (2) ingestion of cysticerci in undercooked pork followed by self-inoculation with eggs from feces.

Clinical presentation   Headache, nausea/vomiting, seizures, altered level of consciousness, focal neurologic signs, and visual changes

Classification   (1) Racemose form—cysts found at base of brain in basal cisterns; associated with formation of hydrocephalus; and (2) *Cysticercus cellulosae* form—with parenchymal cysts; associated with seizures

Differential diagnosis   Bacterial abscess, fungal abscess, *Cryptococcus*, *Coccidiodes*, and tumor

Diagnosis and studies   Serological testing and biopsy of surgical specimen

Imaging   Contrast-enhanced CT/MRI can show single or multiple rim-enhancing cysts. Can occasionally see head of scolex in parenchymal cyst. May see calcifications from old "burned out" cysts.

Treatment   Praziquantel 50 to 100 mg/kg/day for 15 to 30 days; alternative: albendazole 10 to 15 mg/kg/day for 8 days. Some include steroids to help decrease the inflammatory response in the brain parenchyma as the cysts die.

Echinococcus (Hydatid [cyst] Disease)

Organism is tapeworm that infects carnivorous animals (dog is primary definitive host). It is common in the Mediterranean; spread by fecal-oral route. CNS is involved in only 2% of cases.[26] *E. multilocularis* is most common pathogen of the species.

Clinical presentation   Headache, nausea/vomiting, seizures, hemiparesis, papilledema, cranial nerve palsies, and dysarthria

Diagnosis and studies   Serological tests

Imaging   CT/MRI can show cyst with sharp borders, without enhancement or associated edema.

Treatment   Surgical excision; cyst must be removed intact to prevent spilling contents. Treat with albendazole 400 mg bid.

Malaria

All serious infections are caused by *P. falciparum*; infects over 2.5 billion people worldwide, causing 1 million to 3 million deaths annually. It has been eradicated in North America and Europe. Vector transmission is via mosquito. Infection causes capillary vascular obstruction.

Clinical presentation   Fever, chills, anemia, altered level of consciousness, renal failure, jaundice, thrombocytopenia, and seizures

Diagnosis and studies   Examination of blood smear

Treatment   Quinine sulfate 650 mg q 8 hours for 3 to 7 days plus doxycycline 100 mg bid for 7 days. Despite treatment, there is a 20% mortality.

Syphilis

Caused by *T. pallidum*; transmitted by sexual contact. CNS infection develops in 8 to 40% of cases. If left untreated, ~25% will develop tertiary syphilis in 5 to 40 years. Syphilitic gummas are tumorlike lesions primarily involving skin and mucous membranes; can involve the brain.

   Neurosyphilis is divided into four syndromes: syphilitic meningitis, meningiovascular syphilis, tabes dorsalis, and general paresis. Tabes dorsalis is atrophy of the dorsal columns in the spinal cord leading to loss of sensation and proprioception, mostly in lower extremities. It is associated with Argyll-Robertson pupil (no pupillary reaction to light, but accommodation is preserved). General paresis (also referred to as general paralysis of the insane) is the gradual deterioration of mental function with loss of motor control and seizures.

Diagnosis and studies   Test for venereal disease research laboratory (VDRL) in CSF and rapid plasma regain (RPR) in serum.

Treatment   Penicillin G 12 million to 24 million units IV/day divided q 4 hours for 10 to 14 days; if penicillin allergic, doxycycline 200 mg q day for 21 days

Lyme Disease

Multisystem disease caused by deer tick (*Borrelia burgdorferi*); most common arthropod-borne infection in the United States.[27] Three clinical stages: (1) early stage, characterized by a distinctive rash known as erythema migrans; (2) dissemination stage, occurs days to weeks following infection; characterized by flulike symptoms called erythema chronicum migrans, which, if left untreated, can disseminate and involve cardiac and neurologic systems. This consists of a clinical triad of meningitis, cranial neuritis, and radiculopathy.[28] It occurs in 10 to 15% of patients with stage 2 Lyme disease; (3) persistent infection, with symptoms that may not appear until weeks, months, or years after infection. Stage 3 typically involves joint pain. Other symptoms include arthritis and chronic neurologic problems, such as encephalopathy, ataxia, dementia, and neuropathy.

Diagnosis and studies Based on history and the presence of the typical macular rash. Antibody serologies cannot be detected until ~3 weeks postinfection; CSF consistent with aseptic (viral) meningitis.

Treatment Doxycycline 100 mg bid for 3 to 4 weeks. If neurologic abnormalities present, use ceftriaxone 2 g IV daily for 2 to 4 weeks.

Rickettsia/Ehrlichia

Small gram-negative intracellular organisms transmitted by tick bites; can cause systemic infections that can present as encephalitis. Known as Rocky Mountain spotted fever and ehrlichiosis.

Diagnosis and studies Clinical information is based on history of tick bite; also, specialized serological tests are available.

Treatment Empiric treatment with doxycycline 100 mg bid for 10 to 14 days; in children, chloramphenicol 50 mg/kg/day divided into 4 doses. Mortality is 2 to 6%.

Amebic Encephalitis

Uniformly fatal meningioencephalitis caused by *Naegleria fowleri*; found in lakes in warm climates. It is a rapidly progressive encephalitis.

Diagnosis and studies Based on history of swimming in warm, freshwater lakes. CSF shows bacterial or fungal meningitis picture; however, Gram's stain and culture are negative.

Imaging MRI can show frontal lobe involvement.

Treatment Amphotericin B IV and intrathecal tetracycline and rifampin.[29]

Prion Disease, Creutzfeldt-Jakob Disease (similar to "mad cow" disease)

Fatal encephalopathy characterized by rapidly progressive dementia, ataxia, and myoclonus. Also called transmissible spongiform encephalopathy. Can be inherited or acquired (ingestion of infected tissue).

Clinical presentation   Progressive dementia, fatigue, ataxia, myoclonus, tremor, rigidity, and focal neurologic deficits

Diagnosis and studies   CSF is usually normal; EEG can show bilateral sharp waves or periodic spikes.

Imaging   No characteristic findings on CT/MRI; can show atrophy

Treatment   None. Median survival is 5 months; 80% die in first year.

◆ CNS Infections in HIV Patients

Forty to 60% of all patients with acquired immunodeficiency syndrome (AIDS) will develop neurologic complications related to the disease.[30] One third of patients with HIV will have neurologic symptoms as the presenting manifestation of the disease.[31]

Most common organisms   Toxoplasma, primary B cell lymphoma, JC virus (causative agent for progressive multifocal leukoencephalopathy), *Cryptococcus*, and cytomegalovirus (CMV).

Toxoplasma Gondii

Ten percent of the general population of the United States has been infected with *toxoplasma gondii*.[32] The major reservoir is domestic cats, spread to humans by fecal-oral route. Generally asymptomatic except in the setting of severe immunosuppression such as with advanced HIV disease when the CD4 count <200 or when reactivation of infection produces single or multiple abscesses in the brain parenchyma.

Clinical presentation   Headache, fever, altered level of consciousness, lethargy, focal neurologic signs. Can also present with seizures or intracerebral hemorrhage.

Differential diagnosis   Bacterial abscess, fungal abscess, parasitic infection, tumor, lymphoma, viral encephalitis, progressive multifocal leukoencephalopathy (PML), and CMV

Diagnosis and studies   CSF analysis may be similar to that of parameningeal infection; however, there may be an elevated WBC count with neutrophilic predominance. The glucose may be normal and the protein elevated. There should be a serological test for *Toxoplasma* antibodies.

Imaging   Contrast-enhanced CT/MRI will show characteristic round, rim-enhancing lesion, single or multiple, with associated white matter edema; difficult to differentiate from tumor or other types of abscesses radiologically

Treatment   If toxoplasmosis is suspected, start empiric therapy with pyrimethamine 100 mg daily plus sulfadiazine 1 g IV q 6 hours or clindamycin 600 to 1200 mg IV q 6 hours. Alternate regimen: trimethoprin/sulfamethoxazole 160/800 q 6 hours. Treat for 3 to 6 weeks.

Lifelong treatment for AIDS patients: pyrimethamine 25 to 75 mg daily plus sulfadiazine 500 to 1000 mg qid plus folic acid 10 to 20 mg daily. Follow patient clinically, and repeat imaging 10 to 14 days after starting treatment if there is no clinical or radiological response to empiric treatment. Biopsy of lesion may be required to rule out lymphoma and/or PML. Median survival is 15 months.

Lymphoma

Lymphoma develops in ~5% of patients with HIV disease.[33] It is due to Epstein-Barr virus–associated B cell type. Approximately one third of patients will present with CNS disease.[34]

Clinical presentation   Lethargy, confusion, cognitive deficits, focal neurologic signs, seizures, and cranial nerve palsies

Differential diagnosis   Toxoplasmosis, PML, other tumors (primary or metastatic), bacterial abscess, fungal abscess, parasitic infection, CMV, and viral encephalitis

Diagnosis and studies   Routine laboratory tests are not usually helpful; no serological tests for identification. Diagnosis must be strongly considered in patients who do not respond to empiric treatment. For toxoplasmosis, definitive diagnosis requires biopsy.

Imaging   Contrast-enhanced CT/MRI will show white matter lesions, possibly contrast enhancement. The lesion may cross the corpus callosum.

Treatment   Chemotherapy; dexamethasone can cause tumors to "melt" away; whole brain radiotherapy. Median survival is 3 months.

Progressive Multifocal Leukoencephalopathy

PML is a progressive demyelinating disease, primarily seen in immunocompromised patients,[35] such as those with HIV, lymphoma, chronic lymphocytic leukemia, lupus, and diseases caused by JC virus. Antibodies to JC virus can be detected in CSF.[36–38]

Clinical presentation   Progressive focal neurologic deficits and cognitive decline[39,40]

Differential diagnosis   Multiple sclerosis, adrenal leukodystrophy, acute disseminated encephalomyelitis, toxoplasmosis, lymphoma, prion disease, and CMV

Diagnosis and studies   CSF analysis usually normal. JC virus can be detected in CSF by serology and PCR. Definitive diagnosis requires biopsy, which is frequently diagnostic.

Imaging   CT/MRI shows diffuse white matter disease; does not enhance with contrast

Treatment   There is no proven effective therapy. Median survival is 15 months.

Cytomegalovirus

Fifty to 80% of the general adult population in the United States has been infected; most are asymptomatic. In nonimmunocompromised adults, infection is similar clinically to mononucleosis. Seen in patients late in the course of HIV disease: CD4 count <50; most common infection is rhinitis. Can involve spinal cord—characterized by ascending motor weakness, areflexia, and loss of bowel/bladder function.[41] Similar to Guillain-Barré syndrome.

Clinical presentation   Progressive deterioration of mental status and cognitive function, headaches, and seizures

Differential diagnosis   Viral encephalitis, PML, lymphoma, toxoplasmosis, parasitic infection, and prion disease

Diagnosis and studies   CSF is essentially normal; may have elevated protein. May test serology for CMV antigen by PCR. Can also perform specific viral cultures.

Imaging   MRI can show nonspecific hyperintense signal changes on T2-weighted images and FLAIR sequences.[42]

Treatment   Gancyclovir 5 mg/kg IV q 12 hours plus foscarnet 90 mg/kg IV q 12 hours. Subsequently, treat HIV disease with antiretroviral therapy.

HIV Encephalopathy

Most common neurologic involvement in AIDS. Two thirds of patients with HIV/AIDS and one third of AIDS patients will have dementia at time of death.[43] HIV causes diffuse brain atrophy.

Clinical presentation   Altered level of consciousness, cognitive dysfunction, gait abnormalities, postural instability

Differential diagnosis   Viral encephalitis, PML, prion disease, parasitic infection, dementia, and metabolic encephalopathy

Diagnosis and studies   CSF usually nondiagnostic,[44] although patient may have a slight elevation of WBC. Glucose is normal, protein is elevated. HIV antibodies can be detected in CSF.

Imaging   CT/MRI will show generalized atrophy without specific findings. MRI may show hyperintense periventricular white matter abnormalities of T2-weighted images and FLAIR sequences.

Treatment   Antiretroviral therapy. HIV disease can also cause an AIDS-related myelopathy and cranial neuropathies.

◆ Spinal Infections

There are three types of spinal infections: spinal epidural abscess, vertebral osteomyelitis, and diskitis.

Spinal Epidural Abscess

More common in elderly, immunocompromised, and IVDA.[45,46] Most common route of spread is hematogenous; most commonly located in lumbar region.

Risk factors   Osteomyelitis, diskitis, diabetes, cancer, IVDA, alcohol abuse, and chronic renal failure.[47]

Sources of infection (hematogenous): skin infection, endocarditis, bacteremia, urinary tract infection (UTI), dental abscess, respiratory infection, penetrating trauma, and psoas abscess. Can also occur from direct extension from vertebral body, disk space infection, or paraspinal/psoas abscess.[45] With hematogenous spread, abscess usually forms posteriorly in the spinal canal; if direct extension from osteomyelitis or diskitis, abscess usually forms anteriorly.[45,48] Neurologic deficits caused by epidural abscess are thought to be secondary to compression of neural elements combined with vascular thrombosis and infarction.[49–51]

Most common organisms   *S. aureus*, aerobic and anaerobic streptococci, *Pseudomonas*, *Escherichia coli*, and TB (common in chronic form)[47]

Clinical presentation   Back pain, fever; associated with nerve root or spinal cord dysfunction, such as weakness, pain, and loss of bowel/bladder control

Differential diagnosis   Spinal TB, tumor, disk herniation, spinal stenosis, multiple sclerosis, HIV, myelopathy, and spondylotic myelopathy

Diagnosis and studies   Routine laboratory tests are not usually helpful; most common laboratory abnormality is elevated ESR.[52] Blood cultures are positive in 60% of cases.

Imaging   Contrast-enhanced MRI is modality of choice that can demonstrate fluid collection as well as the degree of spinal cord compression. Thorough neurologic exam and MRI localize can the affected area.

Treatment   In patients without neurologic deficits, use vancomycin 1 g IV q 12 hours, rifampin 600 mg daily, and cefotaxime 2 g IV q 8 hours for 6 to 8 weeks. Surgical evacuation is warranted if neurologic deficits are present; if surgical evacuation is done, follow with antibiotics and immobilization in a brace. Bracing is recommended in both cases. If abscess is located posteriorly, can perform laminectomies. If abscess is located anteriorly in the spinal canal, the patient may need corpectomy with anterior and possibly posterior stabilization. Mortality is 18 to 23%. Improvement of neurologic function postoperatively is rare.

Vertebral Osteomyelitis

Spinal infections account for 2 to 4% of cases of osteomyelitis,[53] which is due to hematogenous spread. Fifty percent of cases are located in the lumbar spine.[54]

Most common organisms   *S. aureus* ~60%,[55] gram-negative bacilli (*Pseudomonas*, *Proteus*, *E. coli*), and fungal pathogens

Risk factors   Diabetes, chronic steroid use, dialysis, IVDA, malnutrition, malignancy, advanced age, and immunosuppression[55,56]
    Sources of infection are commonly respiratory, bacteremia, UTI, soft tissue abscess, dental abscess, and postsurgical causes (~2.5%).[57,58] Spinal TB[59] has increased since the AIDS epidemic.

Clinical presentation   Localized back pain unrelated to movement or position, fever

Differential diagnosis   Important to differentiate osteomyelitis from neoplasms

Diagnosis and studies   Most common laboratory abnormality is elevated ESR. Blood cultures are positive in only ~25% of cases. CT-guided biopsy should be performed for identification of organism if blood culture is negative.[55] Open biopsy may be necessary; specimens must be sent for bacterial and fungal cultures.

Imaging   X-rays can show disk space narrowing and end-plate changes. Bone scan and MRI are the most sensitive studies for identifying vertebral osteomyelitis.[60] MRI demonstrates hyperintense signal in the vertebral body on T2-weighted images.

Treatment   Antibiotic therapy for 4 weeks combined with spinal bracing. Treat with anti-TB medications for 12 months if patient has Pott's disease; also treat with spinal immobilization with bracing. Surgery is indicated if patient has neurologic deficit, spinal instability, a poor response to antibiotic therapy, or a nondiagnostic CT-guided biopsy.

Diskitis

Rare infection of nucleus pulposis with secondary involvement of end plate and vertebral body. Can be spontaneous or postprocedure. Risk factors are similar to those for vertebral osteomyelitis; must be differentiated from tumors that preferentially avoid the disk space.

Most common organisms   *S. aureus* (spontaneous), *S. epidermidis* (postprocedure), *Pseudomonas* (IVDA), and *E. coli*

Clinical presentation   Localized back pain, paraspinal muscle spasm, and radicular symptoms, such as pain, weakness, and paresthesias

Diagnosis and studies   Elevated ESR. Blood cultures are positive in ~50% of cases.

Imaging   X-ray can show destruction of disk space as well as end-plate irregularities. MRI can show involvement of disk space and is useful to rule out epidural abscess. CT-guided biopsy may be necessary to make definitive diagnosis.

Treatment   Similar to treatment for osteomyelitis: antibiotics (vancomycin, rifampin, cefotaxime) for 4 to 6 weeks, immobilization with brace. Surgery is rarely required.

◆ Iatrogenic Infections

Main types: ventriculostomy, CSF fistula, CSF shunt infection, and postoperative wound infections

Ventriculostomy

Infection is the most common complication associated with the use of external ventricular drains (incidence 0–27%).[61,62] Prophylactic antibiotics should be directed toward gram-positive organisms.

Risk factors   Hemorrhage, neurosurgery manipulation of drainage system, and duration of use[63]

Most common organism: S. epidermidis[64]

Diagnosis and studies   CSF analysis and culture

Treatment   Empiric antibiotics initially, including vancomycin, as well as broad gram-negative coverage, such as ceftazidime, ciprofloxacin, gentamicin, or piperacillin/tazobactam. Adjust antibiotics based on culture and sensitivity results. May need to include intrathecal vancomycin or gentamicin, depending on culture results

CSF Fistula

Three types: spontaneous, postsurgical, and post-traumatic. Two to 3% of patients with head injury developed CSF fistulas,[65] of which 70% stop spontaneously within 1 week. Common sites of leakage include mastoid air cells, frontal sinus, cribriform plate, and sphenoid sinus.

Most common organisms   S. pneumoniae, S. aureus, P. aeruginosa, and Enterobacteriaceae[66]

Diagnosis and studies   CSF analysis and culture. Coronal CT with thin cuts after intrathecal contrast can be helpful for localizing leaks in the skull base.

Treatment   Elevate head of bed (HOB) >45 degrees at all times. Acetazolamide 250 mg qid to decrease CSF production, as well as lumbar drain, should be strongly considered. Lumbar drain provides excellent CSF diversion and allows easy access to CSF for frequent analysis. Surgical repair is indicated for persistent leaks. For infected fluid, use vancomycin 1 g IV q 8 hours with ceftazidime 2 g IV q 8 hours for 14 days, or use for 1 week after CSF normalizes. Change to nafcillin/oxacillin if not methicillin-resistant S. aureus (MRSA). Add gentamicin, pipericillin/tazobactam, or ciprofloxacin for Pseudomonas.

Shunt Infection

Accepted infection rate is 5 to 7%.[67] There is an increased risk of seizures and mortality after infection. Fifty percent of infections are within 2 weeks, 70% within 2 months. Skin is most common source.

Risk factors   Length of procedure and young age

Most common organisms   *S. epidermidis*—most common, *S. aureus*, gram-negative bacilli, and *Enterococcus*

Clinical presentation   Fever, headache, nausea, vomiting, lethargy, anorexia, irritability, and signs of shunt malfunction

Diagnosis and studies   CSF findings are consistent with parameningeal infection (e.g., WBC mildly elevated, glucose normal to decreased, protein elevated, and Gram's stain positive in 50% of cases). Culture may be negative in 40%. CT/MRI is usually not helpful for diagnosis, but when present, there may be enhancement or hyperintense signal of ependymal lining or ventriculomegaly consistent with shunt malfunction.

Treatment   Empiric antibiotics: vancomycin with or without rifampin, combined with broad gram-negative coverage; continue for 10 to 14 days or after CSF is normal for 3 days.
    Specific antibiotics: *S. aureus*/*S. epidermidis*—IV and intrathecal (IT) vancomycin with or without rifampin; for gram-negative bacilli, use third-generation cephalosporin or aminoglycoside IV with IT gentamicin.
    In addition to antibiotic use, there should be removal of hardware. Most experts recommend either externalization of shunt hardware or removal of entire shunt assembly and the additional placement of an external ventricular drain. There should be replacement of the shunt with a completely new system when CSF is sterile.

Wound Infections

Wound infections represent a 1 to 5% risk after laminectomy.[68] Degree of infection ranges from superficial to full thickness with wound dehiscence.

Risk factors   Increasing age, diabetes, obesity, and chronic steroid use

Most common organisms   *S. aureus*

Clinical presentation   Pain, erythema, and purulent discharge at incision site

Diagnosis and studies   Wound swab, culture, and sensitivity; should include aerobic and anaerobic cultures

Treatment   Superficial infection: use first-generation cephalosporin or antistaphylococcal penicillin. Deep infection: use vancomycin/ceftazidime. Treat 10 to 14 days; adjust antibiotics based on culture and sensitivity results. Need irrigation and drainage of deeper infections with antibiotic pulse irrigation, followed by tension-free closure utilizing retention sutures.

◆ Nosocomial Infections

Nosocomial infections account for >20% of hospital infections.[69] The normal physical and chemical barriers are altered by trauma, surgery, endotracheal tubes, nasogastric tubes, invasive catheters, monitoring devices, and drains.

Most common infections: pneumonia, urinary tract infection, sinusitis, and bacteremia, as well as wound infections[70]

Pneumonia

Most common nosocomial infection in the intensive care unit (ICU).[71] There is increased incidence of pneumonia with prolonged endotracheal intubation and mechanical ventilation.

Risk factors   Endotracheal intubation and aspiration[72]

Most common organisms   In ventilator-associated pneumonia, *S. aureus*.[73] Most common in the neurosurgical population: *Pseudomonas*, family Enterobacteriaceae, *Acinetobacter*.[74]

Treatment   Empiric antibiotics as recommended by the American Thoracic Society: fluoroquinolone, aminoglycoside, or third-generation cephalosporin combined with antipseudomonal and anti-MRSA agents[75]

Urinary Tract Infection

Second most common infection in the ICU.[76] UTI accounts for ~40% of all infections.[77]

Risk factors   Gender (female) and duration of use of catheter

Most common organisms   *E. coli*, proteus, *Pseudomonas*, and yeast[78]

Sinusitis

Sinusitis is associated with mechanical ventilation or use of nasogastric tubes. Bacteria can reach sinuses via facial or basilar skull fractures.

Most common organisms   *S. aureus*, gram-negative bacilli, *Pseudomonas*, and *Streptococcus*.[79] If untreated, can lead to osteomyelitis, subdural or epidural empyemas, meningitis, or abscess.[80]

Bacteremia

Bacteremia represents 13% of nosocomial ICU infections; 90% are related to central venous catheters (CVCs).[81] The alternative to a CVC is a percutaneously inserted central catheter, which decreased the incidence of complications and infections compared with central lines.[82]

Most common organisms   *S. epidermidis, S. aureus, Pseudomonas,* and *Enterobacter*[83]

Treatment   If bacteremia is suspected, replace existing CVC. Empiric antibiotics should include vancomycin plus broad gram-negative coverage.[83]

Case Management

The symptoms of the patient described in the case study are consistent with encephalitis or meningitis. Meningitis can be bacterial, viral, or other. Bacterial meningitis is associated with more neurologic changes; however, because there is no nuchal rigidity, meningitis is less likely than encephalitis. CSF studies are recommended as well as an MRI with and without contrast. The patient must be examined closely for tick bites and other changes. If there are no systemic changes, then the more likely diagnosis is *Rickettsia/Ehrlichia.* This is a small gram-negative intracellular organism transmitted by tick bites; the disease is also known as Rocky Mountain spotted fever and ehrlichiosis. The diagnosis is based on clinical information on the history of the tick bite. There may be positive specialized serological tests. Treatment is with doxycycline 100 mg bid for 10 to 14 days or chloramphenicol 50 mg/kg/day divided into 4 doses.

References

1. Winn HR. Youman's Neurological Surgery. 5th ed. Philadelphia: WB Saunders; 2004
2. Greenberg MS. Handbook of Neurosurgery. 5th ed. New York: Thieme; 2001
3. Gilbert DN, Moellening RC, Sande MA, eds. The Sanford Guide to Antimicrobial Therapy. 29th ed. Hyde Park, VT: Antimicrobial Therapy; 1999
4. Ryan MW, Antonelli PJ. Pneumococcal antibiotic resistance and rates of meningitis in children. Laryngoscope 2000;110:961–964
5. Dawson KG, Emerson JC, Burns JL. Fifteen years' experience with bacterial meningitis. Pediatr Infect Dis J 1999;18:816–822
6. Hayden RT, Frenkel LD. More laboratory testing: greater cost but not necessarily better. Pediatr Infect Dis J 2000;19:290–292
7. Mein J, Lum G. CSF bacterial antigen tests offer no advantage over Gram's stain in the diagnosis of bacterial meningitis. Pathology 1999;31:67–69
8. Maniglia AJ, Goodwin WJ, Arnold JE, et al. Intracranial abscesses secondary to nasal, sinus, and orbital infections in adults and children. Arch Otolaryngol Head Neck Surg 1989;115:1424–1429

9. Dill SR, Cobbs CG, McDonald CK. Subdural empyema: analysis of 32 cases and review. Clin Infect Dis 1995;20:372–386

10. Canale DJ. William Macewen and the treatment of brain abscesses: revisited after 100 years. J Neurosurg 1996;84:133–142

11. Nielson H, Gyldensted C, Harmsen A. Cerebral abscess: aetiology and pathogenesis, symptoms, diagnosis and treatment. A review of 200 cases from 1935–1976. Acta Neurol Scand 1982;65:609–622

12. Garvey G. Current concepts of bacterial infections of the central nervous system: bacterial meningitis and bacterial brain abscess. J Neurosurg 1983;59:735–744

13. Cohen DJ. Lung abscess: back for an encore? Postgrad Med 1982;72:215–218

14. Leib SL, Tauber MG. Pathogenesis and pathophysiology of bacterial infections. In: Scheld WM, Whitley RJ, Durak DT, eds. Infections of the Central Nervous System. 3rd ed. Philadelphia: Lippincott-Raven; 2004:301–304

15. Mamelak AN, Obana WG, Flaherty JF, Rosenblum ML. Nocardial brain abscess: treatment strategies and factors influencing outcome. Neurosurgery 1994;35: 622–631

16. Desprechins B, Stadnik T, Koerts G, Shabana W, Breucq C, Osteaux. Use of diffusion-weighted MR imaging in differential diagnosis between intracerebral necrotic tumors and cerebral abscess. AJNR 1999;20:1252–1257

17. Esiri MM. Herpes simplex encephalitis: an immunohistochemical study of the distribution of viral antigens within the brain. J Neurol Sci 1982;54:209–226

18. Wheat LJ, Batteiger BE, Sathapatayarongs B. *Histoplasma capsulatum* infections of the central nervous system: a clinical review. Medicine (Baltimore) 1990;69: 244–260

19. Vincent T, Galgiani JN, Huppert M, Salkin D. The natural history of coccidioidal meningitis: VA–Armed Forces Cooperative Studies, 1955–1958. Clin Infect Dis 1993;16:247–254

20. Boyza E, Dreyer JS, Hewitt WL, Meyer RD. Coccidioidal meningitis: an analysis of 31 cases and review of the literature. Medicine (Baltimore) 1981;60:139–172

21. Gonyea EF. The spectrum of primary blastomycotic meningitis: a review of central nervous system blastomycosis. Ann Neurol 1978;3:26–39

22. Zuger A, Lowy FD. Tuberculosis. In: Scheld WM, Whitley RJ, Durak DT, eds. Infections of the Central Nervous System. 2nd ed. Philadelphia: Lippincott-Raven; 1997:417–443

23. Traub M, Colchester AC, Kingsley DP, Swash M. Tuberculosis of the central nervous system. Q J Med 1984;53:81–100

24. Barrett-Connor E. Tuberculosis meningitis in adults. South Med J 1967;60(10): 1061–1067

25. Dastur DK, Wadia NH. Spinal meningitides with radiculomyelopathy, II: Pathology and pathogenesis. J Neurol Sci 1969;8:261–293

26. Arana-Inguez R, Lopez-Fernandez JR. Parasitosis of the nervous system with special reference to *Echinococcus*. Clin Neurosurg 1966;14:123–144

27. Nocton JJ, Steere AC. Lyme disease. Adv Int Med 1995;40:69–117

28. Pachner AR, Steere AC. The triad of neurologic manifestations of Lyme disease: meningitis, cranial neuritis, and radiculoneuritis. Neurology 1985;35:47–53

29. Durack DT. Amebic infections. In: Scheld WM, Whitley RJ, Durak DT, eds. Infections of the Central Nervous System. 2nd ed. Philadelphia: Lippincott-Raven; 1997:831–844

30. Levy RM, Bredesen DE, Rosenblum ML. Neurological manifestations of the acquired immunodeficiency syndrome (AIDS): experience at UCSF and review of the literature. J Neurosurg 1985;62:475–495

31. Simpson DM, Tagliati M. Neurologic manifestations of HIV infection. Ann Inter Med 1994;121:769–785

32. Montoya JG, Remington JS. *Toxoplasma gondii*. In: Mandell GL, Bennett JE, Dolan R, eds. Principles and Practices of Infectious Disease. 5th ed. Philadelphia: Churchill-Livingstone; 2000:2858–2892

33. Jean WC, Hall WA. Management of cranial and spinal infections. Contemp Neurosurg 1998;20:1–10

34. Levine AM. Epidemiology, clinical characteristics, and management of AIDS-related lymphoma. Hematol Oncol Clin North Am 1991;5:331–342

35. Rosenblum ML, Levy RM, Bredesen DE, So YT, Wara W, Ziegler JL. Primary central nervous system lymphomas in patients with AIDS. Ann Neurol 1988;23(Suppl): 513–516

36. Koralnik JJ, Boden D, Mai VX, Lord CI, Letvin NL. JC virus DNA load in patients with and without progressive multifocal leukoencephalopathy. Neurology 1999; 52:253–260

37. McGuire D, Barhite S, Hollander H, Miles M. JC virus DNA in CSF of HIV-infected patients: predictive value for progressive multifocal leukoencephalopathy. Ann Neurol 1995;37:395–399

38. Vago L, Cinque P, Sala E, et al. JCV-DNA and BKV-DNA in the CNS tissue and CSF of AIDS patients and normal subjects: study of 41 cases and review of the literature. J Acquir Immune Defic Syndr Hum Retrovirol 1996;12:139–146

39. Astrom K-E, Mancall EL, Richardson EP, Jr. Progressive multifocal leuko-encephalopathy: a hitherto unrecognized complication of chronic lymphatic leukemia and Hodgkin's disease. Brain 1958;81:93–110

40. Richardson EP, Jr. Progressive multifocal leukoencephalopathy. N Engl J Med 1961;265:815–823

41. Eidelberg D, Sitrel A, Vogel H, Walker D, Kleefield J, Crumpacker CS III. Progressive polyradiculopathy in AIDS. Neurology 1986;36:912–916

42. Clifford DB, Arribas JR, Storch GA, Tourtelotte W, Wippold FJ. Magnetic resonance brain imaging lacks sensitivity for AIDS-associated cytomegalovirus encephalitis. J Neurovirol 1996;2:397–403

43. McArthur JC. HIV-associated CNS syndromes. In: Bellman A, ed. Director Course 140 [4/25–5/1/1993, St. Paul, MN]: AIDS in the Central Nervous System. New York: American Academy of Neurology; 1993:5

44. Navia BA, Jordan BD, Price RW. The AIDS dementia complex, I: Clinical features. Ann Neurol 1986;19:517–524

45. Mackenzie AR, Laing RBS, Smith CC, Kaar GF, Smith FW. Spinal epidural abscess: the importance of early diagnosis and treatment. J Neurol Neurosurg Psychiatry 1998;65:209–212

46. Martin RJ, Yuan HA. Neurosurgical care of spinal epidural, subdural, and intramedullary abscesses and arachnoiditis. Orthop Clin North Am 1996;27: 125–136

47. Khanna RK, Ghaus MM, Rock JP, Rosenblum ML. Spinal epidural abscess: evaluation of 5 factors influencing outcome. Neurosurgery 1996;39:958–964

48. Hlavin ML, Kaminski HJ, Ross JS, Ganz E. Spinal epidural abscess: a 10 year perspective. Neurosurgery 1990;27:177–184

49. Obrador GT, Levenson DJ. Spinal epidural abscess in hemodialysis patients: report of 3 cases and review of the literature. Am J Kidney Dis 1996;27:75–83

50. Wheeler D, Keiser P, Rigamonti D, Keay S. Medical management of spinal epidural abscesses: case report and review. Clin Infect Dis 1992;15:22–27

51. Feldenzer JA, McKeever PE, Schaberg DR, Campbell JA, Hoff JT. The pathogenesis of spinal epidural abscess: microangiopathic studies in an experimental model. J Neurosurg 1998;69:110–114

52. Curling OD, Gower DJ, McWhorter JM. Changing concepts in spinal epidural abscess: a report of 29 cases. Neurosurgery 1990;27:185–192

53. Schmorl G, Junghanns H. The Human Spine: In Health and Disease. New York: Grune & Stratton; 1971

54. Khan IA, Vaccaro AR, Zlotolow DA. Management of vertebral diskitis and osteomyelitis. Orthopedics 1999;22:758–765

55. Sapico FL. Microbiology and antimicrobial therapy of spinal infections. Orthop Clin North Am 1996;27:9–13

56. Stausbaugh LJ. Vertebral osteomyelitis: how to differentiate it from other causes of back and neck pain. Postgrad Med J 1995;97:147–154

57. Ozuna RM, Delamarter RB. Pyogenic vertebral osteomyelitis and postsurgical disc space infections. Orthop Clin North Am 1996;27:87–94

58. Klein JD, Garfin SR. Nutritional status in the patient with spinal infection. Orthop Clin North Am 1996;27:33–36

59. Broner FA, Garland DE, Zigler JE. Spinal infections in the immunocompromised host. Orthop Clin North Am 1996;27:37–46

60. Vaccaro AR, Shah SH, Schweiter ME, Rosenfeld JF, Cotler JM. MRI description of vertebral osteomyelitis, neoplasm, and compression fracture. Orthopedics 1999;22:67–73

61. Alleyne CH, Hassan M, Zanbranski JM. The efficacy and cost of prophylactic and periprocedural antibiotics in patients with external ventricular drains. Neurosurgery 2000;47:1124–1127

62. Khanna RK, Rosenblum ML, Rock JP, Malik GM. Prolonged external ventricular drainage with percutaneous long-tunnel ventriculostomies. J Neurosurg 1995;83:791–794

63. Cummings R. Understanding external ventricular drainage. J Neurosci Nurs 1992; 24:84–87

64. Rodvold KA. Therapeutic considerations for infections caused by *Staphylococcus epidermidis*. Pharmacotherapy 1988 8(6 Pt2):145–185

65. Baltas I, Tsoulfa S, Sakellariou P, et al. Post-traumatic meningitis: bacteriology, hydrocephalus, and outcome. Neurosurgery 1994;35:422–427

66. Hand WL, Sanford JP. Post-traumatic bacterial meningitis. Ann Int Med 1970;72: 869–874

67. Yogev R. CSF shunt infections: a personal view. Pediatr Infect Dis 1985;4:113–118

68. Shektman A, Granick MS, Solomon MP, et al. Management of infected laminectomy wounds. Neurosurgery 1994;35:307–309

69. Brown R, Colodny S, Drapkin M, et al. One-day prevalence study of nosocomial infections, antibiotic usage, and selected infection control practices in adult medical/surgical ICUs in the United States. Infec Control Hosp Epidemiology April (Suppl), 1995

70. Emori TG, Gaynes RP. An overview of nosocomial infections, including the role of the microbiology laboratory. Clin Microbiol Rev 1993;6:428–446

71. Edwards J, Jarvis W. The distribution of nosocomial infections by site and pathogenin in adult and pediatric intensive care units in the United States 1986–1990. In: Program and Abstracts of the Third Decennial International Conference on Nosocomial Infections, Centers for Disease Control and the National Foundation for Infectious Diseases; 1990; Atlanta. Abstract B19

72. Sanderson PJ. The sources of pneumonia in ITU patients. Infect Control 1986;7(Suppl 2):104–106

73. George DL. Epidemiology of nosocomial pneumonia in intensive care unit patients. Clin Chest Med 1995;16:29–44

74. Rello J, Ausina V, Castella J, et al. Nosocomial respiratory tract infections in multiple trauma patients: influence of level of consciousness with implications for therapy. Chest 1992;102:525–529

75. American Thoracic Society. Hospital-acquired pneumonia in adults: diagnosis assessment of severity, initial antimicrobial therapy, and preventative strategies. A consensus statement. Am J Respir Crit Care Med 1996;153:1711–1725

76. Paradisi F, Corti G, Mangani V. Urosepsis in the critical care unit. Crit Care Clin 1998;14:165–180

77. Weinstein RA. Epidemiology and control of nosocomial infections in adult intensive care units. Am J Med 1991;91:1855–1915

78. Bergen GA, Toney JF. Infection versus colonization in the critical care unit. Crit Care Clin 1998;14:71–90

79. Westergren V, Lundblad L, Hellquist HB, et al. Ventilator-associated sinusitis: a review. Clin Infect Dis 1998;27:851–864

80. Clayman GL, Adams GL, Paugh DR, et al. Intracranial complications of paranasal sinusitis: a combined institutional review. Laryngoscope 1991;101:234–239

81. Maki D. Infections due to infusion therapy. In: Bennett J, Brachman P, eds. Hospital Infections. Boston: Little, Brown; 1992:849

82. Raad I, Davis S, Becker M, et al. Low infection rate and long durability of nontunneled Silastic catheters: a safe and cost-effective alternative for long-term venous access. Arch Intern Med 1993;153:1791–1796

83. Cunha BA. Intravenous line infections. Crit Care Clin 1998;14:339–346

25
Systemic Complications
Daniel Hutton and John D. Cantando

Case Study

A 69-year-old Hispanic female undergoes craniotomy for evacuation of a traumatic subdural hematoma at a community hospital, and is transferred on postoperative day 2 to a tertiary care trauma center for a higher level of care in the neurosurgical intensive care unit. At the original hospital, her abnormally high glucose level was not corrected, as it was considered a normal reaction to the steroids she was being treated with "for brain swelling." She arrived at the trauma center with a Glasgow Coma Scale (GCS) score of 5 and a blood pressure of 85/50. She was loaded with dilantin at the original hospital, and started on 100 mg doses every 8 hours. No neuroimaging was sent with the patient.

See page 372 for Case Management.

The neurosurgical intensive care unit (NICU) treats a variety of patients with a multitude of pathologies, ranging from aneurysms, both pre- and postop, to head and spinal cord injuries, to brain tumors. The goal of any systemic complication is the prompt diagnosis and return of adequate perfusion and oxygenation to neural tissue. Though focused on the management of neurologic injury, physicians and surgeons must maintain proper perspective of the primary tenets of intensive care medicine.

This chapter reviews the chief systemic complications associated with the NICU patient and offers recommendations to prevent their occurrence.

◆ Electrolyte Disturbances

Aberrant electrolytes are the most common complication seen in the NICU, occurring in 59.3% of the Traumatic Coma Data Bank (TCDB) register.[1] They are primarily in the category of early complications, seen from the time of admission through the first 5 days. It is therefore imperative to monitor fluid status, including total intake and output, daily body weight, and color and specific gravity of urine, so as to avoid unnecessary cerebral edema or volume contraction. Consideration must be made for patients on chronic diuretics, nasogastric or orogastric suction tubes, or with fever or diarrhea. Serum sodium and glucose are principally addressed due to their effects on serum osmolarity. Abnormalities in serum potassium are frequently encountered due to gastric suctioning, diarrhea, and medications. Along with correcting the underlying pathology, normal serum concentrations should be maintained (**Tables 25–1** and **25–2**).

◆ Hyperglycemia

Hyperglycemia usually reflects a stress reaction and can worsen outcome after traumatic brain injury.[2,3] To avoid this complication, serum glucose should be kept <110 mg/dL.

Table 25–1   Hyponatremia

Syndrome of Inappropriate Antidiuretic Hormone (SIADH)

Usually a euvolemic to slightly hypervolemic state, with urine osmolarity greater than serum osmolarity and elevated urine sodium
Diagnosis:
Serum sodium < 135 mEq/L
Serum osmolarity < 280 mOsm/L
Urine sodium > 40 mEq/L
Treatment:
Fluid restriction is paramount. Keep total fluid intake to <1000 mL/day. If volume restriction may be detrimental to other coexisting pathology, demeclocycline may be used. It is an antibiotic that partially blocks the renal collecting duct's response to ADH.
For patients with elevated ICP or actively seizing due to hyponatremia, hypertonic normal saline (3%) may be instituted.

Cerebral Salt Wasting Syndrome (CSW)

Usually a hypovolemic state, with low serum sodium, elevated urine sodium, and elevated urine sodium
Diagnosis:
Urine sodium > 40 mEq/L in the setting of a hypovolemic state
Treatment:
Replacement of intravascular volume with isotonic normal saline (0.9%) is the initial treatment of choice.
If refractory, use hypertonic saline or salt tablet per mouth or feeding tube, depending on level of consciousness.

ADH, antidiuretic hormone; ICP, intracranial pressure.

Table 25–2   Hypernatremia

Diabetes insipidus

Inability to concentrate urine due to insufficient ADH in the circulatory system

Pathophysiology based on damage to the pituitary stalk from increased ICP or shearing injury. May also be seen in patients with recent surgery in the sellar region (pituitary adenoma, craniopharyngioma, aneurysms of the circle of Willis, etc.).

Extremely grave prognostic sign

Diagnosis:

Urine output >200–250 cc/hour for 2 hours

Elevated serum sodium and other signs of volume contraction: increasing hematocrit, creatinine, urine specific gravity

Treatment:

Tenuous, due to the unwanted effect of excessive fluid exacerbating cerebral edema. Judicious doses of exogenous vasopressin are suggested to rapidly decrease the urine output and maintain vascular volume.

ADH, antidiuretic hormone; ICP, intracranial pressure.

◆ Pneumonia

Pneumonia is the second most common systemic complication in severe head injury.[1] It usually occurs 5 to 10 days following injury. It also occurs more frequently due to impaired airway reflexes, leading to greater possibility of aspiration.

Risk factors include the following:

◆ Ventilatory assistance > 24 hours
◆ Use of barbiturates for treatment of increased intracranial pressure (ICP)[4]
◆ Presence of ICP monitor[5]

The diagnosis of pneumonia includes the following:

◆ High index of suspicion
◆ Obtaining routine surveillance sputum cultures
◆ Low threshold to start broad-spectrum antibiotics

To prevent this complication, avoid neutralizing gastric pH. The use of alkaline antacids and histamine type 2 blockers increases the risk of pneumonia.[6] Sucralfate binds to negatively charged ions of damaged gastric mucosa and prevents ulcers without increasing the gastric pH.

◆ Blood Pressure

Hypotension

Patients in the NICU frequently have episodes of hypotension. In multitrauma patients, other etiologies must be entertained, necessitating examination of pulse pressure, oxygen saturation, arterial blood gases, and cardiopulmonary and abdominal compartments. In patients with severe traumatic brain injury (GCS ≤ 8), it has been shown that a single episode of systolic blood pressure (SBP) < 90 mm Hg, from injury to arrival at the hospital, doubles the mortality. In the NICU, eliminating hypotension would reduce unfavorable outcome (Glasgow Outcome Scores 1, 2, and 3) by 9.3%.[1] Additionally, patients with spinal cord injuries are prone to sustained hypotension, which, if not corrected, can lead to infarction.

To limit the effects of hypotension, the following recommendations are made:

◆ Patients with severe traumatic brain injury should have cerebral perfusion pressure (CPP) >70 mm Hg in most cases.
◆ Patients should be kept euvolemic, with a normal central venous pressure (CVP).
◆ Episodes of hypotension/suboptimal CPP should be treated first with fluids, then with vasopressors as necessary.

Spinal Cord Injuries and Hypotension

Patients with spinal cord injuries develop hypotension from a lack of sympathetic input to the vasculature, causing pooling and decreased return to the right heart, as well as unopposed parasympathetic tone to the heart, resulting in bradycardia. The goal of therapy is to maintain SBP >90 mm Hg.

The following general considerations apply to the treatment of spinal cord injuries:

◆ Maintain spinal precautions
◆ Provide adequate oxygenation
◆ Prescribe atropine for bradycardia and hypotension
◆ Continue judicious fluid management
◆ Watch for development of pulmonary edema
◆ Start vasopressors (dopamine is the vasopressor of choice)

Methylprednisolone must be given within 8 hours of injury.[6] The initial dosage is 30 mg/kg intravenous (IV) bolus over 15 minutes (rate [mL/hour] = patient's weight [kg] × 1.92). After a 45-minute pause, the maintenance dose is 5.4 mg/kg/hour (rate [mL/hour] = weight [kg] × 0.0864). The duration of maintenance therapy depends on the timing of the initial bolus. If it is given <3 hours from injury, maintenance steroids should be continued for

23 hours. If the initial dose is given 3 to 8 hours after injury, continue for 47 hours.[7]

Other investigational medications are naloxone, tirilizad mesylate, and lazaroid.[8]

Hypertension

Elevated blood pressure is of particular consequence in the NICU. Patients with unsecured aneurysms, arteriovenous malformations (AVMs), or intraparenchymal hematomas should have strict parameters for hypertension. However, hypertension associated with bradycardia and respiratory depression (Cushing's triad) is symbolic for dangerously elevated ICP pressure and demands immediate evaluation. These symptoms may be easily missed if the patient is on a ventilator or because of autonomic instability.

Intravenous Treatment of Hypertension

Nitrates, specifically, nitroglycerine and nitroprusside, may elevate ICP and should be used cautiously. They preferentially dilate peripheral vasculature, creating a cerebral steal phenomenon. Prolonged use of nitroprusside may lead to thiocyanate toxicity.

Labetalol blocks α_1 and β_1, and β_2 receptors. It has no effect on ICP. Labetalol may be used in controlled congestive heart failure (CHF): no coronary steal effect. It is contraindicated in asthma. The maximum dose is 300 mg/day.

Enalaprilat is an angiontensin converting enzyme (ACE) inhibitor that acts within 15 minutes. Side effects include hyperkalemia.

◆ Thromboembolism

Deep venous thrombosis (DVT) is a common complication in the NICU. Although no hypercoagulable state is usually present, other risk factors, including endothelial damage and venous stasis, are due to immobilization or predisposing trauma. DVT may be as prevalent as 58% if no prophylaxis is used.[9] Other risk factors include spinal cord injury; pelvic, femur, or tibia fractures; surgery; blood transfusion; and older age.[9]

Prophylaxis

Sequential compression stockings and low-dose heparin have been found to decrease the incidence of thromboembolism from 8.98 to 2.9%. Heparin is relatively contraindicated in patients with traumatic brain injury; therefore, compression stockings are generally advocated. Vena cava filters are advocated for first-line prophylaxis. However, with repeated embolization, filters may provide a more reliable means to protect against hypoxia.

◆ Coagulopathy

Serologic markers for disseminated intravascular coagulation (fibrinogen split products) and degree of traumatic brain injury have been positively correlated.[10] The most common site for diffuse intravascular thrombosis is the central nervous system, often resulting in necrosis.[11] Microvascular and radiographically evident petechial hemorrhages and contusions are thought to be the result of disseminated intravascular coagulation.

◆ Anemia

Optimal hematocrit is not well established. Patients with multisystem trauma or prolonged stays in the NICU are at greater risk of developing anemia of various etiologies. All primary sources of bleeding should be aggressively sought. Patients with blunt chest or abdominal injury should be evaluated for hemothorax and retroperitoneal bleeding, respectively. Other rare causes include medication reaction but are usually accompanied by hemolysis. A hematocrit greater than 33% is generally used to optimize cerebral blood flow.[12]

◆ Fever

Fever is a potent vasodilator and can raise ICP and cerebral metabolic requirement for oxygen ($CMRO_2$). Infectious causes should be aggressively sought and treated. Prophylactic antibiotics are generally unwarranted, with the exception of ventricular catheters. Antipyretics and cooling blankets should be used.

◆ Hypoxia

In ventilated patients, common etiologies of hypoxia must be aggressively determined. To maintain adequate cerebral and systemic oxygenation, oxygen-carrying capacity, acid–base balance, and pulmonary pathologies should be determined. The initial evaluation should include hemoglobin/hematocrit, arterial blood gases, chest x-ray, D-dimer, and venous duplex. If there is further suspicion of pulmonary embolism, spiral chest computed tomography (CT), ventilation/perfusion (V/Q) scan, or the gold standard pulmonary angiography should be expedited.

◆ Sepsis

Sepsis is diagnosed by positive blood cultures along with meeting the criteria for systemic inflammatory response syndrome (SIRS). SIRS can result from a wide variety of etiologies, including infections, trauma, and stress. The criteria for the diagnosis of SIRS are heart rate >90, temperature >38°C or <36°C, tachnypnea >20 breaths/minute, and white blood (cell) count (WBC) >12,000 cells/mm^3 or <4000 cells/mm^3.

Sepsis results in a derangement of fluid balance via an array of pathologies. Insensible water loss results from elevated temperatures. Depleted intravascular volume is multifactorial, but principally due to increased microvascular permeability[13] and increased venous compliance, resulting in pooling.

Diagnosis hinges on a thorough examination of the patient and guided laboratory studies. Examination of the patient's skin for decubitus ulcers or infiltrated IVs or central lines is crucial. Removal of all indwelling central catheters, peripheral lines, and Foley catheters with culture is paramount for removing a possible nidus of infection. A chest x-ray should be performed to evaluate for pneumonia or empyema.

Initial empiric treatment should be employed after cultures are taken. Broad-spectrum treatment with two or more antibiotics may be started and tailored once final cultures and sensitivities have returned. Aggressive hydration is also a cornerstone of treatment. When crystalloid fluids are not adequate to maintain perfusion, dopamine is typically the initial vasopressor/inotrope of choice. Depending on the severity of sepsis, a Swan-Ganz catheter is often necessary to assess fluid volume, vascular resistance, and cardiac output.

◆ Gastrointestinal Bleed

Ulceration of gastric mucosa is commonly seen with traumatic brain injury. Although the mechanism is not fully understood, most experts theorize that an excess of gastrin with the resultant increase in gastric acidity weakens the gastric mucosa. Kamada et al[13] found that endoscopic evaluation of gastric mucosa demonstrates damage within the first 24 hours, with 17% of these erosions progressing to systemically significant hemorrhages. The severity of brain injury is directly related to the development of gastric bleeding.[14] Other risk factors for gastric bleeding include respiratory failure, burns >25% body surface area, hypotension, sepsis, jaundice, peritonitis, coagulopathy, and hepatic failure. Prophylaxis includes antacids, which neutralize gastric acidity but are time consuming; histamine type 2 blockers, which block acid production but are potentially sedating and have a possible side effect of thrombocytopenia; and sucralfate, which strengthens gastric mucosa; does not alter gastrin, acid production, or pH; and produces less nosocomial pneumonia association.

◆ Seizures

In those patients with severe head injury, seizures occur in ~15%.[12] At times seizures may be difficult to monitor in the NICU because of sedatives and paralytics. There should be a heightened clinical suspicion to detect and subsequently initiate treatment. Therefore, if clinically warranted, continuous electroencephalography is the method of choice for detection. Though not associated with worse morbidity or mortality, seizures can potentially impair jugular venous oxygen saturation ($SjvO_2$) if cerebral blood flow is already compromised.[13] Prophylaxis against post-traumatic seizures is controversial and should be discontinued after 7 days.[2,15]

Case Management

The surgical evacuation of the subdural hematoma is only the beginning of the sophisticated management of this patient. She needs to have her steroids discontinued immediately, as they have no role in traumatic brain injury. She should have a repeat CT head scan to get a good baseline of her intracranial picture, and because her GCS is 8 or less, she will need a ventriculostomy/intracranial pressure monitor inserted after confirmation that she is not coagulopathic. It is essential that her hypotension be corrected because it is associated with poor prognosis. As hyperglycemia can be damaging to the brain, using an insulin drip, her glucose level should be corrected to an ideal level of < 110 mg/dL. After a dilantin level is sent, the patient should be continued on 100 mg dilantin every 8 hours for a total of 7 days. The patient will need aggressive cerebral partial pressure management, serial CT head imaging, and close follow-up of her electrolyte levels.

References

1. Temkin NR, Dikmen SS, Wilensky AJ, et al. A Randomized, double-blind study of phenytoin for prevention of posttraumatic seizures. N Engl J Med 1990;323: 497–502
2. Cherian L, Goodman JC, Robertson CS. Hyperglycemia increases brain injury caused by secondary ischemia after cortical impact injury to rats. Crit Care Med 1997;25:1378–1383
3. Cherian L, Hannay HJ, Vagner G, et al. Hyperglycemia increases neurologic damage and behavioral deficits from post-traumatic secondary insults. J Neurotrauma 1998;15:307–322
4. Braun SR, Levin AB, Clark KL. Role of corticosteroids in the development of pneumonia in mechanically ventilated head-injured victims. Crit Care Med 1986;14: 198–201
5. Born JD, Albert A, Hans P, et al. Relative prognostic value of best motor response and brain stem reflexes in patients with severe head injury. Neurosurgery 1985;16:595–601

6. Driks MR, Craven DE, Celli BR, et al. Nosocomial pneumonia in intubated patients given sucralfate as compared with antacids or histamine type 2 blockers: the role of gastric colonization. N Engl J Med 1987;317:1376–1382

7. Bracken MB, Shepard MJ, Collins WF, et al. A randomized, controlled trial of methylprednisolone or naloxone in the treatment of acute spinal cord injury. N Engl J Med 1990;322:1405–1411

8. Bracken MB, Shepard MS, Holford TR, et al. Administration of methylprednisolone for 24 or 48 hours or tirilizad mesylate for 48 hours in the treatment of acute spinal cord injury. JAMA 1997;277:1597–1604

9. Geerts WH, Code KI, Jay RM, et al. A prospective study of venous thromboembolism after major trauma. N Engl J Med 1994;331:1601–1606

10. Kauffman HH, Hui KS, Mattson JC, et al. Clinicopathological correlations of disseminated intravascular coagulation in patients with head injury. Neurosurgery 1984;15:32–42

11. Hinshaw LB. Sepsis/septic shock: participation of the microcirculation. An abbreviated review. Crit Care Med 1996;24:1072

12. Jennett B. Early traumatic epilepsy. Incidence and signifigance after nonmissile head injuries. Arch Neurol 1974;30:394–398

13. Kamada T, Fusamoto H, Kawano S, et al. Gastrointestinal bleeding following head injury: a clinical study of 433 cases. J Trauma 1977;17:44–47

14. Brain Trauma Foundation, American Association of Neurological Surgeons, and Joint Section on Neurotrauma and Critical Care. Role of antiseizure prophylaxis following head injury. J Neurotrauma 2000;17:549–553

15. Piek J, Chesnut RM, Marshall LF, et al. Extracranial complications of severe head injury. J Neurosurg 1992;77:901–907

Section V

Specific Diseases

26
Disease-Specific Phenomena

John D. Cantando and Javed Siddiqi

Case Study

A 56-year-old woman of Vietnamese origin presented to the emergency room, complaining of the "worst headache" of her life. Computed tomography (CT) head was suggestive of a right-sided subarachnoid hemorrhage, and a cerebral angiogram confirmed a middle cerebral artery aneurysm. The patient had successful surgical clipping of the aneurysm. Postoperatively, she had a slowly declining sodium level, which continued downwards despite fluid restriction for suspected overhydration during surgery versus a mild case of syndrome of inappropriate antidiuretic hormone (SIADH). The patient remained clinically stable.

See page 383 for Case Management.

◆ Cerebral Vasospasm after Subarachnoid Hemorrhage

Mechanical narrowing or spasm of the lumen of cerebral vessels results in decreased blood flow, leading to ischemia and infarction. It is most commonly seen after aneurysmal subarachnoid hemorrhage (SAH), but it is also seen after traumatic SAH, intraventricular hemorrhage, and SAH of unknown etiology. It is the most significant cause of morbidity and mortality in patients surviving the initial aneurysm rupture. There are two components: clinical vasospasm (delayed ischemic neurologic deficit) and radiographic vasospasm.

Characteristics of Vasospasm

The onset of cerebral vasospasm (CVS) almost never occurs before the third day after SAH and typically will have a peak incidence between days 6 and 10. Clinical spasm usually is resolved by the end of the second week posthemorrhage, although the onset can occur as late as day 17.

Radiographic CVSs are seen in 30 to 70% of angiograms,[1,2] as opposed to clinical spasms, which are seen in ~20 to 30% of patients after SAH. Radiographic spasm may occur in the absence of clinical spasm and vice versa (i.e., patients may have a small vessel spasm, causing neurologic deficit, but an angiogram may not be able to detect it). Mild CVSs are usually reversible, whereas severe CVSs can result in permanent deficits and death in 7% of patients. CVSs that occur early are associated with the worst neurologic deficits.

In 1980, Fisher et al[3] revealed a correlation between the thickness of the subarachnoid blood on CT scan and the risk of developing CVS. Patients classified as Fisher III (localized clot and/or vertical layer >1 mm thick within the subarachnoid space) are at greatest risk of developing symptomatic CVS. Twenty-three of the 24 patients in Fisher et al's study who were grade III developed clinical CVS.

Diagnosis of Vasospasm

Diagnosis of vasospasm is primarily clinical, but it can be confirmed and monitored with various radiologic and neurodiagnostic tests. Clinically, there is usually a gradual worsening of headache, confusion, and meningismus, and possibly focal neurologic deficit. Clinical CVS in the anterior cerebral artery territory is more common than that of the middle cerebral artery (MCA).

Transcranial Doppler (TCD) ultrasound is the most utilized method of diagnosing and monitoring clinical CVSs. It measures blood velocity in major intracranial arteries (ICAs), which is used to determine if there may be arterial narrowing. Not only the actual velocity but also the relationship between the relative velocity of the ICA and the velocity of flow in the internal carotid artery is important. This relationship is referred to as the Lindergaard ratio. It is commonly used to express the difference in velocity between the MCA and the ICA, but it is also used in velocity measurements of all large intracranial vessels. The Lindergaard ratio may help to distinguish vasospasm from hyperemia (**Table 26–1**).[4]

Cerebral angiogram can detect vessel narrowing in larger vessels. Half of the patients with angiographic spasm will be asymptomatic. Angiograms may miss spasm of small arteries in patients who are symptomatic.

Xenon 133, xenon CT, single-photon emission computed tomography (SPECT), and positron emission tomography (PET) scanning are among the other methods used to detect low-flow arterial states. However, these may not be routinely available at many institutions, and they may not be practical

Table 26–1   Transcranial Doppler Ultrasound Velocities[1–5]

100 cm/second suggests initial changes in blood flow.
100–200 cm/second correlates with mild vasospasm.
200 cm/second or greater is associated with severe spasm.
LR 3–6 correlates with mild CVS.
LR > 6 correlates with severe CVS.

CVS, cerebral vasospasm; LR, Lindergaard ratio.

for daily or frequent use. TCD ultrasound is less time consuming, less costly, and can be used daily to monitor CVS and its response to treatment.

Treatment of Vasospasm

Treatment of CVS is aimed at preventing and reversing ischemic insults. Hypovolemia can hasten the onset of CVS, and spasm can be lessened or prevented by ensuring that post-SAH patients are adequately hydrated. Early surgery for clipping of aneurysms can allow for more aggressive hyperdynamic therapy and also can allow for removal of cisternal clot, reducing the incidence of CVS.

Currently, the use of nimodipine as a neuroprotectant and, alternatively, nicardipine has been found to offer protection by improving blood rheology, preventing calcium influx into injured cells, and acting as an antiplatelet aggregator.

Hyperdynamic, or "triple-H," (hypertensive, hypervolemic, and hemodilution) therapy is the mainstay of treatment in patients with surgically or endovascularly treated aneurysms. A mild form of this type of therapy can be used in unsecured aneurysms, but it may cause the aneurysm to rerupture. Hyperdynamic therapy should not be started if there is a new cerebral hemorrhage, a new large infarct, or severe cerebral edema.[5]

Some experts advocate starting therapy prior to the onset of CVS to combat the common occurrence of hypovolemia in patients with SAH.[6] In a randomized control trial, Lennihan et al[7] found that the prevention of hypovolemia rather than the promotion of hypervolemia was critical in the prevention of cerebral ischemia. Induction of hypervolemia can be done with isotonic/hypertonic crystalloids and with colloids (albumin) or blood.

After the ruptured aneurysms have been clipped or coiled, the neurosurgeon has greater freedom to use certain medicines to raise blood pressure. Vasopressors can be used to augment blood pressure to improve cerebral perfusion. In this approach, increase blood pressure in 10 to 15% increments until neurologic function shows improvement. This may require increasing systolic blood pressure (SBP) to 240 mm Hg or mean arterial pressure (MAP) to 150 mm Hg (for clipped aneurysms). Wean pressors upon improvement and allow blood pressure to fall to sustain an acceptable neurologic function. Targets for central venous pressure (CVP) are 6 to 8 mm Hg; pulmonary capillary wedge pressure (PCWP), 16 to 18 mm Hg.

Once a patient has evidence of symptomatic vasospasm, he or she should be treated with hyperdynamic therapy for at least 14 days or until symptoms resolve and there is no angiographic evidence of vasospasm.

Complications of triple-H therapy include exacerbation of cerebral edema, pulmonary edema, intracerebral hemorrhage (ICH), worsened infarctions, rebleeding of unsecured aneurysms, myocardial infarction, and problems related to pulmonary artery catheter.

Transluminal Balloon Angioplasty

Transluminal balloon angioplasty allows the neurosurgeon to direct mechanical opening of a vessel using neuroendovascular techniques. It is reserved for patients with clinical vasospasm not improving using hyper-dynamic therapy and with radiographic evidence of vasospasm. The best results are seen if the procedure is done within 24 hours of neurologic decline.[8–11] Up to 70% of patients can have clinical and lasting improve-ment.

Angioplasty should be avoided if there is a new cerebral hemorrhage or a large area of infarction because of the risk of re-perfusion injury. Furthermore, angioplasty, if clinical and radiologic benefits do not persist, may need to be repeated.

Endovascular use of intra-arterial papaverine is sometimes recom-mended; however, the clinical benefits are short-lived. It is helpful in placing angioplasty balloons and in treating vessels inaccessible to angioplasty catheters.

Recent investigations measuring cerebral lactate to pyruvate ratios and brain tissue oxygen tension before and after balloon angioplasty show data that may be able to provide an early diagnosis of CVS and allow monitoring of threatened cerebral tissue regions.[12]

◆ Cerebral Salt Wasting Syndrome and Subarachnoid Hemorrhage

Hyponatremia is a frequent finding in the neurosurgical intensive care unit (NICU) patient, and it can be a common cause of neurologic deterioration in a patient with aneurysmal SAH, especially in anterior communicating artery aneurysms. In the 1950s, when the condition was first described, NICU patients with hyponatremia were initially thought to have cerebral salt wasting (CSW); but as the description of SIADH became more popular later in that decade, CSW fell out of favor, and many hyponatremic patients with CSW were treated with fluid restriction.[13] CSW is associated with hyponatremia and extracellular volume depletion. Harrigan[14] summarized the evidence in favor of CSW as follows:

1. A negative salt balance is present with hyponatremia in many patients with intracranial disease.
2. These patients were found to be volume depleted, which is incompati-ble with SIADH.
3. They improved with volume and salt replacement.

Clinical manifestations of hyponatremia include confusion, lethargy, seizures, and coma. It is likely that both humoral and neural mechanisms are involved in the renal wasting of sodium. Atrial natriuretic factor involve-ment is likely, but it does not appear to be the primary factor. No solid lab-oratory studies are available to reliably distinguish SIADH and CSW. In fact, laboratory tests may be identical.

Findings in CSW

Laboratory findings include

◆ Hyponatremia
◆ Elevated urine sodium
◆ Increased blood urea nitrogen/creatinine (BUN/Cr) ratio
◆ Serum osmolality normal or increased
◆ Hematocrit normal or increased
◆ Serum uric acid normal

Clinical findings include

◆ CVP decreased (<6 cm)
◆ PCWP decreased (<8 mm Hg)
◆ Negative salt balance
◆ Decreased plasma volume (<35 cc/kg)
◆ Signs and symptoms of dehydration
◆ Decreased weight and orthostatic hypotension

Treatment of CSW

It is crucial to make a correct diagnosis, because treatment plans for CSW and SIADH are opposite. Patients with cerebral injury who are already hypovolemic will be at greater risk of ischemia and infarction. In one study, the administration of normal saline 50 cc/kg/day and oral salt 12 g/day was shown to be effective in restoring serum within 3 days.[15] Three percent saline is also used for severe hyponatremia, especially if the patient is symptomatic. Correction of sodium should occur no faster than 0.5 to 1.0 mEq/L/hour, and maximum correction should not exceed 20 mEq/L in the first 48 hours. Correct initially to a serum sodium level of 130 to 134 mEq/L and the remainder of the salt deficit over 1 or 2 days.

◆ Hyperdynamic Syndrome after Carotid Endarterectomy

Hyperdynamic syndrome following carotid endarterectomy (CEA) occurs in ~0.3 to 1.0% of patients, and usually >24 hours after surgery. Heralding signs and symptoms include ipsilateral frontal headache within the first week (better with sitting), focal motor seizures that are characteristically difficult to control,[16] and etiology thought to be the return of blood flow to areas previously rendered chronically ischemic and with poor autoregulation.[17,18]

Risk factors for hyperdynamic syndrome are

- Carotid stenosis > 90%
- Poor collateral hemisphereic flow
- Contralateral carotid occlusion
- Evidence of ipsilateral chronic hypoperfusion
- Pre- and postoperative hypertension
- Preexisting ipsilateral cerebral infarction (especially recent)
- Preoperative anticoagulation or antiplatelet treatment

CT Findings of hyperdynamic syndrome may show mild edema, petechial hemorrhages, and ICH ipsilateral to the side of the CEA.

◆ Intracerebral Hemorrhage after Carotid Endarterectomy

ICH is the most catastrophic complication of the hyperperfusion syndrome. It occurs in ~0.5 to 0.7% of patients after CEA and accounts for ~20% of perioperative strokes. In one study, all ICHs occurred between days 1 and 10 postprocedure.[19] The cause of ICH is most likely the blood–brain barrier being overcome by a rapid increase in the cerebral blood flow that occurs after CEA. The mortality is ~30%, with the highest risk factor appearing to be relief of high-grade stenosis.

Treatment of ICH after CEA

Once ICH is seen, stop all anticoagulation, and control blood pressure. If ICH is accompanied by mass effect and progressive deficit, and there is an accessible lesion, a craniotomy should be performed with evacuation of the hematoma.

In general, neurologic deficit within the first 12 hours after CEA is almost always due to thromboembolic phenomena from the CEA site. The CEA site should be urgently reexplored. However, deficits occurring 12 to 24 hours after CEA could be from hyperperfusion syndrome and should be investigated with a noncontrasted CT of the brain and cerebral angiography. Anticoagulation or antiplatelet therapy in the latter group of patients could result in catastrophic consequences if started prior to knowing if there is an ICH.

◆ Arteriovenous Malformations and Rebleeding

Cerebral arteriovenous malformations (AVMs) can be treated by open surgical resection, radiosurgically, endovascularly, or a combination of the three. Depending on the size and flow characteristics, there can be various degrees of adjacent brain vascular steal, hemorrhage, chronic hypoperfusion, and low-grade ischemia.

The most common cause for postoperative ICH after AVM surgery is retained AVM, which needs to be meticulously searched for. However, hemorrhagic complications can occur after total extirpation of cerebral AVMs.[20-32] AVMs that are large and with the highest flow rates are at greatest risk. The incidence is 0.01 to 0.10%.

There are two theories to explain rebleeding. The normal perfusion pressure breakthrough theory, as outlined by Spetzler[22] in 1978, says that chronic hypoperfusion leads to impaired autoregulation around the AVM; after excision, the return of normal pressure causes local hyperemia and capillary leakage. The occlusive hyperemia theory, first proposed by al-Rodhan et al[29] in 1993, maintains that the obstruction of the venous outflow system of adjacent brain causes passive hyperemia and a stagnant arterial flow in the former AVM feeders.

Exact pathophysiological and hemodynamic mechanisms are not fully understood, and it is likely that combinations of the above theories in conjunction with a yet unidentified mechanism are at play.

The treatment of ICH after fully resected AVM surgery may require evacuation of ICH, careful blood pressure management, and antiedema medication. Adequate hydration and blood volume since dehydration can promote further venous thrombosis. Serum hematocrit <35 is recommended. If the patient is in poor neurologic condition, barbiturate coma may be helpful by globally reducing blood flow and allowing the normal brain to develop normal autoregulation.

Case Management

While this patient was almost certainly treated postoperatively with hypertension, hemodilution, and hypervolemia (i.e., triple H) therapy, iatrogenic overhydration is an uncommon etiology of hyponatremia in aneurysmal subarachnoid hemorrhage patients. CSW is the most common cause of hyponatremia in this patient population, though SIADH is an important condition to exclude since it can mimic CSW and because the treatments for SIADH and CSW are opposites. The patient should be treated with 3% saline IV, 30 cc/hour, and the sodium level followed closely for correction. If the sodium level does not increase within 24 hours, or if the sodium level continues to drop, a Swan-Ganz catheter may be necessary to assess the patient's fluid status. Hyponatremia in SIADH is associated with fluid retention or hypervolemia; hyponatremia in CSW is associated with euvolemia.

References

1. Kassell NF, Sasaki T, Colohan AR, et al. Cerebral vasopasm following aneurysmal SAH. Stroke 1985;16:562–572
2. Heros R, Zervas NT, Varsos V, et al. Cerebral vasospasm after SAH: an update. Ann Neurol 1983;14:599–608
3. Fisher CM, Kistler JP, Davis JM, et al. Relation of cerebral vasospasm to SAH: visuatomographic scanning. Neurosurgery 1980;6:1–9
4. Grosset DG, Straiton J, McDonald I, et al. Use of transcranial Doppler sonography to predict development of delayed ischemic deficit after subarachnoid hemorrhage. J Neurosurg 1993;78:183–187
5. Shimoda M, Oda S, Tsugane R, et al. Intracranial complications of hypervolemic therapy in patients with delayed ischemic deficit attributed to vasospasm. J Neurosurg 1993;78:423–429
6. Solomon RA, Fink ME, Lennihan L, et al. Early aneurysm surgery and prophylactic hypervolemic hypertensive therapy for the treatment of aneurysmal subarachnoid hemorrhage. Neurosurgery 1988;23:699–704
7. Lennihan L, Mayer SA, Fink ME, et al. Effect of hypervolemic therapy on cerebral blood flow after SAH: a randomized trial. Stroke 2000;31:383–391
8. Newell DW, Eskridge JM, Mayberg MR, et al. Angioplasty for the treatment of symptomatic vasospasm following SAH. J Neurosurg 1989;71:654–660
9. Polin RS, Coenen V, Hansen C, et al. Efficacy of transluminal angioplasty for the management of symptomatic cerebral vasospasm following aneurysmal SAH. J Neurosurg 2000;92:284–290
10. Bejjani GK, Bank WO, Olan WJ, et al. The efficacy and safety of angioplasty for cerebral vasospasm after SAH. Neurosurgery 1998;42:979–986
11. Rosenwasser RH, Armonda RA, Thomas JE, et al. Therapeutic modalities for the management of cerebral vasospasm: timing of endovascular options. Neurosurgery 1999;44:975–980
12. Hoelper BM, Hoffman E, Sporleder R, et al. Transluminal balloon angioplasty improves brain tissue oxygenation and metabolism in severe vasospasm after aneurysmal SAH: case report. Neurosurgery 2003;52:1970–1976
13. Cort JH. Cerebral salt wasting. Lancet 1974:752–754
14. Harrigan MR. Cerebral salt wasting syndrome: a review. Neurosurgery 1996;38: 152–160
15. Sivakumar V, Rajshekhar V, Chandy MJ. Management of neurosurgical patients with hyponatremia and natriuresis. Neurosurgery 1994;34:269–274
16. Kieburtz K, Ricotta TJ, Moxley RT III. Seizures following carotid endarterectomy. Arch Neurol 1990;47:568–570
17. Riles TS, Imparato AM, Jacobowitz GR, et al. The cause of perioperative stroke after carotid endarterectomy. J Vasc Surg 1994;19:206–216
18. Pomposelli FB, Lamparello PJ, Riles TS, et al. Intracranial hemorrhage after carotid endarterectomy. J Vasc Surg 1988;7:248–255
19. Sundt TM. Occlusive Cerebrovascular Disease. Philadelphia: WB Saunders; 1987
20. Batjer HH, Devous MD, Seibert GB, et al. Intracranial AVM: relationship between clinical factors and surgical complications. Neurosurgery 1989;24:75–79
21. Batjer HH, Devous MD, Meyer YJ, et al. Cerebrovascular hemodynamics in AVM complicated by normal perfusion pressure breakthrough. Neurosurgery 1988; 22:503–509
22. Spetzler RF, Wilson CB, Weinstein P, et al. Normal perfusion pressure breakthrough theory. Clin Neurosurg 1978;25:651–672
23. Spetzler RF, Hargraves RW, McCormick PW, et al. Relationship of perfusion pressure and size to risk of hemorrhage from AVMs. J Neurosurg 1992;76:918–923
24. Batjer HH, Purdy PD, Giller CA, et al. Evidence of redistribution of cerebral blood flow during treatment for an intracranial AVM. Neurosurgery 1989;25:599–605
25. Morgan MK, Johnston IH, Hallinan TM, et al. Complications of surgery for AVMs of the brain. J Neurosurg 1993;78:176–182

26. Sekhon LHS, Morgan MK, Spence I, et al. Normal perfusion pressure breakthrough: the role of the capillaries. J Neurosurg 1997;86:519–524

27. Pollock BE. Occlusive hyperemia: a radiosurgical phenomenon? Neurosurgery 2000;47:1178–1184

28. Schaller C, Urbach H, Schramm J, et al. Role of venous drainage in cerebral AVM surgery, as related to the development of postoperative hyperperfusion injury. Neurosurgery 2002;51:921–929

29. al-Rodhan NRF, Sundt TM, Piepgras DG, et al. Occlusive hyperemia: a theory for the hemodynamic complications following resection of intracerebral AVMs. J Neurosurg 1993;78:167–175

30. Young WL, Pile-Spellman J, Prohovnik I, et al. Evidence for adaptive autoregulatory displacement in hypotensive cortical territories adjacent to AVMs. Neurosurgery 1994;34:601–611

31. Young WL, Kader A, Orstein E, et al. Cerebral hyperemia after AVM resection is related to "breakthrough" complications but not to feeding artery pressure. Neurosurgery 1996;38:1085–1095

32. Roost DV, Schramm J. What factors are related to impairment of cerebrovascular reserve after AVM resection? A cerebral blood flow study using xenon enhanced computed tomography. Neurosurgery 2001;48:709–717

27

Unique Pediatric Neurosurgical Intensive Care Unit Issues

Lynn M. Serrano and Dan Miulli

Case Study

A 5-year-old girl falls off a golf cart and sustains what appears to be a minor head injury. She is assessed in the emergency room by neurosurgery and found to have some memory loss and mild confusion. A computed tomography (CT) scan of the head shows minimal frontal contusions bilaterally. She is admitted to the pediatric intensive care unit for observation, and a repeat CT scan of the head the next day. The patient deteriorates neurologically overnight, and a Stat CT scan of the head shows the contusions unchanged, but significant brain edema.

See page 397 for Case Management.

Although many physicians treat children as "little adults," a child's physiological state is different than an adult's, both metabolically and electrophysiologically. It should also be noted that children are in a constant state of growth that disrupts their equilibrium and necessitates adjustments. For these reasons, as well as because of the variety of disease pathologies, the treatment of children, particularly in the pediatric neurosurgical intensive care unit (NICU), requires extensive training and a degree of familiarity and comfort. Comanagement of the patient with a pediatrician or intensivist is recommended.[1] Pediatric neurosurgical procedures, barring an emergency, should preferably be performed with a neurosurgeon well experienced in treating children. There are special neurosurgical considerations when treating the pediatric population in an intensive care situation.[2,3]

◆ General Care Guidelines for Pediatric NICU Patients

The lack of familiarity with and misunderstanding of necessary medical treatment often frighten children and their families. Any child under the age of 16 years should be placed in the pediatric ward. Special visitation should be allowed by close family members to comfort the child. Early involvement of a child life specialist or social worker is encouraged to help with expectations and transitions, as well as to follow up on concerns. Several studies confirm the benefit of a location within the ward of a "safe haven." This is usually the playroom or family room. Within this safe haven there should be no medical conversations, patient care checks, or treatments.[4–6]

◆ Intravenous Fluids and Electrolytes

Intracellular fluid, as a percentage of total body water, is ~30% at birth and increases to 40% by 1 year of life. Adequate fluid and electrolyte maintenance is needed for general health maintenance, as well as for recovery from neurologic injury (**Table 27–1**).[7]

There are two ways to calculate baseline fluid requirements in children.[8] The "kg method" is based on the weight of the patient, as follows:

◆ For the first 10 kg of body weight: 100 mL/kg/day *plus*
◆ For the second 10 kg of body weight: 50 mL/kg/day *plus*
◆ For the weight above 20 kg: 20 mL/kg/day

An alternative method for determining baseline intravenous (IV) fluids in children is the "meter squared method," which is as follows:

◆ Maintenance fluids are 1500 mL/m²/day.
◆ Divide by 24 to get the flow rate per hour.
◆ To calculate the surface area, use the "rule of sixes" (see **Table 27–2**) or a formal body surface area chart or equation (see discussion in Nutrition section).[8]

The healthy and ideal fluid and electrolyte status of any patient is normovolemic with normal chemical balance. Of special consideration is brain injury or parenchymal edema from trauma or disease process. Like adult patients, pediatric patients with brain injury need to stay normal volemic to prevent brain edema. Sodium should stay on the high end of normal and

Table 27–1   Pediatric Electrolyte Requirements

Electrolyte	Requirement
Sodium	3–4 mEq/kg/day
Potassium	2–3 mEq/kg/day
Glucose	100–200 mg/kg/hour

Source: Data from Gomella LG. Clinician's Pocket Reference. Stamford, CT: Appleton & Lange; 1997.

Table 27–2　"Rule of Sixes" for Estimating Body Surface Area in Children

Weight (lb)	Body Surface Area (m²)
3	0.1
6	0.2
12	0.3
18	0.4
24	0.5
30	0.6
36	0.7
42	0.8
48	0.9
60	1.0
Each additional 10 lb	Add 0.1
>100	Treat as adult

Source: Data from Fuhrman BP. Pediatric Critical Care. St. Louis, MO: CV Mosby; 1998.

glucose on the low end to decrease the risk of edema in patients with a broken blood–brain barrier. This rule of thumb does not hold true in endocrinological or systemic comorbidities or in spinal shock patients; these cases should treat the underlying pathology directly.[9]

◆ Respiratory Maintenance

As with adults, pulmonary function and stability must be maintained in the pediatric NICU patient. Data regarding neurologic injury secondary to hypoxia within children are sparse. In general, adult guidelines should be followed, including oxygen saturation maintenance >95% and a minimum hemoglobin and hematocrit levels of 10.0 and 33.0, respectively, realizing that the normal pediatric values vary with age but are not much higher than these minimums. Children are much more sensitive to hemodynamic shifts than adults.[10–13]

The indications for endotracheal intubation are vast. The most obvious, of course, is respiratory distress or failure of any etiology. With pediatric NICU patients specifically, damage to the central nervous system (CNS) from infection, hemorrhage, trauma, hydrocephalus, or mass lesions can lead to the need for mechanical ventilation. Also, uncooperative patients, due to age, disease pathology, or closed head injury, may require temporary intubation to assist in ongoing care, including diagnosis, imaging, and treatment. Patients with cervical spine injuries should be intubated via an inline technique to minimize the risk of additional neurologic deficit. Those patients with possible or diagnosed facial trauma or anterior skull fractures should be intubated with direct visualization through the oral or nasal cavity as appropriate to minimize possible brain penetration, additional damage, or misplacement of the tubing.

Patients with raised intracranial pressure (ICP) regardless of etiology may benefit from intubation. Care should be taken to intubate these patients, as the procedure itself may increase cerebral blood flow and subsequently ICP. Adequate sedation may help alleviate this problem. Under normal circumstances, cerebral oxygen requirements are coupled with cerebral blood flow, and are increased with temperature, activity, agitation, seizure, and injury. Blood flow will increase as the partial pressure of oxygen in arterial blood (PaO_2) falls below 60 or as the partial pressure of carbon dioxide in arterial blood ($PaCO_2$) increases. NICU patients require higher PaO_2 levels and low to normal $PaCO_2$ levels to optimize recovery. In an acute neurologic decline, a temporary period of mild hyperventilation may help minimize edema and provide the necessary time for definitive diagnostic or treatment measures, but it should never be used as maintenance treatment of elevated ICP.[10,11]

A stepwise approach should be taken when intubating pediatric NICU patients. Of course, adequate sedation and pain management are necessary, as discussed earlier. The equipment should be prepared and set up at the bedside. Vital signs should be recorded every 2 minutes. Provide 100% oxygen prior to starting the procedure (and consider assisted hyperventilation if applicable). Assess the patient for a possible difficult airway and familiarize yourself with the patient's cricoid and neck curvature. Always consider the possible need for inline or fiberoptic intubation after traumatic injuries or unknown spinal cord status. If there is associated cardiovascular compromise or hypovolemia, use diazepam or midazolam and/or fentanyl, plus lidocaine and vecuronium or another relaxant. Without these associated conditions, you can replace the diazepam/midazolam and fentanyl with thiopental. When adequate medication effect is achieved, the laryngoscopy or endotracheal intubation can be completed.

Arterial lines should be placed on all intubated patients to provide not only reliable, easily attainable blood pressure parameters but also arterial access for blood gas analysis. Arterial blood gas analysis should be performed with every ventilator adjustment, any clinical change, and as a baseline on intubated patients twice daily.

◆ Intracranial Pressure and Cerebral Blood Flow

Cerebral perfusion pressure (CPP) is the pressure via which blood and nutrients are delivered to the brain. As ICP increases, or mean arterial pressure (MAP) decreases, the CPP will also decrease, which will ultimately decrease cerebral blood flow. Normal cerebral blood flow in adults is 50 mL/100 g/minute. Gray matter blood flow is ~4 times higher than white matter. Newborn blood flow is ~40 mL/100 g/minute. Cerebral blood flow then increases to accommodate growth and learning. By age 4, the average cerebral blood flow is 108 mL/100 g/minute and can remain as high as twice that of adults until 18 years of age.[14-16]

An injured brain requires a fine line of adequate cerebral blood flow to maintain function, perfuse any ischemic penumbra, and heal while not increasing edema. This is where CPP plays a role. According to traumatic brain injury guidelines, CPP > 55 is recommended for children, with an ideal >65. Tight fluid control and pressors may be needed to maintain adequate MAP in the face of rising ICP to achieve this goal.

In children, it is often difficult to measure ICP. Ventriculostomies can be used as a direct measurement; however, an accurate examination can suggest elevated ICP as well. Papilledema is often a late finding of elevated ICP in children relative to adults, whereas vomiting occurs much more regularly and reliably as a predictive symptom. Assessment of fontanelles can also yield pressure data. Note that when children are lying flat or having a Valsalva's maneuver, fontanelles can be bulging and firm without abnormality. However, in the sitting position, a calm child should have soft, non-bulging fontanelles; any firmness or bulge is suggestive of elevated ICP. Another useful clinical gauge of ICP is head circumference. Although head circumference abnormalities can stem from a variety of causes, it can be used to suspect intracranial pathology and possibly high ICP, particularly if augmented by other clinical findings. An estimation of ICP is 1.5 to 6.0 mm Hg in children <2 years of age, equal to the child's age in the 2 to 15 year range, and 8 to 15 mm Hg in children and adults >15 years old.

In the pediatric NICU, ICP and CPP are treated as the fifth and sixth vital signs. Evaluation, early identification of trends, and rapid treatment can prevent additional neurologic decline and improve outcome.

◆ Nutrition

States of physical and/or psychological stress change the metabolic needs of patients. Nutritional support is vital to the management and outcome of pediatric NICU patients. Most clinical research has been directed toward adult patients; however, most concepts carry over to children. In the 1960s, total parenteral nutrition (TPN) became widely used and helped to relieve the metabolic component of the systemic stress response. However, more recently, natural enteral support has been advocated to facilitate gut motility, mucosal healthiness, and natural flora preservation.[8] In particular, neonate patient data have suggested even small amounts of gastrointestinal feedings promote enterohepatic enzyme delivery, reduce mucosal atrophy, and decrease the risk of jaundice.[17,18]

Regardless of the mode of nutrition, the goal should be to maintain fluids, electrolytes, and vitamins, as well as to provide adequate calorie intake for a metabolically stressed and altered system. Some recent literature has suggested the need for an increased amount of protein, but there are conflicting views on this.[8,12] The basal energy expenditures of patients in various states can be estimated by modified normograms based on the Harris-Benedict formula[19] or by respirometry and indirect calorimetry.

Tables 27–3, **27–4**, and **27–5** are examples of normograms used to determine and apply the basal energy expenditure of patients in critical care settings.[8]

Table 27–3 Caloric Requirements for Infants and Children[6]

Age (in years)	Calories (kcal/kg)
<40 weeks' gestation	80
0–1	90–120
1–7	75–90
7–12	60–75
12–18	45–60

Table 27–4 Percent Change in Caloric Requirements in Stressed Conditions[6]

Percent increase in caloric requirement	Pathological condition
12	Every degree temperature > 37°C
20–30	Major surgery
40–50	Sepsis
50–100	Failure to thrive

Source: Data from Farrell MM. Brain death in the pediatric patient: historical, sociological, religious, cultural, legal, and ethical considerations. Crit Care Med 1993;21:1951–1965.

Table 27–5 Basal Metabolic Rates for Healthy Subjects[6]

Age (years)	Males (kcal/m^2/hour)	Females (kcal/m^2/hour)
1	53	53
2–3	52	52
4–5	50	49
6–7	48	46
8–9	46	43
10–11	44	42
12–13	42	41
14–15	42	39
16–17	41	37
18–19	40	36
20–25	38	35

Source: Data from Farrell MM. Brain death in the pediatric patient: historical, sociological, religious, cultural, legal, and ethical considerations. Crit Care Med 1993;21:1951–1965.

Body surface area, which is necessary to complete most basal energy expenditure calculations, can be estimated by the "rule of sixes" or via the equation

Body Surface Area (m^2) = square root of $[(height (cm) \times weight (kg)) / 3600]$

◆ Activity Level

The activity level of children in the NICU setting will vary depending on pathology. The general rule is to mobilize, mobilize, mobilize.

Intubated patients are the exception to this rule, as being intubated can be a traumatic state, misinterpreted by children of any age. These patients should be kept under adequate sedation and pain management. Infectious patients can increase activity within their secured environment, and bed rest patients can adjust the head of the bed. Patients with head of bed alteration limitations due to weight-bearing restrictions, drains, or underlying pathology, such as intracranial edema or spinal fluid circulation considerations, should adjust their activity within the parameters set by their condition but try to keep the head of bed greater than 30 degrees above horizontal if safe.

Cervical collars and spinal braces, depending on the injury or baseline etiology causing the need for support, can be worn out of bed, and patients are still encouraged to increase activity. Braces should be worn snuggly and secured adequately to maximize support and minimize slipping or discomfort during activity. Some patients prefer to have a liner of gauze or piece of material such as a shirt under the brace to prevent skin contact and irritation.

Activity can decrease the risk of comorbidities associated with hospitalization, including deep vein thrombosis, pulmonary embolisms, pneumonia, constipation, and pressure sores. Also, depression has been shown to be decreased among patients with out-of-bed activities and environmental changes. Environmental changes can consist of outside visits, hallway walks, wheelchair excursions, or simply a change in the furniture setup within the room.

Patients with indwelling deep tissue drains or open shunt systems should not be allowed into common areas secondary to the risk of contamination. These patients should still increase activity as tolerated, but the security of the drain system should be monitored.

◆ Pharmacology

Injectable, oral, rectal, and transdermal medications are all used in children. Special attention is paid to dosing, preparation, delivery, and administration. Due to the lack of judgment expressed in children, IV medications are frequently used in the pediatric NICU setting to facilitate compliance and limit discomfort during administration. Dosing is usually by weight and/or therapeutic level maintenance. **Table 27–6** lists several of the medications frequently used in the care of pediatric NICU patients.[20,21]

If medications require piggybacking, the suggested fluid is 0.9% normal saline. The additional osmolarity and sodium, as well as the lack of sugar, will help with edema. An exception to this is in the setting of electrolyte imbalance or endocrine pathology, whether or not related to the neurosurgical diagnosis. In these cases, a risk-to-benefit ratio as well as ease of treatment of the adverse reaction must be weighed when determining the fluid base in which to mix medication.

When giving IV medications, there are five questions that should be asked by administering staff, in addition to confirming the dose of the drug:

1. Is the line large enough to accommodate the drug, and is the line in adequate position?
2. Is the patient's cardiac function strong enough to dilute and circulate the drug effectively?
3. Does the infusion require a pump, or can it be administered directly?
4. Is there a need for titratable or prn (as circumstances may require) dosing?
5. Are there any drug-to-drug interactions or special administration instructions with the drug in question? Can it be given with TPN/tube feeds?

Also, when required to maximally concentrate fluid solutions, the "rule of six" should be applied. The rule of six (not to be confused with the "rule of sixes"; see **Table 27–2**) states that 6 times the patient's weight is equal to the amount of drug (mg) that, in 100 mL of fluid, will result in a solution delivering 1 μg/kg/minute when infused at 1 mL/hour. (Note: For two drugs, epinephrine and isoproterenol, 0.6 should be used.) Stated mathematically:

$$6 \times \frac{\text{(Desired dose in } \mu\text{g/kg/minute)}}{\text{Desired rate (mL/hr)}} = \frac{\text{Amount (mg) of drug}}{100 \text{ mL of fluid}}$$

Studies have shown the most common mistake made with drug administration is carelessness in dosing because of a lack of time to recheck dosage instructions, miscalculations, or presumed familiarity with a particular drug. This problem is preventable.

◆ Medical Imaging

There is a significant overlap between adults and children in regard to medical imaging. As a general rule, if a study is needed for diagnosis, treatment, or follow-up, then it must be done. Unnecessary studies are avoided

Table 27–6   Frequently Used Medications in the Pediatric NICU Patient[7]

Medication	Indication	Dose/Route	Miscellaneous
Acetaminophen	Pain/fever	10 mg/kg/dose PO/PR q 4–6 hours	
Acetaminophen w/codeine	Pain	1 tsp q 4 hours	For >3 years old
Morphine (MSO_4)	Pain	0.1 mg/kg IM/SQ/IV every 1–4 hours	May raise ICP; IV not recommended in children
Midalozam	Sedation or intubation	0.2–0.7 mg/kg IV/PO/IM	
Diazepam	Sedation or intubation	0.2 mg/kg IV or PR	Maximum 30 mg IV
Lidocaine	Intubation	1.0 mg/kg IV	Dysrhythmias
Vecuronium	Relaxant, paralytic	0.1 mg/kg IV	Duration 15–30 minutes
Thiopental	Sedation	4 mg/kg IV	
Ketamine	Anesthetic, sedation	1 mg/kg IV over 1 minute; 4 mg/kg IM	10–20 minutes effect; concurrent atropine minimizes salivation
Fentanyl	Sedation	5 µg/kg IV	
Propofol	Sedation	5–50 µg/kg/minute	
Dilantin	Anticonvulsant	Load 10 mg/kg at <50 mg/minute rate; maintenance 5 mg/kg/day	Not recommended in children for >12 hours Watch levels: age dependent; can cause arrhythmias
Phenobarbital	Anticonvulsant	Load 10 mg/kg at <60 mg/minute rate; maintenance 3 mg/kg/minute PO	
Phenergan	Antihistamine, antiemetic	6.25 mg PO/IV/IM/PR q 6 hours	May raise ICP
Anzemet	Antiemetic	0.35 mg/kg IV q 6 hours; 1.2 mg/kg PO q 6 hours	
Dopamine	Inotrope/pressor	2 mg/kg/minute titrated to effect	Maximum 50 mg/kg/minute; solution = 400 mg in 250 mL D5W
Dobutamine	Inotrope/pressor	2 µg/kg/minute titrated to effect	Maximum 20 µg/kg/minute; solution = 250 mg in 250 mL D5W

D5W, dextrose 5% in water; ICP, intracranial pressure; IM, intramuscularly; IV, intravenous; NICU, neurosurgical intensive care unit; PO, orally; PR, far point of accommodation; SQ, subcutaneous.

in both subsets of patients to prevent unnecessary cost accumulation and radiation exposure, not to mention discomfort, the risk of transport, and systemic difficulties in obtaining the tests. In particular with children is the concern of radiation exposure on their developing system and bone growth. The average chest x-ray radiation exposure is 1.4 mGy, and the average head computed tomography (CT) scan radiation exposure is 8.0 mGy. Most literature suggests adverse effects do not start occurring until after exposure to 100 mGy.[22] Young children also are usually not as cooperative and have difficulty lying still. Frequently, conscious sedation or temporary intubation is required to obtain an adequate study. This then exposes the patient to another set of risks, and the benefit-to-risk ratio needs to be clearly discussed with the legal guardians, as well as with other medical staff involved in the case. Whether sedation is required or not, it should be noted that there are risks to transporting critically ill patients to the radiology department. Risks include environmental exposure, infection, accidental line removal, systemic instability, and positional difficulties. Because of these risks, medically necessary imaging should be portable if possible and of acceptable quality; if transport to the radiology department is pertinent, all necessary studies from all disciplines should be performed during one trip to minimize risks and promote efficiency. This requires effective communication between complex multidisciplinary care plans.

Table 27–7   Modified Coma Scale for Infant[8]

Response	Score
Eye opening	
Spontaneous	4
To speech	3
To pain	2
None	1
Verbal	
Coos, babbles	5
Irritable cry	4
Cries to pain only	3
Moans to pain only	2
None	1
Motor	
Normal spontaneous movements	6
Withdraws to touch	5
Withdraws to pain	4
Abnormal flexion	3
Abnormal extension	2
None	1

◆ The Pediatric Neurologic Exam

Unlike adult examinations, there is no rigid normal baseline in a pediatric neurologic exam. Developmental milestones should be met sequentially and have been well documented; however, minimal timeline variations and personality trends do occur that can affect an exam at any given point.

The examiner should take into account the age of the child. The child should be placed in a comfortable setting with family present if possible. Much of the pediatric exam can be done while observing and interacting with the patient, paying close attention to facial expressions and the eyes, any verbalizations, and motor interactions. The pupils must be examined, even in uncooperative patients: no exceptions. Also, a head circumference and body weight should be documented and trends followed. The remainder of the exam can use a modified Glasgow Coma Scale format. Such standardizations help document exams reliably and reproducibly (**Tables 27–7** and **27–8**).[23]

During infancy, children can exhibit flexor activity while sleeping; this is a normal variant. Also, children can have asymmetric blink and dysconjugate gaze up to 6 months of age without concern. A positive plantar or Babinski's reflex can occur normally up to 1 year of age, as well as areflexia or hyperreflexia of deep tendon reflexes.

Table 27–8   Children's Coma Scale[7,8]

Response	Score
Ocular	
Pursuit	4
EOM intact, reactive pupils	3
EOM impaired	2
EOM paralyzed, fixed pupils	1
Verbal	
Cries	3
Spontaneous respirations	2
Apneic	1
Motor	
Flexes and extends	4
Withdraws from painful stimuli	3
Hypertonic	2
Flaccid	1

EOM, extraocular muscles.

Case Management

The child described in this story has developed malignant cerebral edema syndrome, which is a phenomenon seen in children more commonly than in adults. This kind of cerebral edema can come on very rapidly and has a very high associated mortality. The child needs to be treated aggressively medically to keep cerebral perfusion pressure (CPP) over 60 mm Hg and intracrania pressure (ICP) under 20 mm Hg. This case also illustrates well why children with seemingly minor head injuries should be observed in the pediatric intensive care unit.

References

1. Wexler MR, Nureman A, Umanski P. A decade of experience in craniofacial surgery (Hebrew). Harefuah 1992;122:146–152
2. Lopez PJ, Galvan MM, Rubio ML. Descriptive analysis of neurological disorders in the pediatric intensive care unit of a regional reference hospital (Spanish). An Esp Pediatr 2000;53:119–124
3. Jone HR. Guillain-Barré syndrome: perspectives with infants and children. Semin Pediatr Neurol 2000;7:91–102
4. Cantagrel S. Mortality in a pediatric hospital: six year retrospective study. Arch Pediatr 2000;7:725–731
5. Boldt J, Maleck W. Intensive care research in Germany: an analysis of papers in important international journals. Anasthesiol Intensivmed Notfallmed Schmerzther 1999;34:542–548
6. Farrell MM. Brain death in the pediatric patient: historical, sociological, religious, cultural, legal, and ethical considerations. Crit Care Med 1993;21:1951–1965
7. Gomella LG. Clinician's Pocket Reference. Norwalk, CT: Appleton & Lange; 1997
8. Fuhrman BP. Pediatric Critical Care. St. Louis, MO: CV Mosby; 1998
9. Abbate B. Head injuries in children: consideration of 3715 consecutive cases. Minerva Pediatr 2000;52:623–628
10. Smith ER. Neurosurgical aspects of critical care neurology. Semin Pediatr Neurol 2004;11:169–178
11. Smith ER. Cerebral pathophysiology and critical care neurology: basic hemodynamic principles, cerebral perfusion, and intracranial pressure. Semin Pediatr Neurol 2004;11:89–104
12. Levin DL. Pediatric Intensive Care. 2nd ed. New York: Churchill Livingstone; 1997
13. Andrews BT. Intensive Care in Neurosurgery. New York: Thieme; 2003
14. Suzuki K. Changes of regional cerebral blood flow with advancing age in normal children. Nagoya Med J 1990;34:159–170
15. Raimondi AJ. Pediatric Neurosurgery. New York: Springer-Verlag; 1987
16. McLaurin RL. Pediatric Neurosurgery. Philadelphia: WB Saunders; 1989
17. Merritt RJ. Cholestasis associated with total parenteral nutrition. J Pediatr Gastroenterol Nutr 1986;5:9–22
18. Roche AF. The gastrointestinal response to injury, starvation, and enteral nutrition. Paper presented at: Eighth Ross Conference on Medical Research;1988; Columbus, OH
19. Harris JA, Benedict F. A Biometric Study of Basal Metabolism in Man. Washington, DC: Carnegie Institute; 1919
20. Casella EB. Management of acute seizure episodes and status epliepticus in children. J Pediatr (Rio J) 1999;75:S197–S206

21. Brettfeld C. Evaluation of Ames seralyzer for the therapeutic drug monitor of phenobarbital and phenytoin. Ther Drug Monit 1989;11:612–615
22. It's Your Health Care—Health Canada. Diagnostics x-rays and pregnancy. Available at: http://www.hc-sc.gc.ca/iyh-vsv/med/xray-radiographie_e.html. Accessed September 3, 2006.
23. Allan WC. Neonatal intensive care neurology. Semin Pediatr Neurol 2004; 11:119–128

28
Brain Death

Dan Miulli

Case Study

A 72-year-old female presented with acute loss of consciousness while sitting in a chair at home. Her workup included a computed tomography (CT) scan that demonstrated a complete left hemispheric infarction, causing mass effect, and 2 cm of midline shift. She was admitted to the neurosurgical intensive care unit (NICU), where she was intubated. Her temperature was 32.8°C or 91°F, blood pressure 90/45, and heart rate 65. Her neurologic exam demonstrated no response to pain, her pupils were 8 mm and nonreactive, and there were no corneal reflexes. The family wanted to know if the patient was dead.

See page 413 for Case Management.

◆ History of Death Policy

Individually, states determine the definition of death, as do countries. In the 1950s, medical advancements that included mechanical ventilation made it possible to keep some vital organs viable. Then, with additional advances in medicine, functioning organs could be transplanted into other individuals, and those patients improved. This established the efficacy of transplanted organs from supported bodies over organs from bodies with no functioning circulation and respiration. The hope delivered by transplant surgeons, because of their ability to restore vital organs to patients dying from similar organ failure, led to brain death as a declaration of death. Death can also be characterized as somatic death, which is the complete cessation of cardiac and respiratory function. In 1970, after 10 years of study, the first statute determining death in all circumstances was passed. In 1978, the National Conference of Commissioners on Uniform State Laws completed the Uniform Brain Death Act. In 1980, the same commission drafted the Uniform Determination of Death Act, which is the basis for the majority of death laws in the United States. The Death Act of 1980 sets the general legal standard for determining death, but not the medical criteria for doing so. The medical profession remains free to formulate acceptable medical practices and to utilize new biomedical knowledge, diagnostic tests, and equipment.[1-6]

◆ Definition of Death

According to the Death Act of 1980, for death to be declared, "The entire brain must cease to function, irreversibly." The "entire brain" includes the brainstem and the neocortex. This definition takes into consideration anencephaly, a condition in which an infant is born with the anatomical lack of most cerebral hemispheres but with a functioning brainstem. Such an infant is considered legally alive.[7] Although the Death Act of 1980 established the criterion for death, the definition did not address diagnostic tests and specific medical procedures. This gave the medical and legal profession flexibility to develop diagnostic procedures while leaving the door open for disagreement and the need for judicial review. Then in 1981, the President's Commission for the Study of Ethical Problems in Medicine and Biomedical and Behavioral Research developed standards for the determination of brain death, which, with some modifications, are adhered to worldwide.[3,8]

The consensus on death declaration by way of lack of brain function must include three mandatory parts: (1) there must be no brain and no brainstem function—the person must be apneic; (2) the etiology must be known and irreversible; and (3) there must be no confounding factors. An example of a state law, the State of California Health and Safety Code, Section 7184, is:

A person who is declared brain dead is legally and physiologically dead. An individual who has sustained either (1) irreversible cessation of circulatory and respiratory functions, or (2) irreversible cessation of all functions of the entire brain, including the brainstem, is dead.

A determination of brain death must be made in accordance with accepted medical standards. In 42 states, one licensed physician is required (in a few states, the physician's representative can declare brain death); in the 8 other states, two licensed physicians are required. Hospital bylaws usually provide for criteria to pronounce death by means of a neurologic exam and may add qualifications. In most guidelines, the physician who declares a patient dead can be any licensed physician knowledgeable of and comfortable with performing a detailed neurologic exam and familiar with the procedures to declare someone dead. Uniformly, the licensed physician does not have to be a neurologist or neurosurgeon. The only ethical consideration should be that the physician is not the transplant surgeon, because this may appear as a conflict of interest.

In 48 states, family permission is not required prior to performing a brain death exam. Only in New York and New Jersey can families object for religious reasons.[8]

The opposing opinion to the Death Act is that the entire body must not function for the declaration of death. When the heart and lungs are not functioning, which is the criterion for somatic death, a machine can take over until a new heart and lung(s) are transplanted. The result will be an individual who, after recovery, may resume his or her life. However, after the brain ceases to function, there is, as of yet, no machine that can take over until transplantation. In the future, if transplantation were to occur, the result would be a different person lacking the memories and physical abilities, as well as lacking the hope, love, caring, and spirit, that resided in the brain in the unique individual that died. In essence, the other brain that was being transplanted was simply acquiring a new body.

◆ Initial Criteria

To pronounce a person dead, there must be evidence of irreversible brain damage. The examining licensed physician must personally review the CT or magnetic resonance imaging (MRI) scan; it must be consistent with an irreversible condition incompatible with life, such as sustained negative cerebral perfusion pressure, massive stroke, lack of gray-white junction, edema, shift, and multiple other conditions. To proceed with a complete neurologic exam for pronouncing the patient dead, there must be hemo-dynamic stability; the patient cannot be arresting. It is not unusual for pupils to be fixed and dilated immediately after resuscitation. This nonre-sponsive brain condition can also be seen during seizures, when abnormal brain activity is impeding functional interaction. To declare death, a patient can be on multiple vasopressors.

There are major criteria that must be met before considering a valid neu-rologic exam for the purpose of declaring a patient dead. The body should have a systolic blood pressure ≥90 mm Hg. The body core temperature must be above 32.2°C or 90°F. Below 28°C, there is loss of brainstem reflexes.[1,4,9] In a trauma center, it is not unusual to see hypothermia in patients, such as snow skiers, the winter homeless, addicts, and cold-acclimatized patients who have ingested opioids, barbiturates, benzodiazepines, phenothiazines, tricyclic antidepressants, and lithium.[10,11] The patient cannot be under the effects of skeletal muscle paralytics. Furthermore, there can be no metabolic abnormalities causing coma or loss of brainstem reflexes and no hypoglycemia.

Patients can be declared legally dead if they have ingested drugs; how-ever, the licensed physician has to certify and document that the patient is not toxic on drugs and that the drugs are not preventing brainstem function and are not causing coma. Even in the case of overdose, the pupillary reflex is usually present. However, medications can cause almost any side effects, and there are anecdotal reports that tricyclic antidepressants can mimic brain death. When drug ingestion is suspected, do not rush to pronounce dead; instead, wait and investigate. If the patient is truly dead, he or she will remain that way. Attempt to discover which drug was used, and before proceeding with the neurologic exam, observe the patient for at least 4 or 5 times the excretion half-life, assuming there is no no half-life prolongation due to additional organ dysfunction. Some guidelines provide for specific drugs.[1,12] Excessive intake of alcohol would delay the performance of a death-determining exam. Alcohol (EtOH)–valid levels for brain death determinations are <800 to 1500 mg/dL, whereas the legal intoxication level is 80 to 100 mg/dL.[1] With certain suspected drug and medication ingestion, antidotes may be administered. However, if a medication is being prescribed to reduce the cerebral metabolic rate for oxygenation ($CMRO_2$) or if it is necessary to protect the brain in some form, the benefits of giving the antidote must outweigh the risks, for example, when administering flumazenil 0.2, then 0.3 mg intravenous (IV) for benzodiazepine overdose. When opioid overdose is suspected, administer naloxone 0.2 to 2.0 mg IV. Additional therapeutic cerebral protectant medications are barbiturates, used to reduce increased intracranial pressure (ICP), and $CMRO_2$ by inhibiting brain activity, placing the patient in a medication-induced coma. The clinical diagnosis of brain death can still be made after stopping the medication if the serum levels are less than the therapeutic range. In most laboratories, the level would be <5 to 15 $\mu g/mL$. This is below the level required for burst suppression, 50 $\mu g/mL$. When a drug or poison cannot be quantified but seems highly likely from history, one should not make the diagnosis of brain death.

One criterion for death pronouncement is the consideration of altering neurologic status due to drugs' affect on metabolism. The same consideration of pure systemic abnormalities must also be made; the systemic abnormality must not be causing the coma or loss of brainstem reflexes. Severe abnormalities such as hypoglycemia or hyperglycemia, hyponatremia, hypernatremia, hypothyroidism, panhypopituitarism, or Addison's disease may decrease the level of consciousness and confuse neurologic examination, but a complete loss of brainstem reflexes is seldom observed. The licensed physician must once again document that the systemic abnormalities are not the cause of coma.[1] The many guidelines state that the patient should not be hypoglycemic.

◆ Brain Death Exam

Only after the initial criteria are met can the licensed physician proceed with the neurologic exam. The exam documents the function of the cerebral hemispheres and the brainstem. When it can be performed, it is as sensitive as any technological test for determining global brain function. It will not assess the entire or specific function of the basal ganglia, thalamus, or cerebral cortices. To assume a lack of functional cerebral hemispheres, the patient must be in a coma. An often touted but rare clinical condition that, by exam, may mimic complete and irreversible lack of entire brain function is a "super" locked-in syndrome, when there is profound damage to the brainstem, with the exception of the ascending reticular activating system (ARAS), and intact cerebral hemisphere function. This circumstance is rare and may be excluded easily in most instances. The history, physical, and radiological and physiological review should argue against this condition. The less severe locked-in syndrome is produced by ischemic or hemorrhagic destruction to the descending motor pathways, the corticospinal and corticobulbar tracts of the basis pontis (ventral pons), and the reticular formation of the pontine tegmentum, sparing the ARAS. It is a pure motor paresis, sparing the sensory pathways. In this somewhat less severe condition, the patient still retains vertical eye and eyelid movements. If there is true concern about either type of locked-in syndrome in which the person is conscious but cannot move or breathe, a simple electroencephalogram (EEG) can be performed to determine the function of the cerebral hemispheres.[13]

The main test of cortical, basal ganglia function is conscious interaction and conscious reaction to painful stimuli. Pain reaction does occur without consciousness in brainstem and spinal reflexes. Although brainstem reflexes negate death, pronouncement by detailed neurologic exam can occur if spinal reflexes are present. A viable spinal cord is not an exclusion of death; a person could have spinal cord function such as spinal reflexes and still be dead.

In examining consciousness, the physician must determine if the patient talks or makes any sound. Next, the physician must determine if the patient will open his or her eyes to name, touch, or painful stimuli. The examiner must then determine if the patient follows commands, localizes to pain, withdraws to pain, or has decorticate or decerebrate response to pain. Simply applying pinpricks to the body is not an appropriate stimulation of pain. Pressure on the supraorbital nerve positioned on the medial aspect of the eyebrow ridge is the best place to test for motor response to pain. It can also be elicited with temporomandibular joint compression. Do not use painful stimuli such as sternal rubbing or twisting of forearm or nipples because of the disfiguring and psychological effect that may have on family members or health care workers. Additionally, peripheral stimulation, such as nail bed pressure, may elicit a spinal reflex instead of a central response, often confusing the exam. A spinal reflex is a stereotypical repetitive, nonsustained movement that is usually monosynaptic. A withdrawal brainstem response is more complex because of additional inputs. The difference between high-level withdrawal response and decorticate reflex or spinal reflex can be determined by applying pain to the medial upper arm. The withdrawal response will usually be to abduct the arm away from the chest, whereas the reflex will be to adduct the arm toward the chest. A nonreflex conscious pain response demonstrates some integrity of the spine–brainstem–thalamus–cortical basal ganglion pathway. If there is decreased input from the cerebral hemispheres, decreased input through the cortical spinal tract, a functioning rubrospinal tract, and motor flexor of the distal limb, inhibition of extensor muscles becomes dominant, resulting in decorticate activity.

If there is disruption between the superior colliculi (anterior quadrigeminal bodies) or the decussation of the rubrospinal pathway, the rostral portion of the vestibular nuclei, pain stimulation becomes the major response of the vestibulospinal tract. This results in extensor tone to motor neurons innervating the neck, back, and limbs, and inhibition of flexion of the trunk and limbs. Since the track is uncrossed, the decerebrate activity occurs on the same side of the lesion. Spinal cord responses in addition to the stereotypical repetitive, nonsustained movement at the site of stimulation may also be seen as a slow response in the extremities, brief flexion of the fingers, or minimal eyelid deviation.

As the detailed neurologic exam proceeds down from the cerebral cortex and diencephalons, the function of the midbrain and the nuclei of cranial nerve (CN) II and CN III is probed. The physician examines these structures, testing the pupillary reflex using a bright flashlight, first directed into one pupil so that it hits the retina, and then into the other. Simply opening the eyelid in room light does not qualify. If there is any concern that the pupil may have constricted, it did. Dilated pupils are >4 mm, and asymmetric pupils are >1 mm different. Pupils that are asymmetrical and small are usually a sign of midbrain or pontine injury in a living person. Always err on the side of caution and on the side of life. If orbital or papillary inspection is hampered, use a magnifying glass. This reflex of sensory and autonomic motor response can demonstrate activity even if the patient has been chemically paralyzed.

The corneal reflex indicates the integrity of the midpons, CN V sensory component, and CN VII motor component. It is performed by touching the cornea away from the pupil with a cotton-tipped applicator and observing a blink response. The blink may be slight; however, any movement is an indicator of function and life. For this test, do not use a paper towel, piece of paper, or any material that may be abrasive to the cornea. If the person survives, he or she should not be required to get a corneal transplant simply because the examining physician did not take the time to find a cotton-tipped applicator.

Next, the midbrain to lower pons is tested, investigating the oculovestibular reflex by injecting ice water into the external auditory canal that is known to have an intact unobstructed tympanic membrane. The physician observes the eye movement while stimulating the vestibular system. First, elevate the head to 30 degrees to allow maximum stimulation of the horizontal canal. Then inject 30 to 50 cc of ice water into the external auditory canal and watch 30 seconds or more for the slow movement to the side of the cold-water stimulus. In coma, the quick nystagmus is lost, and the slow component to the side of the cold-water stimulus remains. If there is no brainstem reflex, the eyes will not move. Test one side, wait 5 minutes, then test the other. Testing the other side too soon after the first will inhibit the slow component to the side of the cold-water stimulus. This tests the CN III, VI, and VIII, the medial longitudinal fasciculus (MLF), the paramedian pontine reticular formation (PPRF), and the lower pons. Similar information can be obtained during the oculocephalic reflex. However, if spinal cord injury is suspected, do not perform the test. It would be terrible to have someone survive an ordeal to wake up quadriplegic. The oculocephalic reflex is observed while turning the patient's head. Fast turning of the head to both sides should not produce any eye movement; however, conjunctival swelling sometimes makes this difficult to elicit. This is referred to as the doll's eyes reflex because the patient's eyes, like the painted eyes of a doll, stay fixed forward without movement. This reflex tests the similar components of the oculovestibular reflex: CN III, VI, and VIII; MLF; PPRF; and lower pons.

A cough response should be attempted using a suction catheter inserted into the endotracheal tube and advanced to the level of the carina, followed by deep suctioning to test lower brainstem or medulla function. Do not just move the endotracheal tube. The simple stimulation of the gag reflex is a variable test, as it can be blunted by medication and normal physiology. This test, in which there is a cough or sensation, then elevation of the uvula, monitors the function of CN V, IX, and X and the medulla.

Certain movements are seen in the dead body and do not denote brainstem function. There can be spinal reflex spontaneous movements of the head and limbs; respiratory-like spinal reflex movements of the shoulders, back, and intercostal muscles without tidal volumes; and deep tendon reflexes, superficial abdominal reflexes, triple flexion response, Babinski's reflex, and other spinal reflexes due to stimulation from acidosis or other means. There can also be spinal autonomic responses such as tachycardia, sudden increases in blood pressure, blushing, and sweating. There does not have to be the need for blood pressure control, nor does diabetes insipidus have to be present.[14,15]

Irreversibility

It is a good idea to have two licensed physicians perform the detailed neurologic exam, as is the requirement in 8 states. However, it may not be practical in some settings when there are not enough available licensed physicians who are familiar with that type of exam. It should be determined before the first physician examines the patient whether there is any question that the injury is reversible or not. The CT scan or MRI must be reviewed and be consistent with an irreversible condition incompatible with life, such as sustained negative cerebral perfusion pressure, massive stroke, lack of gray-white junction, edema, shift, and multiple other conditions. If there is a question about irreversibility, then wait some time before the second neurologic exam is performed. Four or more hours is an arbitrary time to wait in an adult; some municipalities wait longer, and in other countries the wait can extend into days. Another licensed physician can repeat the neurologic exam immediately if there is no question about irreversibility, and if required by law, bylaws, or conscience. Once again, it is practical in some instances to have only one detailed neurologic exam to pronounce that a person's life is over.

Apnea Test

After the final detailed neurologic exam, the hallmark of brain death should be performed: the apnea test. Do not perform it before the first detailed neurologic exam. Instead, the apnea test can be performed with the first of two detailed neurologic exams or with the second. It does not have to be performed twice, even in states where two licensed physicians are required to certify death by detailed exam. When a second exam is required, the physician must verify the results of any previous apnea test. It is often practical to perform the apnea test with the first of two required detailed neurologic exams if there is no additional requirement for a waiting period. However, the apnea test may produce a period of relative hypotension or hypoxia, which, with a condition of uncertainty in which the patient may still be alive, is detrimental. Therefore, optimally, the apnea test should be performed with the second detailed neurologic exam (**Table 28–1**).

The apnea exam tests the reticular formation of the caudal medulla. The strongest human drive is to breathe, and the living human will breathe if the by-product of metabolism, CO_2, increases above a certain threshold. Only rarely will the individual not breathe at mildly elevated CO_2 levels, such as a minority with chronic obstructive pulmonary disease (COPD) who function normally with increased CO_2. Although the drive to breathe occurs earlier with hypoxia and later with acidosis, the most reliable drive to determine a lack of brainstem function is rising CO_2. Acidosis will drive respiration; however, the blood–brain barrier is not as permeable to hydrogen ions as it is to CO_2 gas. Therefore, the microenvironment of the medulla is most responsive to escalating CO_2 gas, and brain death is determined by apnea due to the rise of CO_2 above the threshold. Brain death is not determined by hypoxemic or acidemic apnea.

Do not perform the apnea test unless the criteria to proceed with death declaration by neurologic examination have been met; there can be no effect of paralytics, no toxic effects of drugs, and, specific to the apnea test, no high spinal cord injury to prevent ventilation. Before performing the last part of the neurologic exam, the apnea test to investigate the reticular formation of the caudal medulla, the patient must meet additional criteria. The patient should be normothermic, with a core temperature ≥35.0° to 36.5°C or 95° to 97°F. The warmer the body, the quicker the CO_2 will rise. If the body is colder, the apnea test will take longer, leading to possible hypoxia or hemodynamic instability. However, do not attempt to make the patient

Table 28–1 Apnea Test to Declare Death[1–8]

Requirements to do test	When to perform
One required physician and neurologic exam	At the end of the detailed neurologic exam
Two required physicians and neurologic exams, no waiting period or waiting period	At the end of the second neurologic exam. It is acceptable for the second exam to follow the first immediately if there is no reason for a waiting period. Pronouncement of death occurs when second exam is completed

hyperthermic, a condition that will increase $CMRO_2$ should the patient be alive. There should be no hypotension; the systolic blood pressure (SBP) should be greater than 90 mm Hg, although hypotension using 90 mm Hg is an arbitrary number. Young, small women and smaller children have blood pressures normally <90 mm Hg. To decrease the time required off the ventilator, which increases the chance of O_2 desaturation leading to hypotension and cardiac instability, the partial pressure of CO_2 (PCO_2) should be normal, 35 to 45 mm Hg by arterial blood gases (ABG). If COPD is suspected, start with a PCO_2 60 mm Hg or higher. Before beginning the apnea test, the fluids should be running wide open. Vasopressors should be running or hanging and connected to the IV line and able to be given within seconds. SBP in the average adult should be as close to 120 mm Hg as possible but not <90 mm Hg. Vasopressors should be increased as necessary. There should be pulse oximetry, and it should be maintained at 100% to start and without hypoxia throughout the test. The blood pressure and vitals should be monitored continuously; however, if no arterial line has been inserted, monitor the blood pressure with a cuff every minute. Monitoring blood pressure less often will only lead to the arrest of cardiac and pulmonary systems, with the resultant prolonged resuscitation of a patient who would have possibly been pronounced dead 10 minutes later. Hypotension is usually due to acidosis from decreased oxygenation or perfusion. Therefore, high temporary concentrations of O_2 and a hypervolemic state are necessary. If hypotension cannot be controlled, a blood gas should be drawn immediately and the remaining time aborted until measures can be taken to control loss of blood pressure.

The apnea test will measure the ability of the body to take a breath in response to increasing blood CO_2 (PCO_2). The PCO_2 will rise 3 to 6 mm Hg per minute depending on circulation and temperature. Some authors state that PCO_2 will rise 2 to 8 mm Hg; however, these are unusual conditions. The target PCO_2 is 60 mm Hg on an ABG test, although some municipalities use 55 mm Hg. When the patient has COPD, not only should the PCO_2 rise above 60 mm Hg, it must rise at least 20 mm Hg above baseline to prevent any false diagnosis of brain death. To facilitate the levels of CO_2, the ventilator should be adjusted in the COPD patient who is known to be a CO_2 retainer; begin with a PCO_2 of 60 mm Hg before the apnea test. After the increased baseline of 60 mm Hg or higher, the PCO_2 should be allowed to rise at least 20 mm Hg.[4,16–20] Additional concerns may be that the patient has absolutely no CO_2 drive, another unusual condition. Under those circumstances, a cerebral blood flow study should be ordered to confirm the complete absence of brain and brainstem blood flow.

In an attempt to ensure that the apnea test does not lead to cardiac arrest, or that a surviving person does not suffer further injury from hypoxia or ischemia, preoxygenate the patient for 10 minutes with 100% O_2 to eliminate the nitrogen stores, hyperoxygenate tissue to maintain organ viability, and prevent hypotension and cardiac instability. The patient may still develop acidosis during the apnea test from increased CO_2 levels; however, this can be minimized with excellent fluid flow, oxygenation, and blood pressure.

After hyperoxygenation, disconnect the ventilator while maintaining a superadequate O_2 source using a catheter, such as a nasal cannula with the nostril insert cut off, placed at the carina delivering O_2 at 6 L/minute or higher. The alternative is to keep the patient on the ventilator, stopping the breaths administered while maintaining positive pressure support at 10 mm Hg. Be careful: some ventilators have an automatic backup that will deliver 0.5 to 1.0 breath/minute; this fail-safe mechanism must be turned off. Furthermore, the licensed physician must not depend on the ventilator measuring the breaths; instead, he or she must observe the rise and fall of the chest, if present. If using the nasal cannula in the endotracheal tube, verify that both cannulas are at or before the end of the tube. Verify the length before insertion. If the cannulas are too long, they may oxygenate only one lung, and the nasal cannulas may get stuck; neither condition will be known initially. Furthermore, guarantee that there is enough room between the endotracheal tube and the catheter for O_2 to escape so there is no pressure buildup and pneumothorax. Physicians should do no harm, and that includes during the time pronouncing a person dead. The person will be temporarily off the ventilator ~8 to 10 minutes, based on the pretesting PCO_2 level. Under optimal conditions of temperature and blood pressure, after the 10 minutes of apnea multiplied by ~3 mm Hg of arterial CO_2 rise per minute, there should be 30 mm Hg rise from baseline PCO_2 toward the desired target value of 60 mm Hg. During the apnea test, the licensed physician must be present. The apnea test is the last part of the neurologic exam. The physician must observe the abdomen and chest for movements. If there are no movements after 10 minutes, then a new blood gas is drawn. When the arterial blood PCO_2 has reached at least 60 mm Hg, or at least 60 mm Hg plus 20 mm Hg above the patient's elevated normal baseline, if there is a suspected CO_2 retainer, then the apnea test is positive, and the person is pronounced dead. If the PCO_2 has not reached 60 mm Hg on the ABG test, or has not gone 20 mm Hg higher than the minimum 60 mm Hg starting baseline in the CO_2 retainer, the test must be repeated for longer times.

When initial neurologic brain death testing criteria have been met, when there is demonstrated irreversible loss of brain function, when confounding factors are known to not be responsible for coma and absent brainstem function, and when a detailed neurologic exam is completed, including an apnea test, that demonstrates absent brain and brainstem function and reflexes, the clinical diagnosis of death can be made. The patient is pronounced at the time the final detailed neurologic exam and positive apnea test are concluded.

The apnea test procedure involves the following steps:

♦ Disconnect the ventilator, or turn the ventilator to pressure support only, and disconnect the backup breath.
♦ Start the timer.
♦ Place the nasal cannulas with nasal inserts into the endotracheal tube only up to the end of the tube. Be sure that both nasal cannulas slide into the tube without getting stuck and that air is escaping.
♦ Place one hand on the patient's chest, observe, and listen for breath.

- Check blood pressure readings every minute or continuously by ABG. In the average adult, keep as close to 120 mm Hg as possible.
- Check pulse oximetry reading every minute or continuously.
- Be able to increase fluids quickly.
- Be able to increase vasopressors quickly.
- If too hypoxic, abort the test.
- If too hypotensive, abort the test.
- If there are too many cardiac arrhythmias, abort the test.
- After 10 minutes, obtain ABG, place the patient back on the ventilator, and document the time.

Confirmatory Test

A confirmatory test is not needed in adults. The neurologic exam that includes the apnea test must document the lack of brain and brainstem function, must document irreversibility, and must document a lack of confounding factors such as hypothermia and drugs. Only if the entire neurologic exam and complete repeated exam, if applicable, including the apnea test, cannot be performed or is not valid is a confirmatory test required. A confirmatory test cannot replace the apnea test portion of the neurologic exam but is performed when the apnea test or other part of the neurologic test cannot be achieved successfully. It is rare that the patient will not tolerate the apnea test if the above precautions are followed.

If a confirmatory test is mandated, a cerebral angiogram should be performed. The angiogram must include visualization of all remaining anterior and posterior circulation. To diagnose death, there must be no intracerebral filling of the carotid, basilar, or vertebral artery from where it enters the skull. Only the lack of intracerebral arterial circulation needs to be documented. There can be a patent external carotid circulation and delayed filling of the superior sagittal sinus.

EEG does not detect brainstem function and cannot be the sole test to pronounce death. Electrocerebral silence does not exclude the possibility of reversible coma; however, multiple EEGs over an extended time, such as 24 hours, in the absence of medication- or metabolic-induced electrocerebral silence do correlate with a lack of cerebral function. EEG is not the gold standard for diagnosis of brain death, and it does not replace the apnea test, but it is used occasionally. When performing an EEG, there should be no electrical activity during at least 30 minutes of recording. The recording must adhere to the minimum technical standards of the American Clinical Neurophysiology Society (ACNS; formerly the American Electro-encephalographic Society)[21] for EEG recording in suspected brain death. The guidelines include a 16- or 18-channel EEG instrument, with scalp electrodes at least 10 cm apart. The interelectrode impedances should be between 100 and 10,000 ohms. There should be no activity over 2 μV/mm (better determined at 1 μV/mm) for 30 minutes. The high-frequency filter setting should be at 30 Hz, and the low-frequency setting should not be below 1 Hz. There should be no EEG reactivity to intense somatosensory or audiovisual stimuli.[22,23] If cerebral angiogram is not performed, and EEG has to be relied on for confirmation of death, then EEG and repeat EEGs should be combined with brainstem auditory evoked responses (BAERs) to at least examine the brain and brainstem. Both electrical tests have characteristics that can lead to misinterpretation.

Transcranial Doppler (TCD) ultrasonography is now being entertained to assist in the confirmation of brain death. The TCD probe should be placed at the temporal bone above the zygomatic arch or the vertebrobasilar arteries through the suboccipital transcranial window. There should be insonation of at least three separate vessels on each side demonstrating the equivalent findings. However, 10% of people have no temporal insonation windows. Therefore, the initial absence of TCD signal cannot be interpreted as consistent with brain death. TCD utilization must produce a signal at all tested vessels demonstrating small systolic peaks in early systole with a lack of diastolic flow. The posterior cerebral artery (PCA) is usually the first to change, with the middle cerebral artery (MCA) being the last. Other criteria include the pulsatility index, which will be above 2.0 globally, indicating very high vascular resistance associated with greatly increased ICP. If the TCD reveals oscillating flow through the intracranial arteries, then brain death is more certain. Except for oscillating flow, all other criteria can be seen in pentobarbital coma. However, TCD does not detect brainstem flow or flow through small vessels, and it must not be used as meeting criteria to pronounce death.[24-28]

Single-photon emission computed tomography (SPECT) measures brain uptake activity using radio-labeled amphetamine or radionuclide scan using IV technetium 99m hexamethylpropyleneamineoxime (Tc 99m-HMPAO).[29] Tc 99m-HMPAO adequately reflects brain activity and has been used for the determination of brain death. The isotope needs to be injected within 30 minutes of reconstitution and reveals initial dynamic flow images. Then there are important static images of 500,000 counts at several time intervals recorded immediately, between 30 and 60 minutes, and at 2 hours. Tc 99m-HMPAO static images are adequate for demonstrating the posterior fossa and brainstem.[30] During evaluation, there should be no uptake of isotope in intracerebral parenchyma; however, there may be activity in the external carotid circulation that will demonstrate a hollow skull. To have a valid test, correct IV injection needs to be confirmed with additional liver images demonstrating uptake. By comparison to conventional technetium agents, Tc 99m-HMPAO is not dependent on bolus quality and allows evaluation of the posterior fossa and brainstem.[31] The Tc 99m-HMPAO scan is portable, less expensive, and does not require intra-arterial injection.

◆ Brain Death Exam in Children

Before beginning with an examination as part of the declaration of death, the child must meet the initial criteria of irreversibility, no hypothermia, hypotension, or hypoglycemia, and no medications or metabolic changes that would cause coma or loss of brainstem reflexes. The difficult neurologic exam must be completed twice. The nervous system of the newborn is different from the adult because certain physiological functions may not have been developed. However, the same detailed neurologic exam, including the apnea test, must be performed twice. The detailed neurologic exam must be performed before and after the observation period, and the apnea test must be performed only with the second exam.[32]

Some brainstem reflexes are developed late. In children, the pupillary response to light is obtainable only after week 32 of gestation. The grasp response is obtainable after week 36 of gestation. Most importantly, the last part of the detailed neurologic exam, the apnea response to a PCO_2 stimulus, can only be elicited after 33 weeks of gestation. Therefore, in children there need to be additional criteria mandated for the brain death examination. There is a mandatory observation period in children, and the observation is age-dependent. The complete neurologic exam must be completed before and after the observation period. For children ages 8 days to 2 months, the observation period is 48 hours. For ages 2 months to 12 months, the observation period is 24 hours. For ages 12 months and older, the observation period is 12 hours. An infant must be at least 8 days old to be evaluated for clinical brain death.[32–36]

Children's Confirmatory Test

Because the complete neurologic and repeat neurologic exams after the appropriate observation period may not be reliable, as the functions tested may not have developed, confirmatory tests are mandatory. A cerebral angiogram is the gold standard. An EEG should be performed in accordance with ACNS[21] standards, adjusting the 10 cm inter-electrode distance proportional to the head circumference. Because children <1 year old can survive longer periods of electrocerebral silence without cerebral death, EEGs must be repeated. In children ages 8 days to 2 months, there should be two EEGs and two complete neurologic exams (including an apnea test), 48 hours apart. Two EEGs and complete neurologic exams 24 hours apart or the combination of two complete neurologic examinations 24 hours apart, an EEG showing electrocortical silence, and a Tc 99m-HMPAO radionuclide test showing no cerebral uptake are required in children ages 2 months to 1 year, the rationale being that, in addition to the complete neurologic exams, the radionuclide scan will demonstrate no metabolic brain activity, as well as no electrical activity. Some criteria state that the waiting period is not necessary in children ages 2 months to 1 year if there is a complete neurologic exam, an EEG showing electrocortical silence, and a Tc 99m-HMPAO radionuclide test demonstrating no cerebral uptake. Children's brains demonstrate an ability to recover substantial function after much more significant damage than do adult brains; therefore, the observation period is longer. It remains questionable why the cerebral arteriogram as the sole test has not been incorporated into published criteria for pediatric brain death.

◆ After the Declaration of Brain Death

Brain death is dead. According to Youngner et al, "First and foremost, brain death is irreversible. Patients who are brain dead have permanently lost the capacity to think, be aware of self or surroundings, experience, or communicate with others."[37]

Death must be recorded in the medical record chart when the complete neurologic exam, including the apnea test, is finished. The brain dead patient does not remain alive only to die once the ventilator is removed; the person is dead. There is no need for a physician to return to the body and pronounce the body dead again when the heart stops beating. Death is at the time of the completed full neurologic exam; it is not recorded as the time when the body is removed from the organ-supporting ventilator or when cardiopulmonary function ends.

Health care workers must not state that a patient will be kept alive on the ventilator until organs are recovered. The patient is not alive; only the organs are supported with ventilation. After death is pronounced, the ventilator is turned off if no organs are being donated. The family can visit with the body after removal of the remaining organ support. They should be notified that the patient is dead. The family will naturally ask about the beating heart and should be told that the brain, which contains the memories, activities, joys, love, kindness, and spirit of life, has died and will not return; only the body remains. The heart will continue to beat for an unknown length of time, and most of the organs will function if given support; however, the person is gone. The hospital staff policy must address the length of time that the body can remain in the NICU after the declaration of brain death until a decision about organ donation or until the ventilator is stopped. This short period lasting minutes to a few hours should be offered to allow grieving to begin but should not be so long as to provide false hope. Allowing many hours or, worse, days for out-of-state relatives to visit is not in the best interest of the family. An unusually long length of time only prolongs the family's agony and inhibits the healing process.

After the declaration of death, when there is no decision to donate organs, the ventilator is discontinued. During this time until minutes after complete cessation of cardiac function, there may be acidosis, ischemia, and a sympathetic surge. This surge can trigger multiple simultaneous muscle contractions leading to opening of the eyes, elevation of the arms, and sitting up. This is called the Lazarus syndrome. Therefore, the family should be counseled should they decide to remain with the body from the time of ventilator discontinuation and extubation until removal to the morgue.

◆ Organ Donation

Sometimes the body remains in the NICU while the family decides if the dead individual had wanted to donate organs. It is best to discuss with the family the gift of organ donation with the organ donation workers prior to death.[38–40] The organ donation agency should be contacted anytime the patient has a Glasgow Coma Scale score of 5 or less. The agency could then decide if the individual meets the criteria for donation. If questions from the family arise about organ donation prior to the arrival of organ donation workers, the family may be asked about the wishes of the patient. If the patient is pronounced dead by a complete neurologic exam and the family has consented on behalf of the individual to organ donation, the ventilator continues, and the care of the body should be turned over to the organ transplant agency. The agency coordinators will assume care, write orders, and attempt to maintain the adult parameters of $PO_2 \geq 100$ mm Hg, $SBP \geq 100$ mm Hg, and PCO_2 35 to 45 mm Hg.

Case Management

The patient described in the case study is hypothermic and cannot meet initial criteria to be declared brain dead. The patient must be warmed slowly, must not be comatose from medication, must not be hypoglycemic, and must not have severe metabolic abnormalities that would cause coma and loss of brainstem reflexes. If the initial criteria are met and there is an irreversible lesion on CT scan, then the licensed physician may proceed with a brain death exam.

References

1. Wijdicks EFM. Determining brain death in adults. Neurology 1995;45:1003–1011
2. Whole-brain criterion of death first proposed by the Ad Hoc Committee of the Harvard Medical School to Examine the Definition of Brain Death. JAMA 1968; 205:337–340
3. Guidelines for the determination of death: report of the medical consultants on the diagnosis of death to the President's Commission for the Study of Ethical Problems in Medicine and Biomedical Behavioral Research. JAMA 1981; 246(19):2184–2186
4. Practice parameters for determining brain death in adults in 1995 by the Quality Standards Subcommittee of the American Academy of Neurology. Neurology 1995;45:1012–1014

5. Wijdicks EF. The diagnosis of brain death. N Engl J Med 2001;344:1215–1221
6. Curry PD, Bion JF. The diagnosis and management of brain death. Curr Anaesth Crit Care 1994;5:36–40
7. Medical Task Force on Anencephaly. The infant with anencephaly. N Engl J Med 1990;22:669–674
8. Wijdicks EFM. Brain death worldwide accepted fact but no global consensus in diagnostic criteria. Neurology 2002;58:20–25
9. Byrne PA, Nilges RG. The brain stem in brain death: a critical review. Issues Law Med 1993;9:3–21
10. Danzl DF, Pozos RS. Accidental hypothermia. N Engl J Med 1994;331:1756–1760
11. Gilbert M, Busund R, Skagseth A, Nilsen PA, Solbo JP. Resuscitation from accidental hypothermia of 13.7 degrees C with circulatory arrest. [letter] Lancet 2000;355:375–376
12. Kennedy M, Kiloh N. Drugs and brain death. Drug Saf 1996;14:171–180
13. Patterson JR, Grabois M. Locked-in syndrome: a review of 139 cases. Stroke 1986;17:758–764
14. Ropper AH. Unusual spontaneous movements in brain-dead patients. Neurology 1984;34:1089–1092
15. Saposnik G, Bueri JA, Maurino J, Saizar R, Garretto NS. Spontaneous and reflex movements in brain death. Neurology 2000;54:221–223
16. Marks SJ, Zisfein J. Apneic oxygenation in apnea tests for brain death: a controlled trial. Arch Neurol 1990;47:1066–1068
17. Benzel EC, Gross CD, Hadden TA, et al. The apnea test for the determination of brain death. J Neurosurg 1989;71:191–194
18. Benzel EC, Mashburn JP, Conrad S, Modling D. Apnea testing for the determination of brain death: a modified protocol. J Neurosurg 1992;76:1029–1031
19. Belsh JM, Blatt R, Schiffman PL. Apnea testing in brain death. Arch Intern Med 1986;146:2385–2388
20. Van Donselaar CA, Meerualdt JD, Van Gijn J. Apnea testing to confirm brain death in clinical practice. J Neurol Neurosurg Psychiatry 1986;49:1071–1073
21. American Electroencephalographic Society. Guideline 3: minimum technical standards for EEG recording in suspected cerebral death. J Clin Neurophysiol 1994;11:10–13
22. Silverman D, Saunders MG, Schwab RS, Masland RL. Cerebral death and the electroencephalogram: report of the Ad Hoc Committee of the American Electroencephalographic Society on EEG Criteria for Determination of Cerebral Death. JAMA 1969;209:1505–1510
23. American Electroencephalographic Society. Minimum technical standards for EEG recording in suspected cerebral death. J Clin Neurophysiol 1994;11:10–13
24. Report of the American Academy of Neurology, Therapeutics and Technology Assessment Subcommittee. Assessment: transcranial Doppler. Neurology 1990;40:680–681
25. Payen DM, Lamer C, Pilorget A, Moreau T, Beloucif S, Echter E. Evaluation of pulsed Doppler common carotid blood flow as a noninvasive method for brain death diagnosis: a prospective study. Anesthesiology 1990;72:222–229
26. Petty GW, Mohr JP, Pedley TA, et al. The role of transcranial Doppler in confirming brain death: sensitivity, specificity, and suggestions for performance and interpretation. Neurology 1990;40:300–303
27. Jalili M, Crade M, Davis AL. Carotid blood flow velocity changes detected by Doppler ultrasound in determination of brain death in children: a preliminary report. Clin Pediatr (Phila) 1994;33:669–674
28. Newell DW. Transcranial Doppler measurements. New Horiz 1995;3:423–430
29. Bonetti MG, Ciritella P, Valle G, Perrone E. ^{99m}Tc HM-PAO brain perfusion SPECT in brain death. Neuroradiology 1995;37:365–369
30. de la Riva A, Gonzalez FM, Llamas-Elvira JM, et al. Diagnosis of brain death: superiority of perfusion studies with 99Tcm-HMPAO over conventional radionuclide cerebral angiography. Br J Radiol 1992;65(772):289–294

31. Laurin NR, Driedger AA, Hurwitz GA, et al. Cerebral perfusion imaging with technetium-99m HM-PAO in brain death and severe central nervous system injury. J Nucl Med 1989;30(10):1627–1635

32. American Academy of Pediatrics Task Force on Brain Death in Children. Report of special task force: guidelines for the determination of brain death in children. Pediatrics 1987;80:298–300

33. Ashwal S, Schneider S. Brain death in children: part I. Pediatr Neurol 1987;3:5–11

34. Ashwal S, Schneider S. Brain death in children: part II. Pediatr Neurol 1987;3:69–77

35. Ashwal S. Brain death in the newborn: current perspectives. Clin Perinatol 1997;24:859–882

36. Bernat J. A defense of the whole-brain concept of death. Hastings Cent Rep 1998;28:14–23

37. Youngner S, Landefeld CS, Coulton CJ, Juknialis BW, Leary M. "Brain death" and organ retrieval: a cross-sectional survey of knowledge and concepts among health professionals. JAMA 1989;261:2205–2210

38. Franz HG, DeJong W, Wolfe SM, et al. Explaining brain death: a critical feature of the donation process. J Transplant Coord 1997;7:14–21

39. Chabalewski F, Norris MK. The gift of life: talking to families about organ donation. Am J Nurs 1994;94:28–33

40. Medicare and Medicaid programs; hospital conditions of participation; provider agreements and supplier approval. 62 Federal Register 1997;42 CFR Part 482

Section VI

Nursing Issues

29

Nursing Issues

Paula Snyder

The performance of a thorough neurologic history and physical examination is of paramount importance and will enable the neuroscience team to diagnose the patient with neurologic disease rapidly and will expedite definitive treatment.

◆ Obtaining a Neurologic History

An accurate history may be difficult to obtain because of the patient's neurologic status. Family members or a significant other may need to be called on for the patient's history. Old charts and records may also need to be consulted. A detailed history should include the chief complaint, a history of the present illness, and a past medical history. A chief complaint includes a brief statement or response to the question, What brought you to the hospital today? A history of the present illness includes a description of the signs and symptoms, onset, location, severity, duration, frequency, and aggravating and/or alleviating factors. The past medical history should include the patient's medical and medication history, substance use and abuse, sexual history, and family and social history.

The neurologic history should include assessment of pain, headaches, seizures, and changes in eating or sleeping patterns. It should attempt to derive answers to the following:

- Is the patient experiencing weakness, numbness, or tingling; loss of sensation; or strange sensations in his or her arms, legs, or other areas?
- Is there a loss of bowel, bladder, or sexual function?
- Are there cerebellar signs, such as difficulty with gait, balance, coordination, and speech?
- Are there changes in mood, memory, concentration, and understanding of written or spoken language?
- Is the patient experiencing problems with swallowing, choking, or aspiration?

- Are there changes in vision, such as diplopia, blind spots, and decreased acuity?
- Are there problems with hearing or ringing in the ears?
- Are there changes in or loss of sense of taste or smell?
- Has the patient been experiencing dizziness, vertigo, syncope, or nausea/vomiting?
- Does the patient have a history of neurologic disease or injury?

It is important to ascertain the mechanism of injury in trauma patients. Acceleration-deceleration, rotation, flexion-extension, and axial loading may cause specific brain or spinal cord injuries. These injuries may include coup/contrecoup brain injury, diffuse axonal injury, and spinal injuries. "Down" times and extrication times are also important. When did the trauma occur? How long was it before medical assistance was given? Discerning the patient's hypoxia or hypotension at the scene of the injury may give clues to its severity or long-term prognosis. Finding out if there was vomit at the scene, for example, or if the patient had gurgling respirations can alert you to whether or not the patient has been predisposed to respiratory complications such as aspiration pneumonia.

◆ Components of the Neurologic Exam

Mental Status

The mental status exam is a brief assessment to test higher levels of cortical function. Asking simple questions regarding persons, places, time, and reason assesses orientation and attention. Is the patient able to answer questions during the interview, or is he or she distracted, needing to be redirected frequently? Assessment of remote and recent memory is tested with such questions as, What did you have for breakfast? and, Where did you grow up? or by asking the patient to recall three words told to him or her earlier in the exam. Have the patient name objects, such as a pen, paper clip, and comb, and their function or purpose. Have the patient read, write, and copy figures. Test abstract reasoning and judgment by asking the relationship between word pairs (cat–dog, comb–brush, hot–cold) or the meaning of a saying or proverb (e.g., "A stitch in time saves nine"). Refer the patient for neuropsychological evaluation if deficits are present.

Level of Consciousness

The Glasgow Coma Scale (GCS) is the most frequently used tool to assess the level of consciousness (LOC). The patient is scored on a scale of 3 to 15 in three areas based on his or her best responses (**Table 29–1**).[1]

Table 29–1   Glasgow Coma Scale[1]

Eye Opening	Verbal Response	Motor Response
4: opens eyes spontaneously	5: oriented	6: obeys commands
3: opens eyes to sound	4: confused	5: localizes to pain
2: opens eyes to pain	3: inappropriate words	4: withdraws to pain
1: no eye opening	2: incomprehensible sounds	3: flexes/decorticates to pain
	1: nonverbal	2: extends/decerebrates to pain
		1: no response to pain

The patient should be approached quietly (not silently) when assessing for spontaneous eye opening. Several spheres should be checked when assessing for orientation (person, place, time, and reason). The patient should not be overly coached in his or her answers or motor responses. Time should be allowed for the patient to answer questions and follow commands. The same command should be simply repeated to avoid confusing the patient. When assessing pain response, central pain stimulation should be used. Nail bed pressure may elicit a spinal reflex and be confused with withdrawal by the examiner. A purposeful response can be differentiated from flexion by observing if the patient crosses the midline in response to pain.

A patient who is awake, alert, oriented, and obeying commands receives a GCS of 15. A patient who is completely unresponsive to painful stimulation receives a GCS of 3. Patients with a GCS score of 8 or less are comatose[1] and are at high risk for respiratory compromise. These patients are usually intubated and cared for in the neurosurgical intensive care unit (NICU).

Care should be taken when using one-word descriptions of a patient's LOC. It is best to describe the response to stimulation and the kind of stimulation needed to elicit the response (**Table 29–2**).

Table 29–2   Describing a Patient's Level of Consciousness[1–3]

Good	Better
Alert	Responds immediately
Confused	Disoriented to person/time/place/reason
Lethargic	Requires increased or frequent stimuli to be awakened
Obtunded	Minimal response to stimuli; one-word answers
Stuporous	Aroused only by vigorous, continuous stimuli
Comatose	No voluntary, purposeful response

Table 29–3 Pupillary Assessment[1-3]

Pupil	Reaction	Possible Causes
Pinpoint	None or minimal	Pontine injury or narcotic overdose
Midposition	Reactive	Normal response
	Nonreactive	Midbrain injury
Dilated	Reactive	Stimulant use, autonomic dysfunction
	Sluggish/nonreactive	Unilateral: pressure, swelling, hemorrhage, tumor, herniation, aneurysm, or orbital trauma
		Bilateral: brain anoxia, herniation, or death

Pupillary Assessment

Pupillary response is a function of the autonomic nervous system via cranial nerve (CN) III. Parasympathetic and sympathetic control causes the pupils to constrict and dilate. Before beginning the pupil exam, dim the room lights to prevent missing a minimal reaction.

The following steps are followed in a pupillary assessment:

1. *Direct light reflex:* Shine the light directly into one eye. The pupil should immediately constrict to light. When the light is removed, the pupil should immediately dilate.

2. *Consensual response:* Shine the light in one eye while watching for constriction of the opposite pupil. Observe for dilation when the light is removed (**Table 29–3**).

Speech and Language Assessment

Communication incorporates four functions: the ability to listen, read, speak, and write.[1] Disturbances in these functions can be categorized as shown in **Table 29–4**.

Table 29–4 Disturbances in Speech and Language[1-3]

Type	Description
Aphasia	Inability to speak due to disturbances in the dominant hemisphere
Dysphasia	Difficulty in communication
Expressive aphasia (Broca's)	Inability to correctly form thoughts and communicate information; comprehension is relatively preserved
Receptive aphasia (Wernicke's)	Inability to correctly comprehend written (alexia) or verbal language

Cranial Nerve Assessment

There are 12 pairs of cranial nerves. The cranial nerves are numbered I to XII according to the order in which their nuclei connect to the brain (**Table 29–5**).

Motor Assessment

Motor assessment includes a general assessment of

♦ Symmetry
♦ Muscle bulk
♦ Atrophy
♦ Tone: spasticity, rigidity, and flaccidity
♦ Strength
♦ Reflexes

Muscle strength is graded on a scale of 0 to 5, as shown in **Table 29–6**.

The nurse should be vigilant in his or her assessments. Frequent neurologic assessment by the bedside nurse is imperative to detect subtle changes in LOC. It is helpful if nurses who are changing shifts assess the patient's GCS, pupils, and a brief focused motor and sensory exam together. This will help decrease interrater variability and prevent missing significant neurologic changes.

Vital Signs

Vital signs should be documented at least hourly. Careful attention should be paid to trends or gradual changes in vital signs and neurologic responses. These changes may not be noticeable on an hourly basis, but they are significant over time. A decrease in GCS of 2 points is significant and should be reported to the attending physician, as it may signal increasing intracranial pressure (ICP) or tissue hypoxia. Other hourly observations should include pupillary responses, extraocular movements, focused motor and sensory exam, strict intake and output, blood pressure, heart rate and rhythm, temperature, central venous pressure, and pulmonary artery pressures when available.

Changes in vital signs are often late; earlier signs of neurologic deterioration are increasing headaches, agitation, nausea/vomiting, and a sense of impending doom. You may also see cranial nerve changes, such as facial drooping or asymmetry, dysconjugate gaze, and pupillary changes. There may be increasing pronator drift, muscle weakness, and posturing. Brainstem reflexes (gag, cough, and corneal reflexes) should be noted upon initial assessment and during interim assessments, every 4 hours or more often as indicated. Seizure may also indicate neurologic deterioration. Acute changes in LOC may be a sign of silent seizure and should be evaluated by electroencephalogram (EEG).

Table 29–5 Cranial Nerve Assessment[1-3]

Cranial Nerve	Sensory	Motor	Function	Assessment/Test	Comments
I Olfactory	X		Sensory: sense of smell; helps food flavor	Test one nostril at a time with coffee grounds, mint, or lemon	Do not test with alcohol, ammonia, or other noxious solutions that stimulate pain fibers
II Optic	X		Vision	Tested by visual acuity, visual fields, and fundoscopic exam	
III Oculomotor	X	X	Upward, inward, downward, and outward eye movement Parasympathetic: pupillary constriction	Extraocular movements; tested with CN IV and VI Pupillary constriction to direct light and consensual response	Pressure from swelling, hemorrhage, or supracellar tumors can cause herniation of temporal lobe or direct pressure on CN III resulting in pupillary dilatation
IV Trochlear		X	Downward and inward eye movement	Extraocular movements; tested with CN III and VI	Disturbances result in inability to look down at feet and difficulty climbing stairs
V Trigeminal	X	X	Facial sensation and mastication Ophthalmic branch: cornea, conjunctiva, upper lid, forehead, and scalp Maxillary branch: cheek, jaw, hard palate,	Test by touch, pain, and temperature assessment, comparing one side to the other Test by touching with a cotton-tipped applicator, as in cornea test	Trigeminal neuralgia is associated with intense sharp, shooting or electric paroxysmal pain related to stimulation by seemingly benign activities, tumor of the middle fossa or cerebellar-pontine angle, or

			Function	Testing	Abnormal Findings
			nasopharynx, nasal cavity, tongue, upper teeth Mandibular branch: lower teeth, gums, jaw, and mouth; ear and sides of tongue Motor: mastication	Assessed by asking patient to clench jaw, move jaw from side to side against examiner's hand	irritation by atherosclerotic vessels
VI Abducens		X	Moves eye outward	Extraocular movements; tested with CN III and IV	Diplopia when tries to look to side
VII Facial	X	X	Motor: muscles of the face, facial expression Sensory: taste to anterior two thirds of tongue, sensation to the ear Parasympathetic: secretory to nose and mouth, lacrimal glands	Test for ability by having patient raise eyebrows, wrinkle forehead, close eyes, purse lips, puff cheeks Taste with salt and sugar on anterior two thirds of tongue	
VIII Vestibulocochlear	X		Cochlear: hearing Vestibular: sense of balance	Test by whispering in patient's ear, rubbing fingers together near patient's ear Rapid alternating movements; finger to nose test, patient's finger to examiner's finger	Disturbances in equilibrium, vertigo; hearing loss
IX Glossopharyngeal	X	X	Sensory: taste posterior one third of tongue; touch,	Tested with CN X	

(Continued)

Table 29–5 Cranial Nerve Assessment (*Continued*)

Cranial Nerve	Sensory	Motor	Function	Assessment/Test	Comments
			pain, and temperature of palate and pharynx		
			Motor: muscles of swallowing	Assess for voice quality, pitch, hoarseness, and difficulty swallowing	
			Parasympathetic: salivary glands and carotid reflex	Observe for elevation of pharynx and symmetry when patient says "ah" or when posterior pharynx stroked	
X Vagus	X	X	Motor and sensory: pharynx and larynx Swallow, phonation, cough, and gag Visceral sensation of the esophagus, bronchi, abdominal viscera Parasympathetic: respiratory and digestive tract, carotid reflex, and sinoatrial node of heart	Observe for elevation of pharynx and symmetry when patient says "ah" or when posterior pharynx is stroked	
XI Spinal accessory		X	Shoulders and neck	Have patient shrug shoulders and turn head against resistance	
XII Hypoglossal		X	Motor: tongue	Assess for asymmetry, atrophy, fasciculation, deviation, and decreased strength	

CN, cranial nerve.

Table 29–6   Assessment of Muscle Strength[1–3]

Grade	Character
0	No muscle contraction
1	Trace contraction
2	Movement with gravity eliminated
3	Movement against gravity
4−	Slight resistance
4	Moderate resistance
4+	Strong resistance
5	Normal/full strength

Cushing's Response

Cushing's response is the body's reaction to increased ICP and resulting cerebral ischemia. It is characterized by bradycardia, elevated systolic blood pressure (SBP), respiratory irregularities, and widening pulse pressure. As the pressure within the brain nears the cerebral arterial pressure, the vagal and sympathetic nerves are stimulated, resulting in increased cardiac output, bradycardia, and shunting of blood flow from other body organs to the brain. Arterial blood pressure rises in an attempt to restore cerebral perfusion. Cushing's response is a late sign of increased ICP and is associated with irreversible brain damage. It may be transient or not be present in all patients experiencing neurologic deterioration.[1]

Patients who have suffered a direct injury or bleed to the brainstem may exhibit the same signs and symptoms found in increased ICP with normal ICP.[2] Brainstem injuries carry a poor prognosis for recovery.[1]

Blood Pressure

Hypotension associated with head injury is usually a sign of a terminal event. In the NICU patient with signs of life, it is probably attributable to another cause, and it should be evaluated aggressively. In trauma patients, it may be caused by bleeding in the chest, abdomen, or pelvis, or associated with blood loss in long bone fractures, or it may be a result of spinal cord injury (SCI). Hypotension in high SCI is usually accompanied by bradycardia. Hypertension not associated with increased ICP may be caused by pain, fear, and anxiety. The patient may also have a known or unknown history of hypertension.

Heart Rate

Tachycardia in the neurosurgical or head-injured patient may be a result of injury to the hypothalamus or may signify a terminal neurologic event, such as brain herniation or death. Other causes of elevated heart rate may include fever, dehydration, hypotension, and shock. Agitation and pain may also cause tachycardia. A catecholamine "storm," or stress response in a head injury, may also cause a high heart rate.[1] The nurse must be a good detective when looking for the root cause of tachycardias. Just remember to keep the patient calm and comfortable.

Respirations

Respiratory changes may not be as evident in the NICU patient, who often comes to the unit already intubated on mechanical ventilation. Changes can still be observed, though. Respirations may become rapid and deep, as in central neurogenic hyperventilation. This type of hyperventilation serves to lower ICP by lowering partial pressure of CO_2 (PCO_2), thus causing cerebral vasoconstriction, but it may worsen tissue hypoxia. Cheyne-Stokes respirations may precede cerebral herniation. Agonal respirations often occur when death is imminent. Rapid respirations may result from hypoxemia. Inadequate oxygenation of the brain will result in secondary brain injury in the NICU patient. Respiratory monitoring should include continuous assessment of oxygenation status to prevent hypoxemia. The routine O_2 titration order "keep SpO_2 [pulse oxygenation saturation] greater than 97%" will not ensure optimum brain tissue oxygenation. SpO_2 and partial pressure of oxygen in arterial blood (PaO_2) should be correlated with arterial blood gases.

Temperature

Fever should be prevented and treated promptly if it occurs. Cerebral metabolism is increased ~10% with each degree of Celsius temperature. Increased O_2 consumption results in brain tissue hypoxia and secondary brain injury.[1] Hypothermia occurs frequently in SCI patients due to loss of autonomic function and thermoregulation. They are poikilothermic, meaning their temperature changes with environmental temperature changes. The room, therefore, must be kept at a constant temperature. Injury to the hypothalamus may also cause hypothermia. Cooling and/or warming measures should be employed as appropriate.[2] Remember that steroid use may inhibit a patient's ability to mount a fever in the face of infection.

◆ Imaging

It is better to get a computed tomography (CT) scan than to guess whether or not a patient is deteriorating or just waxing and waning. Generally speaking, if the patient does not look as good postop as he or she did preop, you probably need to rule out postop bleeding. Do not just chalk up a change in neurologic status to the patient's being "sensitive" to anesthesia. Subdurals do reaccumulate, epidurals do rebleed, and hematomas can develop in postop hematoma cavities. There may be delayed bleeding in trauma or stroke patients. Be aware and report changes to the physician promptly.

◆ Intracranial Pressure Monitoring

ICP should be monitored in patients with a GCS of 3 to 8 via a ventricular catheter. Guidelines set forth by the Brain Trauma Foundation[3] discuss the high chance of having increased ICP in patients with severe head injuries and with a GCS of 3 to 8 and intracranial findings on CT or GCS of 3 to 8 and two of the following: >40 years of age, posturing, or SBp < 90 mm Hg.[3] Those patients with a GCS of 3 to 8 and not meeting the above criteria still risk having an increased ICP. Some of the benefits of ICP monitoring with a ventriculostomy include the following:

1. Allows identification of elevated ICP before clinical signs and symptoms appear
2. Allows drainage of cerebrospinal fluid (CSF) to treat or prevent increased ICP
3. Allows identification of the patient's tolerance to routine nursing and medical procedures
4. Allows judgment of the patient's response to therapeutic measures, treatments, and medications

Whether you are using the traditional gold standard external transducer system or a fiberoptic catheter for ICP monitoring, remember that it is a potential source for contamination. Strict aseptic technique should be observed when handling and changing tubing and drainage bags. CSF output is monitored every 1 to 2 hours for amount, color, and clarity.

Nursing management of increased ICP is directed toward prevention and early identification of factors that precipitate increased ICP. The simplest maneuver to lower ICP is to increase venous drainage from the brain. The best way to do this is to elevate the head of the bed. Use the reverse Trendelenburg's position for those patients in spinal precautions. Keep the head in the midline position, with minimal or no hip flexion. Prevent abdominal distention by maintaining patency of gastric tubes and by monitoring feedings for high gastric residuals. Titrate sedation to prevent agitation, but by the same token do not oversedate NICU patients. Oversedation can confound the neurologic assessment. Sedation should be held each shift and periodically during the day to allow for neurologic assessment as long as ICP is responsive to resedation.

◆ Stimulation and Family Interaction

How much stimulation is too much? Is the patient's ICP and tissue oxygenation stable while family members are visiting? Watch what they are saying to the patient. Instruct them to speak positively to the patient, with encouraging words. Ask them to tell the patient about things that are important to him or her. Let the patient know that the children and pets are safe and well cared for. Warn the family against telling the patient to "fight," as this may cause increased agitation in the patient. Instruct them not to ask questions when the patient is intubated and/or unable to speak, unless the patient is able to nod his or her head in response; even then, questions should be limited to "yes" "no" types. Music, taped voices of children, get well cards, and pictures may help with the patient's recovery. A few personal items from home also may help comfort the patient.

Recruit the patient's family members. Make them your allies. Teach them the basics of patient care, and involve them in their loved one's daily routine. When the patient has a neurologic disease or injury, he or she is probably going to need family assistance for activities of daily living, at least on a short-term basis, if not for the long term. Teaching family members early will help in their transition to caregivers. An added benefit is that they will not be calling you to the bedside constantly because they are anxious about every gurgle or alarm. Families are often the best alternative to restraint use in agitated patients. However, you must first observe the interaction between the family members and the patient. Do they have a soothing effect on the patient? Are they responsible and attentive to the patient? If they are, you may be able to reduce restraint use while improving the patient's comfort level.

Family members need some distraction when their loved one is in the hospital. After the patient has passed the critical phase of his or her NICU stay, it is a good time to ask the family to begin compiling a "memory book" for the patient. It should include clearly labeled photos of family members, friends, pets, home, cars, and anything else of importance to the patient. This will help the patient remember and/or relearn who was in his or her life and what his or her life was like.

◆ Mobility

It is important to mobilize the patient as soon as possible. Sit the patient up in bed as soon as you can get an okay from the physician. Let the patient dangle his or her legs from the bed. The longer a person lies on his or her back, the harder it will be to move him or her. Use elastic support hose, and change positions slowly to help prevent orthostatic hypotension. Abdominal binders may also be helpful in SCI patients. Involve physical therapists as soon as the patient has passed the initial critical phase of his or her hospitalization. In the meantime, turn the patient frequently (every 2 hours or more frequently). If the patient is on prolonged bed rest, suggest some form of rotational therapy bed.

◆ Discharge Planning

Begin discharge planning when the patient is first admitted. Assess his or her family situation. Are family members available and supportive? Do they have the resources necessary for posthospital care if the patient needs assistance at home? Work with your facility's case managers and social service workers, and begin planning for discharge or placement as soon as possible. Many NICU patients have suffered life-changing illness or injury and will need support to plan and cope. Educate them regarding their injury, prognosis, and potential. Give them the tools they need to adjust to their new life situations.

References

1. Barker E. Neuroscience Nursing: A Spectrum of Care. 2nd ed. St. Louis, MO: CV Mosby; 2002
2. Hickey JV. The Clinical Practice of Neurological and Neurosurgical Nursing. 5th ed. Philadelphia: Lippincott Williams & Wilkins; 2003
3. Guidelines for the Management of Severe Traumatic Brain Injury. New York: Brain Trauma Foundation; 2000

30

Restraints and the Neurosurgical Intensive Care Unit Patient

Paula Snyder

The neurosurgical intensive care unit (NICU) faces unique challenges when it comes to providing patient safety. Patients are often confused, impulsive, restless, and agitated. They may lack the ability to make sound judgments regarding their medical care. Frequently, NICU patients are unaware of their physical limitations. We as health care workers are charged with the responsibility of protecting our patients from physical harm, while at the same time preventing psychological distress.

◆ Guidelines for Restraint Use

Restraint usage reduction is the primary intent of the Joint Commission on Accreditation of Healthcare Organizations' (JCAHO) patient care initiatives.[1] Guidelines from the Centers for Medicare and Medicaid Services (CMS; formerly the Health Care Financing Administration) also emphasize restraint reduction. Both institutions regard restraints and seclusion as last-resort measures and encourage acute care hospitals to use them only when less restrictive means fail.

Restraint use must be guided by state and federal law and by hospital licensing or accreditation requirements at your facility.

A restraint can be defined as any device or method used to restrict a person's movement, mobility, or access to his or her body.[2] Medical restraint can be applied in a variety of settings for a variety of reasons. When a restraint is used to promote medical treatment, such as intravenous (IV) therapy and medications; to prevent pulling lines and therapeutic tubes, such as endotracheal tubes, indwelling catheters, intracranial monitors, or drains; or to prevent disturbing surgical dressings and incisions, it is considered medical restraint, no matter the hospital setting. All other alternative means of preventing the undesired behavior should be exhausted before application of restraint. That being said, if we allow our patients to harm themselves by self-extubation or by pulling out their subdural drain or other medically necessary tubes and lines, then we have not helped them.

Patient safety must be foremost in our minds when using restraints. A JCAHO sentinel event alert from 1998 reports 20 deaths in the previous 2 years of patients in restraints.[3] These deaths had various root causes. Death by strangulation occurred in geriatric patients with vest restraint, half of whom made their way between split side rails. Forty percent of deaths occurred as a result of asphyxiation, and the remainder were due to cardiac arrest and fire (while the patient was attempting to burn off the restraints). The JCAHO identified potential contributing factors as

1. Restraint of smokers
2. Restraint of patients with physical deformities that prevent proper application (especially vests)
3. Supine position predisposing patients to aspiration
4. Prone position predisposing patients to suffocation
5. Not continually observing patients in restraints

Care should be taken to decrease the risk of problems, such as those listed above. All smoking supplies should be removed from the patient's person and environment, and visitors should be advised of restriction due to fire risk. A thorough assessment of appropriateness of planned restraint device, considering the patient's unique physical needs, must be performed prior to application. Proper positioning and observation of the restrained patient are imperative. A nonintubated patient with an altered level of consciousness should not be restrained flat on his or her back because of the risk of aspiration. The head of the bed should be elevated whenever possible. Rarely, if ever, will an NICU patient need to be restrained in the prone position, but if the prone position is used, the airway must be kept unobstructed at all times. The prone position is not recommended for obese, elderly, and pediatric patients.

JCAHO's Provision of Care, Treatment and Services (PC) PC.11.10 through PC.11.100 delineate the appropriate measures for restraint use in hospitals.[1] These standards establish that assessment and reassessments of need for restraint, and alternatives to use are performed according to hospital policy. Additionally, hospital leaders must set forth the institutions's philosophy regarding and standards for restraint use and define the situations in which restraint use is allowable based on clinical evidence. Hospital policies will direct appropriate, safe use of restraint. Restraints must be either ordered by a licensed independent practitioner (LIP) or applied upon specific order according to a hospital-approved protocol that defines clinical criteria for use. Patients are to be monitored while in restraint, and restraint use is to be thoroughly documented in the patient's medical record according to hospital policy. The hospital works via its performance improvement process to find ways to prevent use, develop alternative measures, and improve processes to decrease the risks related to restraint use. These standards are not intended to address behavioral restraint. Restraint is never used as a disciplinary measure.

◆ Procedures for Application of Restraints

Let's put the above information to practical use.

1. Use of medical restraints should be limited to situations with appropriate clinical justification and reserved for patients at risk of self-harm, such as self-extubation, pulling or disturbing medically necessary lines and tubes, and disturbing wounds and dressings, as well as for patients who attempt to ambulate when medically unable to do so. A thorough assessment of risk must be completed for all patients.

2. A written order by an LIP is required upon initiation of restraint. A person qualified by education and experience, according to hospital policy, may initiate restraint in an emergency. The LIP must be notified of initiation and must sign the order within 8 hours. Nurse practitioners or physician's assistants may be allowed to order restraints in some institutions. Some hospitals may elect to allow application of restraints according to a hospital-approved protocol by persons qualified by education and experience, if allowed by state and federal law, and by hospital licensing or accreditation requirements at the facility.

3. The order should be timed, dated, and time limited, not to exceed 24 hours. Type, number of points, and reason for restraint must be included in the order. Restraints must be reordered daily after face-to-face evaluation by LIP. Restraint use should be discussed in a multidisciplinary care conference at regular intervals where alternative measures to restraint are explored.

4. The patient must be closely monitored. Visual observation should take place continually, as defined by your institution. Physical and psychological needs must be attended to no less frequently than every 2 hours. These include skin and circulation assessment, assessment of comfort or agitation levels, toileting and hygiene, hydration and nutrition, and position changes with range of motion. Continuous observation should be considered for highly agitated patients, as they are at increased risk for injury in spite of or resulting from restraint. Ongoing assessment of continued need for restraint and/or trial out of restraint should also be addressed.

5. The patient and his or her family should be educated as to the reason for restraint, the criteria required for release of restraint, and the steps taken to maintain safety while in restraint.

6. All restraint occurrences should be thoroughly documented in the medical record. Clinical justification, alternative measures, response to restraint, physician notification, patient/family education, and patient care should be recorded according to hospital policy.

7. Staff members should be educated regarding the hospital's restraint policies and also in the practical application of restraint. Competency should be demonstrated and maintained by in-service and/or skills

testing at intervals specified by policy. Education regarding the hospital's performance improvement process in respect to restraint reduction and alternatives, as well as hospital statistics compiled on restraints, should be ongoing and disseminated via unit and department meetings at regular intervals.

Important alternatives to restraint use are adequate pain relief to prevent the confused patient from disturbing a wound or dressing, allowing the patient's family to remain at the bedside to prevent or decrease anxiety and fear, and reorienting the patient frequently. Using bedside sitters to monitor the patient's behavior and prevent him or her from pulling tubes and lines or wandering may also be beneficial. Diversional activities such as games, drawing, and television may be helpful for some patients. When an NICU patient has an altered level of consciousness and is intubated on a ventilator, however, the only safe method of preventing self-harm is increased vigilance along with wrist restraint.

References

1. Joint Commission on Healthcare Organizations. Comprehensive Accreditation Manual for Hospitals. The Official Handbook. Oakbrook Terrace, IL: Joint Commission Resources, Inc.: 2007
2. Wigder HN. Restraints [Emedicine website]. June 4, 2004. Available at: http://www.emedicine.com/emerg/topic776.htm. Accessed March 7, 2007
3. Sentinel event alert [Joint Commission on Accreditation of Healthcare Organizations website]. November 18, 1998. Available at: http://www.jcaho.org/ about+us/ news+letters/sentinel+event+alert/print/sea_8.htm. Accessed March 7, 2007

Section VII

Family Issues

31
Family Communication

Theresa Longo and Dan Miulli

Care of the neurosurgical intensive care unit (NICU) patient is more than managing the clinical situation. There are numerous areas that are just as important and must be attended to, particularly communication. Communication should not be left for the health care worker to figure out; it must be part of the neurosurgical curriculum. The recommendations in this chapter have been developed over time, using the expertise of countless clinicians.

The chapter outlines the definition of communication in the NICU setting, along with the goals of communication and its role in relationship building. It offers suggestions on dealing with barriers to communication, including hostile patients and their families. Scenarios are presented depicting challenges in communication between medical and allied health professionals and NICU patients and their families. Additionally, circumstances requiring specialized protocols for communications are discussed.

◆ Definition of Communication

The broadest definition of communication in this setting is the exchange of information between and among physicians doing neurocritical care, their colleagues, multidisciplinary health care specialists, and patients and their families.

Physicians cannot function in the NICU outside the bounds of their relationships with staff. The physicians and the multidisciplinary staff of caregivers in the hospital are one unit in a dyad. The cohesiveness of that unit and its ability to converge on a goal in an organized battle array are a matter of planning, dedication, mutual respect, and practice.

Regardless of the patient's level of consciousness and capacity, the patient cannot be managed and communication cannot be said to occur if the available family members are not taken into account. The patient and his or her family are the other unit in the dyad. The cohesiveness of this unit is subject to patterns of functioning that began before the crisis centered attention on the patient and will continue, in some manner, irrespective of the patient's outcome.

The narrow scope of communication for this chapter is the exchange between physicians and the patient and his or her family. This is the familiar stage for the relationship between the dyads. Communication encompasses all manner of conveying information, but this chapter will focus on verbal communication and unspoken behaviors that convey feelings encountered during conversations.

The milieu in which the communication occurs, that is, the medical setting, the emergency room, and the NICU, indelibly colors the information conveyed, how it is remembered, and how it is used to make decisions both for patients/families and physicians/health care team.

Communication does not occur in a vacuum. The doctor–patient relationship is the basis for communication. The patient and his or her family give and receive information in the context of this relationship, extended to include all of the health care team.

◆ Goals of Communication

Communication can be said to be achieved when the patient/family and physicians/health care team create a dialogue between each other for the patient's sake in which questions are asked and answered truthfully, wisely, and respectfully and the unanswerable questions are acknowledged with compassion, patience, and trust. One-sided conveyance of information devoid of human context may, in some circumstances, seem necessary and appropriate, even if painful, but it is not communication unless it is acknowledged and assimilated.

The goal of communication is fundamentally the exchange of information that might lead to saving the patient's life or salvaging the disabled patient from ruin, but this goal is accomplished or derailed by the quality of the relationship that develops between patient/family and physicians/health care team as a result of the quality of their communication.

It is not enough to know what has or will happen or to be able to say it out loud. The quality of each party's contribution to communication depends as much on presentation, timing, delivery, and receptivity to feedback as it does on the accuracy of the factual data presented.

If no one is pausing to listen, then speech is meaningless, regardless of its content. Silence can be the ultimate in communication if it is shared. **Tables 31–1** and **31–2** outline the premises underlying communication and the type of information needed by the patient and his or her family. **Table 31–3** lists the three main sources of stress—the environment, the patient, and family factors.

Table 31–1   Premises Underlying Communication between the Health Care Team and Patients and Their Families

All communication is filled with concerns for the risks of death or disability.

A common vocabulary, shared context, and shared set of expectations between physicians and patients and their families must be crafted, not assumed.

Medically logical priorities are unlikely to match family priorities.

Opinions concerning goals, values, and quality of life must be explored, not assumed.

Trust and respect between physicians and patients and their family have to be reciprocal; they must be earned and returned.

Communication begins with the staff member the patient and his or her family sees: there is no second chance to make a first impression.

Table 31–2   Patient Situation Preventing Meaningful Communication

Loss of identity/loss of control/altered future/dependency

Coma

Paralysis

Death

Table 31–3   Sources of Stress for NICU Patients and Their Families

Environment
Unfamiliar sights/sounds, unfamiliar activities and fast pace, isolation, separation, waiting, friction with staff/changing staff assignments, communication failures and delays, hunger/thirst, sleep deprivation, hygiene, lack of privacy, no place to store things

Patient
Altered appearance of patient by trauma, disease, or surgery; unfamiliar behavior of patient; unfamiliar tests and procedures, loss of identity; loss of recognition by family; concerns about the future

Family factors
Siblings'/other family members' demands, parental role revision, conflicts for control between spouses and parents, role revisions within the family, career concerns, travel concerns, financial stresses, geographic distance from support systems, discharge planning, future family economic and support issues

Table 31–4   Initial Family Information to Gather

Coping mechanisms the physicians want to encourage versus coping strategies patient/family already use
Health and emotional condition that the patient/family arrives in, including the presence of family members with disabilities
Patient's/family's immediate resources for self-care (psychological, social, monetary, and access to transportation)
Socioeconomic and educational background of patient/family
Cultural and religious precepts/prejudices/preconceptions
Availability, dedication, proximity, and strength of extended support system, including sympathetic employers
Chemical dependency of both patient and family members, including tobacco

◆ Factors Affecting How Information Is Transmitted and Received

Communicating with the patient and family begins and grows by getting to know them. This applies to the health care team as much as it relates to the patient and his or her family.

Data gathering that may hold the key to reaching a patient or family member begins on the first meeting, is supported by the impressions and information gathered by the remainder of the health care team, and continues to expand as the relationship with the patient and his or her family deepens. Some considerations to assist with data gathering should be documented in the nurse's intake sheet. **Table 31–4** outlines the basic information that should be gathered in the first meeting. **Table 31–5** lists the positive and negative coping mechanisms that can be anticipated. **Tables 31–6** and **31–7** give examples of charged words and behaviors, respectively.

Table 31–5   Coping Mechanisms the Family Is Likely to Use

Positive	Negative
Leaning on others for support	Clinging to the patient/refusing to leave the bedside
Reliving the events that led to the crisis	Probing events/questioning information/intellectualizing
Acting strong and competent	Putting on a show of confidence and strength
Blaming themselves or others	Focusing on trivial issues to avoid greater issues
Comparing their plight to those in worse straits (relief)	Exaggerating their circumstances to see themselves as heroes or martyrs
Rehearsing for death	Clinging to inappropriate hope

Table 31–6 Words That Can Be Misunderstood

Death/dying	Coma	Disability
Dependence	Consciousness	Paralysis
Pain/suffering	Communicate	Rehabilitation
Anxiety/fear	Control	Vision/hearing/speech

Table 31–7 Charged Behaviors That Take on Enhanced Significance for Patients and Their Families

Behavior	Significance
Looking	Eye contact or equivalent denotes focus, connectiveness, attentiveness, respect
Listening	Nodding, facial expressions, taking notes (and looking up) denote receptiveness
Touching	Refraining from examining or touching or carrying out other activities while listening denotes focus and implies that what is being heard matters to the one listening
Posture/position	Sitting down and taking steps to ensure privacy or to protect the conversation from interruption indicate commitment to listening and receptiveness to what is said; standing implies a time limit unless it is at the bedside

◆ Techniques for Dealing with the Hostile Patient/Family

Appropriate professionals should address any threat of violence and make preliminary efforts to resolve the conflict. The physician may be dealing with the aftermath of others' interventions or with patient's or family members' refusal to proceed with needed care/procedures. **Table 31–8** outlines actions and suggested approaches to dealing with the hostile patient or family members.

◆ Barriers to Communication

Language differences can cause many problems in communication, both with patients and with their families. This should be addressed by hospital policy using available translators/services in the hospital, the community, or the Internet before the communication problem arises. Communicating

Table 31–8   Approaches to Dealing with Hostile Patients and Their Families

Action	Patient and family present	Family present without patient
Act quickly	Find out precipitating factors from others first; call for help if violence is threatened.	Same; delegate other commitments quickly to limit interruptions.
Find privacy	If the patient is stable, unite the angry patient or family members with <10 key family members.	If patient cannot be included, unite <10 key family members separately in a private place.
Enlist support	Have another health care professional present while defusing hostility.	Have a staff member listen in; enlist key family members to assist.
Acknowledge the anger, then redirect to focus on the patient	Opening ploy acknowledges the stressor, validates the patient's or family's feelings without admitting fault, then diverts attention back to the patient.	Indicate willingness to deal with the trigger for the hostility after the patient/family has been updated and the patient's acute needs are addressed.
Avoid the quarrel	Use nonverbal cues to give impression of openness. Use words to confirm your authority and dedication to the patient's critical medical needs.	Same. Postpone issues not directly related to the patient's survival (e.g., visitation) to be handled as promptly as possible by others more appropriate to the task.
Commit the time; leave an impression of focus, competence, and caring	Limit discussion of what provoked the hostility to information gathering. Defer negotiation about those circumstances to appropriate channels. Avoid making promises or "bribing." Lead by example, away from hostility and away from unreasonable demands.	Detach from the problem, not the people. Display willingness to incorporate their concerns into how things are done (without agreeing to favors/privileges that are not your purview to permit).

via signs and single words by health care providers unfamiliar with a patient's native language may be all that is possible in a crisis, but this practice is to be avoided and never accepted as a habit.

The chronic absence of family members for meetings may be addressed by social workers and discharge planners; in a crisis, law enforcement agencies may need to be contacted.

The hospital should have protocols to facilitate two-physician consent for emergency procedures. This should include involvement of social services and hospital administrators for documentation purposes.

In some cases, families impose demands for special favors that present unique challenges to hospital staff and social services. Physicians can become part of the problem if they make promises to the family that others must cope with keeping. "Bribes" and "rule bending" for patients and families reinforce the family's worst fears about the severity of illness and undermine the family's confidence in the health care team to solve the patient's difficulties. Nothing is as reassuring as "business as usual."

◆ Challenges in Communication: Scenarios

There are certain situations that reveal the challenges to communication between health care workers and NICU patients and their families. **Tables 31–9** through **31–14** offer practical applications of communication skills. **Table 31–9** gives pointers on what to expect at the first meeting between the physician and the patient's family. **Table 31–10** presents the scenario of a patient's death and what the medical team can do to ease the situation. **Table 31–11** gives the case of a patient presenting in decompensation. **Table 31–12** offers suggestions on possible interventions when a patient arrives unstable and worsens. **Table 31–13** distinguishes among situations in which needs are not being met and gives basic suggestions on how to meet those varied needs. Finally, **Table 31–14** addresses the situation in which a patient's recovery is prolonged by further complications.

The role of physicians and the health care team in relationship building with NICU patients and their families can be complicated. **Table 31–15** lists what is needed of physicians and nursing staff from the perspective of the patient and his or her family. These needs should be the focus of the health care team.

◆ The Health Care Team

It would be ideal if physicians and nurses could meet all of the needs of patients and their families. In real life, though, no one can be all things to all patients at all times. Physicians and other members of the health care team, working together, can create a composite, well-orchestrated program to fulfill the needs of most people. **Tables 31–16** and **31–17** address the team approach to communication.

It is the responsibility of the primary service, from attending physician to intern, to establish the credibility and importance of the entire network of health care providers in the critical care setting as sources of information for the patient and his or her family.

Nurses need to hear what the family hears. At least daily, the physicians guiding minute-to-minute care in the unit should define, with the chief bedside caregivers, the content to be shared with the family by all health care team members. Nurses will choose how to transmit information according to gravity and complexity of data and by competency of the communicating

Table 31–9 Initial Meeting between the Health Care Team and the Patient and His or Her Family

The doctor says…	The patient/family hears…
The doctor approaches the family and engages the attention of all before speaking.	Something important is about to be said by a person of authority who cares about whether he or she is heard.
The doctor introduces himself or herself by name and demands the identities of his or her audience, sets the stage for a family spokesperson to emerge, or appoints one.	Distinguishing who is listening and the physician's relation to the patient is a way of acknowledging authority in the family and can be seen as respect; where there is already dissension, this may polarize family members.
The doctor summarizes the patient's state (2 sentences) and interrupts himself or herself to gather baseline data, enlarges on the patient's likely diagnosis and prognosis, then opens the floor to questions. OR	Family will infer that crisis is under control and will respond to overture to tell about the patient and themselves in ways depending on their level of stress and past functioning as a family.
The doctor launches into a summary of the patient's status and current, emergent needs, postpones questions, gets consents for ongoing procedures, indicates what is likely to occur shortly, and leaves. OR	Family will infer that patient's crisis is not contained. If vocabulary is kept simple and the choices offered are straightforward, the family may accept data at face value. If the family hears condescension or is culturally or historically conditioned to expect neglect and exploitation, the family may be angered.
The doctor summarizes the patient's status, current needs, and likely progress; introduces other staff members who will report to the family; estimates when the family can see the patient, gets consents for needed procedures; and departs. OR	Same as above, but the family is likely to respond positively to the promise of ongoing reports by people that the physician approves and the hope of seeing the patient at some specified time in the future.
The doctor or representative uses terminology that the family cannot comprehend, does not introduce or condone liaison personnel, and leaves without ascertaining if he or she is understood.	Family may assume that the patient's crisis is so severe, the physician or representative has no time for them or that the physician does not care about them or the patient. Families with past trust issues may become hostile. Families will conjecture and reinforce erroneous assumptions to cover knowledge deficits.

caregiver, and share the responsibility with respiratory therapists and others. Ideally, there will be planned (weekly) and impromptu multidisciplinary rounds, with and without the patient and family in attendance, in which the team as a whole assimilates and adapts to the patient's changing

Table 31–10   Communication Approaches When the Patient Dies

The family sees…	The medical team sees…	Possible interventions
Family arrives after the patient is pronounced dead. Family confronts outcome with shock.	The patient is assessed, and appropriate management is offered. Physicians and staff disperse to care for others. Appropriate agencies are contacted.	Emergency room liaison personnel succor family while waiting for physicians to return to the scene; the family sees the patient after being updated and after staff has prepared the patient for viewing.
Family members arrive during resuscitation but are denied access to the patient. They confront the outcome with shock and rage.	The patient is assessed, and appropriate management is offered. Liaison personnel are not present to facilitate involving family or a communication failure occurs, so the team is unaware that the family has arrived, or the family's presence is deemed unwise.	Best case: Physicians and liaison personnel meet the family first, re-create events, answer the answerable, and empathize with the loss. Referrals to appropriate agencies are made. Worst case: Family members are exposed to the dead patient without preparation and without ready access to those best able to explain what happened.
Family arrives during resuscitation and has access to the bedside before the patient dies. Family is exposed to the resuscitation process. They confront the outcome with varying degrees of shock.	Constraints imposed by the family's presence do not excessively hinder a practiced team. Resuscitation proceeds with all team members performing as best as possible.	Ideally, staff liaison is continuously present and attends to the family's needs while preventing interference with resuscitation efforts. Worst case: Family members intrude, pose a threat to resuscitation providers, and are removed.

condition, then formulates a presentation to share the information with the family.

Nurses, therapists, and others with the greatest access to the patient and family have the burden of ongoing education and minute-by-minute reinforcement of information already provided to the patient/family. Nurses and others with bedside care responsibilities will not act as independent entities but as contributing members of an organized whole whose opinions will be assimilated into the overall plan discussed with the patient/family.

All health care providers should feed back patient-related information to the primary physician team and wait for the team's directions regarding sharing that data with the patient/family.

Table 31–11 Communication Approaches When the Patient Presents in Decompensation

The patient/family sees…	The medical team sees…	Possible interventions
Catastrophic injury/illness make shocking changes in self or loved one.	Disease or trauma impacts on patient's immediate chances of sustaining life.	Staff and physicians share a duty to describe what they see, what they want to change, and how they will go about it.
Assessment and resuscitation look chaotic to the already frightened family and patient.	Systematic application of protocols by a professional team working under pressure	As above. Use "Good/better/not as good" to update and avoid statistics or interrupting care to explain. Use liaison personnel.
Initial damage and uncertain progress in self or loved one inspire fear of lethality or permanent disability.	Results of examinations, indicating diagnosis, current status, response to treatment, and ultimate prognosis, are obvious.	As above. Ask family for opinions, then counter with accuracy. Give frequent updates, and quickly introduce senior physicians and staff.
Family has one person or a few people who appear in charge and worth listening to.	A hierarchy of authority is based on training and skill set; many are capable of providing information.	Team defers to leader, and leader reinforces confidence in team.
Unexplained delays/unexpected changes in plans/inadequate explanations seem evasive.	Resuscitation is carried forward in a setting where many compete for the same resources and the attention of the same staff.	Avoid excuses; explain delays as soon as possible. Provide reassurance. Staff should give family a role in supporting the patient.

The burden of telling all and the responsibility for coordinating and ameliorating the patient's/family's exposure to dissenting opinions are privileges earned by the primary team of physicians through their responsiveness to new data, new questions, and new concerns brought to their attention by their physician consultants, by nurses, and by all other representatives of caregiving disciplines ·contributing to the patient's ultimate outcome.

The burden of absorbing and acting on the implications of the patient's current and future status belongs to the patient and family: the greatest gift the medical team may offer is to influence how that burden is conferred (**Tables 31–18** and **31–19**).

Be prepared to supply family members with a frame of reference to help them assimilate the information they are about to receive. Reinforce that

Table 31–12   Communication Approaches When the Patient Arrives Unstable and Worsens

The patient/ family sees...	The medical team sees...	Possible interventions
Limited access of the patient to his or her family is offered.	An unstable patient is isolated for his or her protection.	The health care team repeatedly explains to, empathizes with, but always protects the patient.
Strangers converge and do inexplicable or painful things to the patient.	Necessary procedures are done to preserve life by people who should but may not identify their purposes to the family.	Physicians respond with increased opportunity for the family to vent and for doctors to update. The team shares the opportunity to assess pain control needs with the family.
Contradictory information or no information is conveyed to the family; the "wrong" person is contacted, making the information conveyed suspect; information conveyed is too technical to be absorbed; communication with a recognized authority is too sparse or contaminated by the family's hostility; and individual dynamics foster denial.	Confusion follows when caregivers fail to communicate with each other; when individuals communicate who incorrectly assume a common knowledge base; when information changes as it passes between staff or family members; when the patient deteriorates so rapidly that it is impossible to adequately prepare and sustain the family. The foregoing is exacerbated by preexisting family dysfunction and socioeconomic or cultural considerations. Further complications from unrelated stressors are imposed on the staff.	Impromptu multidisciplinary rounds with available staff and key family members are done so that "everybody is heard and everyone hears the same thing." A family spokesperson and team spokespersons are identified. Referrals are made to appropriate support specialists. Ongoing multidisciplinary rounds are made with the family present, and increased scheduled opportunities are provided for the family to connect with attending physicians. The chain of command is reinforced. Physicians validate the staff.

frame of reference as a foundation for continuing communication throughout the patient's course of treatment (**Tables 31–20**, **31–21**, **31–22**, and **31–23**).

It is assumed that all appropriate medical workup has been done to confirm the diagnoses and prognoses leading to this decision point. For purposes of this discussion, it is assumed that there is no advanced directive, no living will, and no written documentation of the patient's wishes. The approach to the family is then predicated on agreement or acceptance that withdrawal of support or withholding cardiopulmonary resuscitation (CPR)

Table 31–13 Communication Approaches When Needs Are Not Being Met

The patient/ family sees…	The medical team sees…	Possible interventions
Emotional needs are not being met.	Lack of leadership, failure to accommodate between specialists, lack of team cooperation Staff members recognize the probable grim outcome and distance themselves from patient/family; the staff withdraws from the increasingly dependent, demanding family; the family exhausts the staff's emotional reserve.	Same as in **Table 31–12**, but increase the frequency of family updates.
Physical needs are not being met.	The hospital is unable to provide food, sleeping accommodations, and privacy to meet family demands, whether appropriate or not.	Emphasize role of authority figures in all disciplines. Physicians in authority must demonstrate confidence in bedside caregivers.
Spiritual needs are not being met.	Staff lacks direction and cohesiveness; gives the impression of lost hope, lost motivation, or dissension among themselves; is unable to hide the same from the family; and is exacerbated as the family spirals out of control.	The health care team must meet separately to support themselves, cope with the looming loss of the patient on their own terms, and recover lost momentum in dealing with the patient's and family's crises.
Patient and family are dissatisfied regardless of the outcome.	Physicians and staff caregivers are dissatisfied regardless of the outcome.	Social services representatives appeal for funds to sustain an indigent family in crisis. The family is counseled regarding available resources. The hospital regains a limit-setting role for the safety of patients and staff. The family is treated with respect but with appropriate limit setting. Physicians lead by example, supporting both the team and the family realistically. Focus groups, including physicians, are appointed to alleviate any remaining tensions and to help participants learn from the experience.

Table 31–14 Communication Approaches When a Patient's Recovery Is Prolonged by Further Complications

The patient/ family sees…	The medical team sees…	Possible interventions
The patient/family is dissatisfied with the patient's rate of improvement and/or prolonged NICU stay due to complications.	The patient's and family's reserves are depleted emotionally, physically, spiritually, and financially.	Physicians insist on and staff facilitate a "timeout" for the family.
The family "settles in," regaining some control and predictability in their lives measured in the services they can convince others to provide. Family looks to find fault or place blame: something is owed them because "this shouldn't have happened in the first place" and "why can't this be over?"	A dependent relationship becomes ingrained. The family is perceived as ungrateful and increasingly demanding because they assume ongoing privileges granted earlier when the patient was more acute, or because they manipulate relationships that divide the staff, or because they impose preferences on patient care that increase staff work, or because they require reassurance very frequently or at inappropriate or inconvenient times.	Senior staff chair multidisciplinary meeting first without, then with, the family to address the new structure with new privileges, new responsibilities, and new roles for family members. Physician involvement is key to helping predict patient progress and to better assist bedside caregivers in redefining the family's relationship with the health care team.
"Someone is not telling us something"	Staff perceives that communication is treated with suspicion, that the family exploits any discrepancies in communicated content or communication delivery, that there may be dissension in the family; that the delay in good news is leading staff to avoid confrontation and perpetuating family's impression that they are being left out	
"Something finally gets better."	Best case: Events lead senior nursing staff and physicians to resume a leadership role, confirm patient's status and progress in unambiguous terms, set limits on special privileges demanded by the family in supportive fashion, and recover mutual respect.	
"Something gets worse."	Worst case: Whether or not the patient worsens, the family attitude worsens, the family withdraws or behaves with hostility toward the staff, and the hospital administration steps in to arbitrate.	

Table 31–15　Perspective: What Patients and Their Families Need from Physicians and Nurses

Honesty: tell the truth; tell it when you know it; admit it when you don't
Predictability, dependability, availability
Compassion
Open-mindedness and a willingness to learn
Knowledge, wisdom, and a willingness to teach
Skill

Table 31–16　Communication: It Takes a Team

Foundation	The team approach is hierarchical, discriminatory, and privileged.
Authority	The chain of command begins with the attending neuro- or trauma surgeon, descends through resident physicians, ramifies through physician consultants, and burgeons to involve nurses, respiratory therapists, and specialists and technicians of ancillary disciplines, inclusive of appropriate hierarchies per discipline.
Sourcing for dissemination of information	The NICU team sets the tone and controls the flow of information through all contributing health care providers by making sure that the information they want communicated is disseminated to the health care providers with the greatest, most frequent access to the patient. Daily rounds are done with nursing staff. A chart or phone contact is kept with consulting physicians.
Choreography for emergencies	Communication during resuscitation should begin via trained liaison personnel who educate and support families per protocol and by rote according to stages of resuscitation identified by the resuscitating physicians.
Postresuscitation	There should be impromptu, frequent meetings between neurosurgeons, consultants, and family at bedside or with nursing staff, including ongoing support from liaison personnel.
Routine care program	Daily updating of staff and family will be by bedside rounds with nursing and multidisciplinary meetings that involve the neurosurgeons, physician consultants, nurses, respiratory therapists, rehabilitation and other services, the patient, and his or her family.

Table 31–17   Team Approach to Communication: Guidelines for Team Members

Individual members represent the team; the team incorporates all; what each one says should reflect what the team is conveying as a unit.

Information disseminated by team members should conform in content and implication: the patient/family should not get mixed or conflicting messages.

The ultimate resource should be the primary physician service; dissension should be shared within the team, not the patient or the patient's family.

Substantive information conveyed should be restricted by scope of practice. Any team member should be able to convey empathy and concern.

When confronted with a question he or she cannot answer, the team member should admit it and refer the question to the appropriate resource.

All team members owe mutual respect and respect for the team as a whole; promoting confidence in the team is the job of every team member.

Table 31–18   Practitioners Who Should Be Incorporated into the Health Care Team

Discipline	Sphere of influence
Physicians	Ultimate information source; center for assimilation of new data from other disciplines; the "authority" that the patient/family will recognize
Nurses (and trained liaison personnel)	Ultimate implementers of any treatment plan; ultimate disseminators of information because of their greater access to patients and families; primary resource for monitoring; the first and the last to touch the patient and family; the "authority" that the patient and family needs to recognize
Therapists: respiratory, physical, occupational, speech, nutritional, and, to lesser degree, technical specialists throughout the hospital	More limited scope of access and practice but convey information relevant to their areas of concern; the harbingers of change in the patient's condition, the "authority" that the patient and family will look to for new hope
Social workers, case workers, discharge planners, child life specialists, clergy, hospital administrators	Ultimate implementers of plans that hinge on family participation; the authorities that patients look to for their future and families look to for support

Table 31–19 Communication Approaches Assuming Patient/Family Duress

Assume the patient/ family at risk for…	What the health care team member can do…
Fear and anxiety leading to preformed conclusions	Be prepared with appropriate facts.
Attention spans that are likely to be short	Watch for wandering; redirect if needed; be brief.
Poor retention of information	Repeat what matters most and confirm that it is heard.
Distraction by side issues	Ask questions that refocus attention.
Having a secondary agenda focused on comfort, security, and control over their immediate surroundings	Leave time to address appropriate concerns. Show you care. If needed, set the stage for limit setting for inappropriate requests.

Table 31–20 Making a Frame of Reference

Begin by describing the patient's baseline appearance to himself or herself and his or her family in simple, easy-to-remember words. Use the primary survey of resuscitation but in layperson's terms.

Tell the family how you make an assessment (what characteristics and in what order) and what changes would indicate improvement or deterioration. Point to features of the patient that the family can see for themselves.

Introduce the family to medical terms they are likely to hear. Use all of what you've taught them to update the family whenever you get a chance.

Table 31–21 Establishing a Relationship

The Gulf between patient/ family and health care team	Bridging the gulf
Assume ignorance of proper use of medical terms.	Avoid medical terms, or define them every time.
Expect a demand for statistics regarding outcome.	Clearly state that statistics refer to population, then explain what they tell us about the patient.
Assume preconceptions about status.	As simply as possible, explain what parameters are assessed and what conclusions have been made concerning the patient's status; set the stage for the future use of labels "good," "better," "worse," and "unchanged," and avoid discussing numeric values or monitored data that can frighten family members if they misinterpret them. Avoid the word *stable*.
Assume a need to "do something."	Validate the family's roles as historians, as assistants in ongoing assessments, and as decision makers.
Assume a need to find hope, whether you see it or not.	Remind family members that "everyone knows what normal looks like" and that if something they think is an improvement is real, it will be evident in time.

Table 31–22   Situations Requiring Special Communication Obtaining Informed Consent

Physicians and nurses should know departmental policy and apply it.

The patient/family should know from the outset that the purpose of the update is to obtain consent for a procedure needed to save the patient's life/restore functioning/hasten recovery, etc.

Initial approach to the patient/family will be to update them on the patient's progress.

The need for the procedure should be apparent to the patient/family from the update.

A description of the procedure, including use of visual aids, if available, should follow.

The specific benefits that will be mentioned in consent documents should be discussed next.

A discussion of possible ill effects from the procedure should follow departmental policy and should be comprehensive, but they should be presented in the context of how likely the patient is to experience these difficulties.

Patient discomfort should be addressed, including consent for conscious sedation, if needed.

Patient and family need to know where the procedure will be done, when it will be done, who will do it, how long it will take, and what the arrangements will be to update the patient/family after it is done.

Always remind the patient/family that there are "no guarantees."

seems ethical, legal, reasonable, respectful, and compassionate to the members of the health care team. It is assumed that all proceedings will be in keeping with hospital policies regarding bioethics committees, and so on. If consent is sought to withhold resuscitation or deny CPR, the procedure with the family then follows the pattern outlined in **Table 31–24**.

Table 31–23   Situations Requiring Special Communication: Withdrawal of Support/Do Not Resuscitate

Patient status	Examples
Illness or trauma has led imminently and unavoidably to a terminal condition.	Intracranial hypertension after severe head trauma
Criteria are met for irreversible coma.	Head injury, near-drowning, asphyxia, stroke
Incurable, progressive illness exists entailing intractable suffering and unacceptable quality of life.	Lou Gehrig's disease, multiple sclerosis
Illness or trauma has led to such severe disability with such poor quality of life that there is no reason to continue artificial means to prolong life or resuscitate from cardiac arrest.	End-stage pulmonary disease in a profoundly brain-damaged patient, as seen in ventricular hemorrhage due to prematurity; brain tumor; stroke; near-drowning

Table 31–24   A Protocol for Obtaining Consent to Withdraw Support or Withhold CPR

A team of doctors, nurses, therapists, social workers, clergy, and so on, discusses the case in advance and arranges to meet with the family as a group. (Some or all of the team members should attend. Do not send only one person.)

The family is approached by a representative of the group to make an appointment to discuss the consent, with the family arranging for appropriate attendance of its members.

The physician reviews the patient's case, including the factors leading to the present discussion.

The family and health care team discuss the implications of the patient's history.

The health care team solicits the family's feelings about the patient's likely outcome, about death and dying in general, about what they think the patient would want, about what they would want for themselves, and about how they will want to remember their actions and decisions 10 years in the future.

The health care team answers questions about what the patient will feel and do if support is withdrawn or resuscitation is denied, the mechanics of the process, and how it will appear to the family. The hospital's documentation for consent for DNR status, including the options to choose some but not all aspects of resuscitation, can be discussed with the family at this point. The family's wishes on how withdrawal of support should be conducted, whom they wish to have present, and so on, can also be discussed now.

The family is given a time frame in which to carry on the discussion in privacy and return a decision. Meetings are arranged and repeated with appropriate/selected members of the health care team until the family delivers a decision.

CPR, cardiopulmonary resuscitation; DNR, do not resuscitate.

A patient who is declared "brain dead" per protocol (see Chapter 28) is removed from life support because he or she is dead. No consent is necessary. The family should be informed with all possible compassion and sensitivity. The timing may be set to accommodate family wishes within reason.

◆ Summary

No illness or injury carries a greater potential for loss of one's identity and perspective on one's environment than injury or illness of the brain or spinal cord. A patient whose critical illness arises from damage of the central nervous system is a person at risk of dying, but also at risk of never being the person he or she was again, or at risk of never being the person he or she could have been. Every interchange between the physician and patient or the patient's family in this setting will be overshadowed by these implications. Attempts by the physician or layperson to focus on any finite detail and exclude the greater context is likely to lead to confusion and friction between and among physicians, other health care providers, family members, and the patient.

The physicians trying to save the patient's life and preserve his or her abilities have a duty to explain what they are doing, why, and what is likely to happen next as best they can. The duty is shared with the remainder of the health care team to a degree in keeping with the potential to affect outcome that accompanies their skills, knowledge, or authority. All share the complementary duty to acknowledge, process, and respond to what the patient and family express after they hear what the prognosis and progress are likely to be.

The patient and his or her family have a duty to provide a history that will help delineate the cause of the patient's catastrophe, and they have a duty to convey what the patient was like before his or her illness or injury occurred. Most of all, they have an obligation to listen, process what they hear, and provide feedback on what they have heard. Ultimately, they will be responsible for coping with the aftermath, including death or disability.

Neither the physicians nor the patient and his or her family will see the patient's illness in the same context. It is up to the physicians and the team of health care providers surrounding and supporting the patient's care to bridge the gap in understanding between themselves and the patient/family.

The patient and family are one: the patient's crisis separates him or her from the life to which medical care endeavors to return the patient. This goal cannot be accomplished unless the context of the patient's life before his or her crisis is fully appreciated.

32

Spiritual Care of the Neurosurgical Intensive Care Unit Patient and Family

John R. Spitalieri

There can be no more completely upsetting and frightening event than to find that a loved one has become critically ill or severely injured and has been taken to the hospital and admitted to the neurosurgical intensive care unit (NICU). Suddenly, everything that was stable before has now changed, and the question of our own mortality, as well as that of our loved one, is brought to the forefront. What may have started off as a normal day has had a surrealistic change, as if looking at a drama on television. Expressed thoughts begin to echo: "This can't be happening, there must be a mistake; either you have the wrong family or the wrong patient, or the wrong diagnoses." Inevitably, the truth starts to sink in as the physical and emotional pain associated with loss and separation takes hold. These are the times when many questions are asked and few pleasant or satisfying answers are given. The emotional strength of a family is put to task, and its members begin to search for solace and understanding.

◆ The Role of the NICU Team

Many patients have been admitted into the NICU, and many of these patients have had good outcomes. The NICU team meets patients as they come into the hospital and then adopts them. The team becomes part of each patient's life as the patient goes from the initial computed tomography (CT) scan, to the operating room or the NICU. Patients are followed daily, not merely seen once a day. Each patient becomes the mission of the NICU team until he or she goes home, is transferred to a rehabilitation facility, or passes away. When patients leave the hospital, their care is not ended; only then does the amount of care change slightly, becoming surpassed by those patients who remain in the hospital. The NICU team is committed to each and every patient, providing each with optimal care. However, given similar circumstances, some patients do better than others.

◆ The Role of the Family

The common denominator in those who do well is support from family. There really does not seem to be a common denominator for those who do not. If a patient's injury or illness is too great, then their destiny is out of the health care team's hands. Though sharing in the patients' lives, regardless of outcome, the NICU team can make the experience more comfortable and less harsh. There are ways to identify the suffering of patients and their families, to help with major life transitions, such as recovery, permanent disability, and death. Perhaps addressing the spiritual needs of patients and families could hold another modality of treatment that needs to be explored. At the heart of the spiritual distress of the sick and dying is suffering, and it is this spiritual distress that is often not addressed adequately.[1–8] Health care providers have taken on a responsibility to relieve physical pain and suffering. This duty should also include spiritual suffering.

Even though spirituality is becoming more recognized and accepted as a part of treatment, not many established guidelines exist for physicians in the NICU for inquiring about the spirituality of patients and their families.[9–14] In fact, a survey of leading neurology textbooks showed minimal guidelines for the care of patients at the end of life and in the NICU. Additionally, none of the textbooks had a chapter on end-of-life care.[14] There is a need to discuss the approaches for inquiring about a patient's and family's spirituality, the importance of spirituality in medical decision making, the role of suffering, and the effects on health care. Those requirements must be tailored to patients in the NICU.

◆ The NICU Setting

NICUs are specially equipped hospital units that are organized to give highly specialized care to patients who suffer from serious brain and spinal cord injury or illness. The NICU team coordinates with other specialized services, such as trauma, cardiology, and infectious disease. The combination of these specially trained services provides a high level of care, continuous observation, and monitoring with the help of nurses and therapists.

There are no specific admission criteria for the NICU. Admission is based on a physician's finding that close observation or specialized monitoring and/or therapy is necessary. There are several broad categories of patients who present to the NICU: trauma, tumor, hemorrhage, and stroke. Although many patients present with one initial finding, they may have an underlying disease, such as a brain tumor. In any event, there are hard realities that patients and their families have to confront.

Unique experiences associated with a stay in the NICU include round-the-clock observation with frequent neurologic exams, intracranial pressure monitoring, electroencephalography, and frequent trips to the radiology department for CT or magnetic resonance imaging (MRI) scans. Families will see their loved ones on complete life support, with monitors and other equipment making their own special noises. This can be very frightening and overwhelming to families whose last memory of their loved one was someone walking and talking. Immediately, the stress level of families is high, and the NICU team must be watchful for signs of that stress. At this time, the different specialty teams should introduce themselves and identify the family's spokesperson. Also, the patient's current condition and overall plan of treatment should be discussed. The time should be taken to explain the situation in simple, concise, and accurate terms.

◆ Spirituality

Spirituality has been defined as "that which allows a person to experience transcendent meaning in life. This is often expressed as a relationship with God, but it can also be about nature, art, music, family, or community—whatever beliefs and values give a person a sense of meaning and purpose in life (p. 129)."[13] Many people identify themselves as being spiritual.[7–9] They feel that, on some level, their life has meaning and purpose. Illness and injury can cause a threat to the individual's spirituality.[7,9] Patients admitted to the NICU may not even have the strength or ability to care for themselves, even on the most basic levels. Here there may only be an attempt at survival. The meaning and purpose of their lives may be lost to them, leading to emotional distress in the patients, as well as in their families. At this time, spiritual counseling can benefit patients and families the most by allowing them to express their concerns for the future while helping them to cope with their suffering.[8,11]

Patients and families may not think of the possibility of bad things happening to them, or they may think that once bad things do happen, a miracle will occur that will deliver them from their suffering. It is human nature to have hope, and hope affects health.[8] Hope reflects faith in and anticipation of a better future. As an extension of this hope, the NICU team enters into a relationship with each patient that commits physicians, along with other members of the health care team, to doing the most to return the patient to a state of health. This relationship takes on the properties of a covenant and includes shared hope, shared risk, and mutual respect.[13]

The era is approaching where spirituality is having more clinical relevance, for example, when coping with illness and death. Patients and families are basing health care decisions on their religious beliefs.[4,7,8] Medical science is still uncertain if spirituality has an effect on health, but several sources are investigating the psychological-neurologic-immunologic axis and how spirituality or religion can be a factor in the treatment of those who are critically ill or injured.[1,4] This involves the personal concerns of the individual patients. Some patients' concerns involve only their faith in God and the pursuit of heaven. Others are most concerned with interpersonal relationships with families and friends. These are things that are not tangible, but give hope and reassurance to those who are so troubled. Their spirituality, in what ever form it takes, is what gives people meaning and purpose in life.[4,7]

In addressing purpose and meaning, large gains can be made with small efforts by the health care providers. For all of the complex treatments of a patient's illness, there does not have to be a complex course for spiritual treatment. Even simply providing access to spiritually oriented activity can be uplifting to individuals and also help in healing. Studies show that for families who had recent deaths and are in mourning, adding religious support in the form of scriptural readings, along with standard grief counseling, can help these families to recover sooner than if given only grief counseling.[4] Allowing patients' families the freedom to seek solace in scripture can reintroduce purpose and meaning when personal values are skewed by grief. This illustrates once again the importance of addressing the spiritual needs of families when in critical care situations.

◆ The Patient and Family's Spiritual History

In the pursuit of a particular patient's health and alleviation of suffering, spirituality needs to be addressed, not just once at the beginning of care but throughout the patient's stay. It is important to ask questions to help understand and anticipate the needs of the patient. Although inquiries should be welcomed, the health care professional should be careful not to impose his or her own beliefs; this is best done by keeping an open mind to other cultures and religions. Also, respecting a patient's and family's wishes and values, especially when it comes to end-of-life matters, will help with this goal. Ask if a patient wants a visit from a chaplain; do not wait for the patient to inquire, as he or she may be unsure whom to ask or how.

Health care providers may feel odd discussing spiritual matters, or they may think that these types of discussions are out of the scope of treatment. Some may feel questions regarding spirituality will be seen as too personal or be interpreted as prying. Numerous studies have showing that such are actually welcomed by patients and families, and that they also help the patient–family–physician relationship.[4,6,7,12,13] In fact, many patients describe themselves as being religious but also report that, the majority of the time, their doctors have not asked questions of spirituality as it pertains to medical decision-making.[4] The NICU team should also be on the lookout for certain phrases that imply spiritual influence in their patients and families. Patients who speak, for example, of being "blessed" or "tortured" may actually be giving clues to their religious nature.[7]

In essence, it is helpful to take a spiritual history of the patient and family. Like most other aspects of the patient's history, there are aids for the efficient gathering of the spiritual history. A screening tool, developed by Puchalski and Romer, helps the health care provider explore the spirituality of patients and families.[13] The acronym FICA represents the types of questions to ask patients: faith in general (F), the importance of the patient's individual faith (I), the patient's identification with a community of faith (C), and how the patient wishes health care providers to address spiritual issues (A).

Other questions that are helpful and comforting include those related to hopes and expectations, as well as fears of the near future that are centered on issues of palliative care and end-of-life issues. These particular types of questions are actually aimed at the spiritual suffering of patients and their families.[4]

Screening questions, as suggested by Dunn,[7] that can be used during the spiritual assessment include the following:

- Do you consider yourself a religious or spiritual person?
- What sustains your hope?
- Do you have religious or spiritual beliefs that help you through difficulty?
- What gives your life meaning?
- How important is your faith or belief in your life?
- Dose your faith influence your feeling about your illness? Your surgery?
- Do you see any possible conflicts between your health care and your beliefs?
- Do you belong to a community of faith?
- Is there a group of people particularly important to you?
- How is your faith working for you today?

◆ The Role of Health Care Providers

Nurses have the most exposure to patients and families and form bonds with them. These bonds can be drawn on to elicit communication and cultural information. Nurses are the "ambassadors" who relay information between individuals in the patient–family–physician relationship.[4,10,15,16] As described by Buchman et al, "When patient, family, and caregivers share common perceptions and goals, this particular role is often simplified to that of translator, ensuring that communication is timely, accurate, and consistent. In contrast, when the perceptions and goals are dissonant, the brokerage role often requires nurses to assume additional responsibilities of arbitration and diplomacy (p. 667)."[4]

◆ Suffering

In an attempt to identify the subtleties of suffering, Hinshaw[9] describes four domains of pain: physical pain, psychological or emotional pain, social pain (pain associated with fear of separation from loved ones), and spiritual pain. These are four areas of potential suffering for patients in the NICU, and integral to treatment is the easing of their suffering no matter what form it takes.[5] What may prove daunting to health care providers is effectively treating spiritual pain when encountered because it is not identified, and often health care workers are ill prepared to treat this type of suffering when discovered. The NICU team has to identify the forms of distress and suffering in patients and their families to provide well-rounded care.[9]

Research is showing that a patient's spirituality can play an important role in ameliorating the sequelae of severe illness.[2] Spiritual suffering is ever present in the sick and dying, and, if not looked for, it will not be recognized when it manifests itself.[5,7] Those who suffer spiritually may be losing hope, may be losing the meaning of their lives and self-worth, and may be doing this in silence and unnecessarily.[7] Much of a patient's suffering begins with worry about an uncertain future. For example, patients fear their physical and emotional symptoms may become too much to bear.[5] Also, families do not want their loved ones to suffer and often inquire about pain medications, specifically asking the dosing and frequency of administration. Key to this is understanding that suffering is different from patient to patient; what causes suffering in one patient may not be a cause of suffering in another.[5]

Suffering is a state of distress that can occur in all patients, but this distress is even more severe when it occurs in NICU patients. Patients suffer when they feel their integrity and autonomy are threatened and feel that their end is near. This is easily understood when considering the thoughts of patients on ventilators, when they have intravenous lines and electrical leads all over their bodies. This is frightening to both patients and their families. Patients will continue to suffer until the threat is ended or their integrity is restored.[5,9] It is part of the NICU team's duty to restore patients' sense of autonomy and to calm their fear and thus reduce their suffering.

Comforting the Patient

A goal of treatment is comfort. The level of pain is asked on a regular basis and rated on a scale from 0 to 10, with 10 being the worst. Pain medication and sedation are used to help make patients more comfortable. Doctors and nurses try to use the least amount necessary to alleviate patients' symptoms so as to not overmedicate, which could potentially mask the neurologic exam. At times, especially in patients who are intubated, sedation is kept so high as to make a patient unresponsive. Intubated patients with severe head injuries may be unresponsive regardless of the level of sedation. This may be upsetting to family members, and it is therefore important to reassure them of the necessity for treatment, as well as the quantity of treatment. Using narcotics and sedation for pain management may be insufficient to relieve all of a patient's suffering. These medicines can help control the physical symptoms of the severely injured or terminally ill, but they may not relieve all of their suffering.[9]

Addressing the issues of suffering may allow patients to feel that they are regaining some control over their condition and empower them to ease their own suffering.[4] A scale from 0 to 10 can also be adapted for stress and worry. Patients and families can be asked simple and direct questions to diagnose sources of pain, such as, Are you suffering? What are your concerns and fears? and What is it that worries you the most?[5] Even just the simple effort of asking the questions and listening to the answers can soothe suffering.[5,9]

◆ The Role of Prayer and the Clergy

There are specialists in the hospital who routinely handle spirituality and religious aspects of patient care. The hospital chaplains are sources of guidance, comfort, and support to the critically ill and their families. There will often be requests for chaplain and prayer services for the ill. Many families believe in the power of prayer.[4,8,13] There are chapels for families to go to and reflect, and chaplains are available in every hospital. Clergy are also available from the communities. Pastoral care is an integral part of health care facilities. Hospitals offer patients the spiritual services of prayer, sacraments, a listening presence, and assistance in dealing with the emotions and questions that come with sickness. These services are provided for both patients and families. Experienced staff chaplains offer sacraments, assist with spiritual care, regardless of faith or religious tradition, strive to visit inpatients and make outpatient visits upon request, and will notify a patient's own pastor upon request. Many patients turn to their own religious leaders for comfort. There are times when health care is not enough for restoring health. This should be presented to the families succinctly and directly so there will be no misunderstanding. Respectfully and in a supportive manner, patients must be permitted to express their spirituality.[4,8,13]

◆ Closure

Health care workers are aware that, ultimately, no matter the collective effort, patients sometimes die. Those who are terminally ill may die in weeks to years; those who are critically injured may die in minutes to days. Yet there is still potential for healing in the face of death, for both patient and family, and even for the health care team.[11] Healing does take place during the process of dying when families gather and can find some meaning to their loved one's life. Important factors in this process include hope, reconciliation, and assurance that suffering and pain will be controlled for the patient.[9,11,16] A critically injured or ill patient who still has his or her faculties is comforted with the assurances of not being abandoned, along with knowing pain and suffering will be treated and minimized. Frequently, family members and patients feel the need for forgiveness or reconciliation, which can be facilitated or mediated by chaplains.[9,16] As a patient's death approaches, the NICU team can shift their priorities from sustaining life to bringing comfort.[16] As for terminally ill patients, hospice offers death with dignity and assists with the change in priority to comfort.[9] Hospice also can comfort the dying in knowing they will not be a burden to their loved ones and that their life and suffering will not be prolonged.[16]

◆ Suggestions for Families

It is important to remember that, although NICU patients may not be able to respond to a voice or touch, they may still be able to hear and feel. Families should be encouraged to talk to their loved ones, to hold their hands, and to let them know they are loved. This gives comfort to family members by restoring some sense of control, allowing them to contribute to their loved ones' comfort. It is also important to help orient patients by telling them who is holding their hand, what day it is, and to update them on the current events of the family. It is best to advise family members to maintain a "good news only" policy, not to relay any distressing information. It is appropriate, for example, to withhold information about the foreclosure on the house or a favorite pet running away. Families who are feeling too emotional should be encouraged to take a break from visiting. Family members should always be informed that there are chaplains available for them and the patient.

◆ Suggestions for the NICU Team

Spirituality is hard to quantify or qualify. Who is to say how families should react or to what extent they should show emotion? Who can predict how health care workers will respond when placed in similar situations? Patients and their families may not be able to comprehend the new and undesirable realities forced upon them, or to understand the limitations of modern medicine. For these reasons, the NICU team is obligated, as soothers, to be serene and understanding. They must explain, in detail, the complexities involving the patients' state of health and the level of care being presented.

Because it can be particularly important to patients with terminal or chronic diagnoses, the support of hope should fall within the clinical purview of the skilled physician. In times of severe disabling illness, hope may be mediated through ritual, meditation, music, prayer, and traditional sacred narratives or other inspirational readings. Spiritual care in hospice skillfully redirects hope toward caring relationships and higher meaning.[4]

The NICU team should not pass judgment on patients or their families when it comes to spiritual issues, nor should they try to persuade anyone to change or subscribe to their own beliefs. They should not form opinions or prejudices.[7,16] Instead, they should ask often about the importance of faith, any religious issues, and how the team of caregivers can help with these issues.[7]

The "Principles Guiding Care at the End of Life" were developed by the American College of Surgeons Committee on Ethics and were approved by the board of regents at its February 1998 meeting.[3]

- Respect the dignity of both patient and caregivers.
- Be sensitive to and respectful of the patient's and family's wishes.
- Use the most appropriate measures that are consistent with the choices of the patient or the patient's legal surrogate.
- Ensure alleviation of pain and management of other physical symptoms.
- Recognize, assess, and address psychological, social, and spiritual problems.
- Ensure appropriate continuity of care by the patient's primary and/or specialist physician.
- Provide access to therapies that may realistically be expected to improve the patient's quality of life.
- Provide access to appropriate palliative care and hospice care.
- Respect the patient's right to refuse treatment.
- Recognize the physician's responsibility to forgo treatments that are futile.

◆ Summary

Spirituality and the assessment of a patient's spirituality are becoming important features in the care of patients in the NICU. Health care workers must adopt the duty to ease spiritual suffering for patients and their families. Very simple questions can be asked, and the mere asking can show patients a level of compassion in a highly mechanized, alien, and somewhat frightening environment. The NICU team can bring surcease from suffering to persons in need with timely attentiveness to these details.

References

1. Baggs JG. Intensive care unit use and collaboration between nurses and physicians. Heart Lung 1989;18:332–338
2. Baggs JG, Schmitt MH, Mushlin A, et al. Nurse–physician collaboration and satisfaction with the decision-making process in three critical care units. Am J Crit Care 1997;6:393–399
3. American College of Surgeons. Principles guiding care at the end of life. Bull Am Coll Surg 1998;83(4):194:665–673
4. Buchman TG, Casell J, Ray SE, Wax ML. Who should manage the dying patient? Rescue, shame, and the surgical ICU dilemma. J Am Coll Surg 2002;194(5):665–673
5. Cassell EJ. Diagnosis of suffering: a perspective. Ann Intern Med 1999;131(7):531–534
6. Cassel EJ. The nature of suffering and the goals of medicine. N Engl J Med 1982;306:639–645
7. Dunn GP. Patient assessment in palliative care: how to see the "big picture" and what to do when "there is no more we can do." J Am Coll Surg 2001;193(5):565–573
8. Ehman JW, Ott BB, Short TH, et al. Do patients want physicians to inquire about their spiritual or religious beliefs if they become gravely ill? Arch Intern Med 1999;159:1803–1806
9. Hinshaw DB. The spiritual needs of the dying patient. J Am Coll Surg 2002;195(4):565–568
10. Jezewski MA. Do-not-resuscitate status: conflict and culture brokering in critical care units. Heart Lung 1994;23:458–465
11. Parker-Oliver D. Redefining hope for the terminally ill. Am J Hospice Palliat Care 2002;19:115–120
12. Post SG, Puchalski CM, Lasson DB. Physicians and patient spirituality: professional boundaries, competency, and ethics. Ann Intern Med 2000;132(7):578–583
13. Puchalski C, Romer AL. Taking a spiritual history allows clinicians to understand patients more fully. J Palliat Med 2000;3:129–137
14. Rabow MW, Fair JM, Hardie GE, et al. An evaluation of the end-of-life care content in leading neurology textbooks. Neurology 2000;55(6):893–894
15. Simpson SH. Reconnecting: the experiences of nurses caring for hopelessly ill patients in intensive care. Intensive Crit Care Nurs 1997;13:189–197
16. Singer PA, Martin DK, Kelner M. Quality end-of-life care: patients' perspectives. JAMA 1999;281(2):163–168

33

Medical-Legal Issues in the Neurosurgical Intensive Care Unit

Dan Miulli, Silvio F. Hoshek, and Rosalinda M. Menoni

Case Study

The police bring into the emergency room an adult Asian male patient, seemingly in his 40s, who was detained for wandering the streets partially clothed and confused. He is initially placed on a psychiatric 72-hour hold as a result of a mental disorder. While in the emergency room, the patient is observed having complex repetitive movements prior to a grand mal seizure. The patient is taken to the radiology department for a computed tomography (CT) scan. In the meantime, the police produce his passport, indicating that he is most likely a visitor from China. The CT scan reveals a left temporal lobe lesion with edema. The patient awakens after the seizure; he is deaf and appears to be acting appropriately, but no one, including the telephone translation service, speaks his dialect. What should be the next steps taken by the hospital and the neurosurgical intensive care unit?

See page 475 for Case Management.

Neurologists and neurosurgeons attempt to treat the systems of the body that make the individual a unique person. If a person suffers almost any permanent neurologic deficit, he or she is usually changed forever. The person may not be able to hold the same employment position, make the same income, or relate to his or her family; be an interacting family member, caregiver, or productive member of society; or may die. Not only does the patient change, but the patient's family changes. Therefore, neurologists and neurosurgeons continually face health care situations that put them at the highest medical-legal risks.

Being admitted to the NICU may indeed be an intense and tumultuous time for the patient and his or her loved ones. This is especially true if an emergency trip to the hospital was necessary as opposed to being part of an elective procedure. It is therefore of paramount importance to create an atmosphere of security, confidence, and respectfulness through caring multidisciplinary professionalism. The primary goals should include an effort to minimize confusion and doubt during this very stressful period while providing free flow of communication and education. This is best achieved through a holistic team approach, which clearly identifies all treating members of the team and their individual areas of expertise. Most important is communication. During the period of patient and family stress, physicians and other health care workers must remain close. They must not back away because of difficulty in care, in family dynamics, or with patients and families relating to the situation. This is even more necessary if complications have occurred.

◆ Health Care Teamwork

All health care workers must present a united front for the patient and family. There must be clear communication about diagnosis, prognosis, and care. It is the physician's responsibility to discuss the patient's condition with the nurse, the primary patient advocate. It is the nurse's responsibility to ask any questions so that he or she may understand all the care provided. It becomes severely problematic when the nurse dismisses or belittles any treatment options. If such a situation exists, then changing the lead health care provider should be discussed with the charge nurse and care transferred. Patients and their families, although under great emotional and physical stress, can perceive the discord and will turn that discord into frustration with and a lack of confidence in the health care provided. This situation leads to medical-legal claims.

At times, patients in the NICU require care from multiple specialties. Although mandatory, it once again provides an opportunity for confusion in communication to patients and their families. The members of the health care delivery team may include trauma service, orthopedists, surgical subspecialists, intensivists, internists, pulmonologists, neurologists, infectious disease specialists, and physiatrists. The hierarchy within the ranks of a service should be delineated as well, appropriately identifying residents, physicians' assistants, and attending physicians. Besides the doctors involved in the patient's care, the patient and/or the family should be able to recognize the nursing staff, respiratory therapists, social workers, therapists from the physical, occupational, and speech services, dietitians, clinical pharmacists, and clergy. The best care of the patient involves much input and coordination; everyone should be of one mind and plan. Such coordination is accomplished through the guidance of regularly scheduled interdisciplinary meetings, during which information is updated and shared so that daily treatment plans can be formulated.

◆ Health Care Workers–Patient/Family Communication

Most legal claims result from a lack or misunderstanding of information. Most patients state that they were not told about an unexpected outcome. This can only be defended by careful communication in the presence of a witness and documentation in the medical record. Health care witnesses need to be present. The situation for the patient and family is complex, with emotions often drawing concentration away from discussions. In most circumstances, the primary service should discuss the coordinated care with the patient and family, often relying on attendance by a consultant. In the NICU, the captain of the team is usually the neurosurgeon, who should be the primary spokesperson, unless deferring to the expertise of another colleague individually or in a conference setting. References to colleagues and ancillary staff should always be made with professional decorum in mind, as a misinterpretation may undermine the credibility of the unit.

The key to achieving the primary objective of an environment of trust and security is the demonstration of regard for preserving the patient's dignity and displaying sensitivity and compassion while making time for daily briefings, particularly when the news is discouraging. It is vital to verify that successful communication has been accomplished. This can be quite challenging when attempting to convey the complexity of the natural history of a disease process or the risks and benefits of an intervention to patients and families from various cultural and socioeconomic backgrounds. The communication to the patient and family must be that the team recognizes the importance of their participation in the treatment plan and eventual outcome.

The patient and family must pick a spokesperson for the group, the main contact for the patient and family. Patients and family members will not understand everything told to them. As expected, they will absorb what they understand most. Every person has a different background, and therefore the information that he or she takes away from any conversation will be different. If each person communicates at separate times with the NICU staff, there will be numerous interpretations of what has been told. When that interpretation is transmitted among the family, there will be opportunities for discrepancies. These discrepancies will be turned into stress, hostility, and lack of confidence in the health care team.

During conferences and discussions with the patient and his or her family, it is necessary not only to convey information but to educate. Many people are visually oriented and benefit from seeing pertinent radiographic studies, such as x-rays, CT and magnetic resonance imaging (MRI) scans, and angiograms, while encouraging and soliciting questions. At times, patients and families overcome with shock and grief understandably hesitate to ask questions; they should then be invited to write down questions for the next discussion. The importance of establishing and maintaining this rapport cannot be underestimated, as it can prove to be sustaining, even in the face of a bad outcome or inevitable complications. Striving to create and maintain this type of atmosphere may actually foster trust and may prevent the formation of misunderstandings and misgivings that lead to discontent and possibly litigation.

Documentation

Detailed documentation of all discussions with patients and their families should always be noted in the medical record, preferably dictated as well. This is strongly recommended in addition to any institutional forms requiring signature.

Despite best efforts, certain situations involving consent, advanced directives, right to privacy, abuse, and declaration of death may require additional diligence lest they lead to polarization or true confrontation. Should such situations occur, the risk management officer must be informed.

Documentation of communication takes the form of many types, from handwritten notes, collaborating nurses and ancillary staff notes, to dictations and hospital forms. Each one should document that communication took place. Each member of the NICU team must learn to communicate and exist in harmony, not only with patients but also with other members of the team. Physicians cannot and should not stand alone. The duty of the NICU team is to eliminate shame; encourage hope; communicate with respectful, unselfish caring any emotions and by logic; build bonds; and teach and inspire others to feel the same. People are different; however, differences build a better and stronger world. The NICU team must ask for opinions and try to empathize with what others are feeling.

Obtaining Consent

Consent is communication about and understanding of a treatment that the health care team is providing to the patient. It is not just about surgery but about many treatments, such as line placements, blood transfusions, ventriculostomy, chest and feeding tubes, and other tube and ostomy procedures. According to the California Hospital Association,

> Every competent adult has the fundamental right of self-determination over his or her body and property. Individuals who are unable to exercise this right, such as minors or incompetent adults, have the right to be represented by another who will protect their interests and preserve their basic rights.[1]

It is paramount that the physician providing the proposed care discuss and obtain consent. Only the health care provider can know what information is material to the decision-making of the patient (**Table 33–1**).[2–4]

When a neurosurgical intervention is performed with implied consent, it is important to discuss the treatment with the patient, if capacity is restored, and with the family as soon as identification of next of kin is established.

The patient and family must understand the risks, benefits, and alternatives to the treatment, as well as the sequelae of the perioperative period. In reference to the initial intervention, this may include infection, rebleeding, further neurologic deterioration, and the need for reintervention. The inherent risks should not be trivialized. The physician must also discuss the nature and goals of alternatives or specific adjunctive medical treatment regimens such as medications that have known side effects or complications. A dictated example of supratentorial surgery follows.

> The risks and benefits of craniotomy for tumor resection have been discussed with the patient and family in extensive detail. I mentioned diagnosis and decompression as the major benefits. I emphasized that risks of surgery include, but are not limited to, bleeding, infection, [cerebrospinal] leak, stroke, seizure, cognitive deficits, speech problems, bowel/bladder dysfunction, visual

Table 33–1   Medical Issues of Consent[2–4]

Issue	Description, who determines or who consents
Implied consent in a medical emergency	Patient unable to consent; no surrogate available; no evidence that patient or surrogate would refuse the treatment; patient would consent if able.
Capacity	Patient's ability to understand nature and consequences of decision, to make and communicate a decision, and to understand its significant benefits, risks, and alternatives. Unless otherwise specified in a written advanced health care directive, the primary physician should make the determination that a patient lacks capacity.
Incompetence	Judicial determination; person lacks the capacity to perform a specific act, needs a conservator to make those individual decisions; consent deferred to other surrogate decision makers. A family member or significant other is the most common surrogate.
Nonconsent	Patient refuses recommended care. The patient has a right to know the consequences of refusing care so that the refusal is also informed. The physician has a duty to inform the patient of the risks of refusing to undergo a recommended simple and common procedure. A court order should be considered if motives are suspect.
Emancipated minor	Married or divorced, active duty with U.S. military, and 14 years of age and older by court order
Self-sufficient minors	15 years of age or older, living separate and apart from parents, and managing own financial affairs. Providers can notify parents if not dealing with sensitive services, such as reproductive services, sexual assault, rape care and treatment, infectious reportable conditions, and some select behavioral health issues.

(Continued)

Table 33–1   Medical Issues of Consent *(Continued)*

Issue	Description, who determines or who consents
Minors	Consent obtained from adult parent or legal guardian, such as either of married biological parents, adoptive parents, a divorced parent with legal custody, or unmarried parents (the father may have to prove paternity if the mother disputes his role). Parents under 18 years of age still have capacity. Other possible consent givers include foster parents, same-sex partners, registered domestic partners, stepparents, grandparents, surrogate parents, and a temporary party with delegated authority, such as a coach or camp director.

deficits and/or diplopia, hemiplegia, and death. Any possible risk may occur. There may be additional pain, and the current pain may not resolve. General risks of pneumonia, [urinary tract infection], [deep venous thrombosis], cardiac arrhythmias, and pulmonary embolus were also discussed. The possibilities of incomplete resection, no benefit, repeat surgery, and need for adjuvant therapies such as radiation and/or chemotherapy were discussed. The seriousness of the patient's condition, and of the planned intervention, was emphasized. I answered all questions and explained it was not possible to foresee all possible complications or adverse outcomes. No guarantees were given. Patient and family wished to proceed with surgery [Siddiqi, personal communication].

◆ Reporting Abuse

Reporting child, elder, and domestic abuse and violent crime is mandated by state and federal statutes. Legally mandated reporters can be criminally or civilly liable for failing to report suspected abuse. The penalties can be 6 months of incarceration or a fine of $1000. Any legally mandated reporter has immunity when making a report. Confidentiality laws do not apply in suspected abuse cases. The statutory duty to report supersedes the confidentiality privilege.

◆ Recording Accidents

When accidents or mistakes happen that result in adverse outcomes, report them to the patient, family, and hospital administration.

When incidents happen, fill out an incident report that is meant to be a confidential communication within the hospital. The report is intended solely to be transmitted to the hospital attorneys for their information and their use in the preparation, investigation, and defense of the health care worker in litigation or potential litigation. It should not be photocopied or made part of the medical record or referenced in the medical record. The incident report should contain a one-sentence summary, a description of the type of incident, including where it occurred, who was involved, any witnesses, contributing factors, the severity of outcome, what changes could be made to reduce the risk in the future, analysis and actions taken, who completed the form, departmental manager review, and quality assurance review. The form should be completed within 24 hours.

◆ Components of a Lawsuit

For a lawsuit to be successfully completed and neglect proven, four areas have to be involved in the conduct between two parties:

1. There must be duty between individuals.
2. There must have been breach of duty by violation of the standard of care as determined by a reasonable physician.
3. There must be injury due to breach of duty.
4. There must be proximate cause.

Once all parts have been proven, the case is settled or judgment is made. Most physicians will be sued. Medical malpractice cases flooded the United States court system by the 1930s and such suits have continued unabated. The cultural, social, ethical, and economic system determines the probability of a lawsuit; however, communication between the doctor and the patient/family is paramount. The lead physician and the NICU team must be united and must communicate and educate patients and their families.

The time in the NICU is emotional and stressful. Those emotions either can be soothed by the NICU team or manipulated and twisted. There are individuals who tend to prey on the emotions of individuals, inventing or reestablishing baseline emotional confusion. Adding more energy to them, reigniting smoldering emotions renews the intensity that may have dissipated. These individuals may even fabricate new emotions for the patient and family, based on their interpretation of a previous foundation. Thus plaintiffs' cases are generated by creating an emotional response. To prevent this, empathize, communicate, teach, and console.

One exception to consent being voluntary is found in the mental health acts that specify that a person can be involuntarily held and transported, assessed, and admitted for up to 72 hours for mental health evaluation and treatment if, as a result of a mental disorder, that person is a danger to himself, a danger to others, or gravely disabled. A related provision[5] provides that any physician providing emergency services to a patient shall not be civilly or criminally liable for detaining the patient (without consent) for up to 8 hours, pending transportation to a mental health facility.

An exception to the aforementioned rule stating that the primary physician determines capacity was ruled on by the California Supreme Court,[6] which found that in the case of a patient on an involuntary 72-hour hold who refuses medication, the determination of capacity shall be made pursuant to a judicial proceeding.

Case Management

The psychiatry and neurosurgery departments are consulted. The Chinese consulate provides an interpreter, and the patient's history and physical examination are completed. No dysfunction in understanding is present using equipment for the hearing impaired. The patient is assessed to have the capacity to consent for medical care, comprehending the risks and benefits germane to the options of treatment. The patient is offered craniotomy for diagnosis and excision of the lesion. The risks and benefits are communicated thoroughly through the official interpreter. All steps are documented in the medical record, including the participation by the interpreter. The patient is amenable and undergoes surgery to excise the lesion. The postoperative course of treatment is uneventful, and he returns home.

References

1. California Hospital Association. Consent Manual. 33rd ed. Sacramento, CA: California Hospital Association; 2006
2. *Cobbs v Grant*, 8 Cal 3d (1972)
3. *Truman v Thomas*, 27 Cal 3d 285 (1980)
4. California Probate Code sections 4658, 4657, 4609
5. Health and Safety Code 1799.111
6. *Riese v St. Mary's Hospital and Medical Center*, 259 Cal 2d 698 (1989)

34

Discharge Planning in the Neurosurgical Intensive Care Unit Patient

Paula Snyder

Discharge planning in the neurosurgical intensive care unit (NICU) should begin upon admission.

Neurologic patients often have increased needs for discharge. Their functional capacity may be significantly decreased because of cognitive and/or physical impairments. These patients may have tracheostomy or gastrostomy tubes, and limited or no bowel and/or bladder control. They may be at increased risk for injury due to cognitive impairment, recent memory deficits, and judgment and impulse control issues and may require constant supervision. Most inpatient rehabilitation programs require that the patient be able to participate in at least 3 hours of therapy each day. Some patients with complex medical problems may not be able to tolerate intensive rehabilitation; others may be medically stable but may not be able to participate in intensive rehabilitation due to the severity of their neurologic injury. Many of these patients may need subacute rehabilitation or skilled nursing with less intensive physical therapy. Generally, the more severe the injury or the longer the NICU/hospital stay, the longer the recovery period and the greater the need for more intensive rehabilitation or long-term care. Patients with only cognitive impairments may not qualify for inpatient rehabilitation.

Early identification of the patient's resources, community resources and outpatient rehabilitation programs, home situation and adaptability, and family support system is imperative for patients not meeting inpatient rehabilitation criteria. Patients rehabilitated on an outpatient basis will need careful evaluation and planning by the multidisciplinary team. Identification of caregivers among a patient's family and friends is essential to a smooth discharge plan. Other areas to be assessed include (1) where outpatient therapies will be received; (2) transportation availability to and from therapies and physician visits; (3) whether home therapy is needed and, if so, whether it is covered by insurance; (4) evaluation of the home environment to identify needs for assistive devices, such as a hospital bed, commode, and a shower chair, as well as supplies (for tracheotomy care, feedings, etc.).

The nurse/case manager, in concert with the multidisciplinary team, assesses the anticipated needs of the patient for discharge. The team usually consists of the nurse, physician, physiatrist, physical therapist, occupational therapist, speech pathologist, dietitian, respiratory therapist, and social worker, along with the patient and his or her family. Each team member has a specific area of responsibility related to discharge planning.

Areas of particular concern when evaluating a patient for potential rehabilitation needs include motor dysfunction, alteration in sensory perception, altered communication patterns, behavioral issues, altered respiratory function, cranial nerve impairment, and cognitive impairment (**Tables 34–1**, **34–2**, and **34–3**).[1]

Table 34–1   Evaluating Patients for Potential Rehabilitation Needs[1]

Alteration	Associated with/demonstrated by
Alteration in motor function	Associated with spinal cord injury, traumatic brain injury, and stroke resulting in paresis, paralysis, incoordination, apraxia, spasticity, and abnormal reflexes
Alteration in sensory perception	Blindness and visual disturbances and defects, loss or disturbance in pain, temperature, and pressure perception, position sense, agnosia
Altered communication patterns	Receptive, expressive, and global dysphasias, aphasia, motor dysphasia
Alteration in behavior	Demonstrated by mood disturbances, depression, poor impulse control, dysinhibition, anger, aggressive behavior
Alteration in cranial nerve function	Swallowing and speech defects, ptosis, diplopia, disruption of taste, smell, hearing, cranial nerve (CN) VII palsy
Alteration in cognitive function	Confusion, altered level of consciousness, impaired memory, judgment, concentration, problem solving, higher thought processes

Table 34–2   Potential Discharge Destinations Based on Diagnosis and/or Deficit[1]

Condition/situation	Discharge destination
Spinal cord injury (SCI)	Acute rehabilitation
Stroke with hemiplegia	Acute rehabilitation
Brain injury with paresis, paralysis, apraxia, ataxia, inability to ambulate	Acute rehabilitation vs skilled nursing facility with physical therapy vs home with outpatient therapy
Ventilator dependent (excluding SCI)	Subacute placement with rehabilitation/physical therapy
Persistent vegetative state	Skilled nursing facility vs subacute facility
Mild cognitive impairment	Home with outpatient therapy
Moderate cognitive impairment	Acute rehabilitation vs home with outpatient therapy
Severe cognitive impairment	Acute rehabiltiation vs skilled nursing facility
Sensory impairment: Blindness	Acute rehabilitation
Communication deficits: aphasia, dysphasia	Home with outpatient therapy
Behavioral issues	Home with outpatient therapy and supervision vs skilled nursing facility

Table 34–3   Team Member Responsibilities for Discharge and Rehabilitation Planning[1]

Team member	Initial assessment	Eligibility and needs evaluation	Environmental assessment	Patient and family education
Case manager	Communicates with insurance/HMO	Determines covered services and rehabilitation options	Communicates with potential rehabilitation facilities	Educates patient and family regarding treatment and discharge plan
Social worker	Family support system and home resources	Determines covered services and rehabilitation options; assists in applications for funding	Communicates with potential rehabilitation facilities	Educates patient and family regarding treatment and discharge plan
Physician	Assesses medical needs and stability	Assesses prognosis for recovery		Educates patient and family regarding treatment and discharge plan
Physical therapist	Assesses physical limitations and functional capacity	Recommendation re: need for assistive devices and ongoing therapy	Explores home environment and related needs	Educates patient and family regarding treatment and discharge plan
Occupational therapist	Assesses physical limitations and functional capacity	Recommendation re: need for assistive devices and ongoing therapy	Explores home environment and related needs	Educates patient and family regarding treatment and discharge plan
Speech pathologist	Assesses cognitive and physical limitations as related to speech, swallowing, and cognition and functional capacity	Recommendation re: need for assistive devices and ongoing therapy	Explores home environment and related needs	Educates patient and family regarding treatment and discharge plan

(Continued)

Table 34–3 Team Member Responsibilities for Discharge and Rehabilitation Planning (*Continued*)

Team member	Initial assessment	Eligibility and needs evaluation	Environmental assessment	Patient and family education
Dietitian	Assesses nutritional status and physical limitations	Recommends nutritional program based on assessed needs		Educates patient and family regarding treatment and discharge plan
Respiratory therapist	Assesses respiratory status and associated needs	Recommends respiratory program based on assessed needs		Educates patient and family regarding treatment and discharge plan
Physiatrist	Assesses physical, cognitive, and social needs and limitations	Designs patient specific medical and rehabilitation program	Facilitates entry into appropriate rehabilitation program	Educates patient and family regarding treatment and discharge plan
Nurse	Assesses physical, cognitive, and social needs and limitations	Communicates perceived need to appropriate team members	Coordinates care and activities of team members	Educates patient and family regarding treatment and discharge plan

HMO, health maintenance organization.

◆ Implications

Determining discharge destination early in the acute hospital phase can facilitate treatment decisions, resource allocation, family education, and counseling. It enables families and discharge planners to choose appropriate posthospital facilities or prepare the home environment. Case management increases patient and family understanding of posthospital needs and promotes the family's ability to meet those needs confidently. It also decreases the length of hospital stay and costs.

Reference

1. Barker E. Neuroscience Nursing: A Spectrum of Care. 2nd ed. St. Louis, MO: CV Mosby; 2002

Index

Page numbers followed by *f* and *t* indicate figures or tables, respectively.